Nursing Management of Pediatric Disaster

Catherine J. Goodhue · Nancy Blake
Editors

Nursing Management of Pediatric Disaster

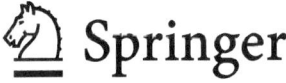 Springer

Editors
Catherine J. Goodhue
Division of Pediatric
Surgery/Trauma Program
Children's Hospital Los Angeles
Los Angeles, CA
USA

Nancy Blake
School of Nursing
University of California Los Angeles
Los Angeles, CA
USA

Chief Nursing Officer
Harbor-UCLA Medical Center
Torrance, CA
USA

ISBN 978-3-030-43427-4   ISBN 978-3-030-43428-1   (eBook)
https://doi.org/10.1007/978-3-030-43428-1

This Springer imprint is published by the registered company Springer Nature Switzerland AG
The registered company address is: Gewerbestrasse 11, 6330 Cham, Switzerland

Contents

Introduction

Nancy Blake

1.1 Introduction

Nurses need to be prepared to respond to disasters any time. Since it is estimated that more than 25% of the population is in the pediatric age range, it is important that all nurses have some competency in the care of pediatric disaster victims, irrespective of their place of work. In a disaster, victims may be transported by police, family-owned private vehicle, or even Uber; so, there is no guarantee that pediatric patients will be transported to health care facilities designated for pediatric care. In fact, during the Route 91 Harvest Festival incident in Las Vegas, a large number of victims were transported by good samaritans and Uber, who relied on the mobile navigation system on their cellular phones to find the closest hospital. The closest hospital was not a trauma center that victims would be sent to if the same patients were transported by first responders. Almost all of the victims of this mass casualty incident (MCI) were adults. The Aurora movie shooting victims were also transported by private vehicles and police cars. During the incident, the pediatric victims ended up being transported to the University Hospital and the adult victims to Denver Children's Hospital. There is no guarantee that adult nurses will not be caring for pediatric victims.

This book is a review of all aspects of care of pediatric disaster victims and pediatric disaster nursing, including day care centers, schools, hospitals, pediatric offices, and communities. It includes a background of disaster nursing, regulations and policies, all aspects of natural and technological disasters, unique vulnerabilities in children, decontamination, and disaster shelters.

N. Blake (✉)
School of Nursing, University of California Los Angeles, Los Angeles, CA, USA

Harbor-UCLA Medical Center, University of California Los Angeles, Torrance, CA, USA
e-mail: nblake@dhs.lacounty.gov

© Springer Nature Switzerland AG 2020
C. J. Goodhue, N. Blake (eds.), *Nursing Management of Pediatric Disaster*,
https://doi.org/10.1007/978-3-030-43428-1_1

All nurses, regardless of where they work, should have a basic understanding of the care of pediatric patients. Disasters can strike anytime and anywhere, and, therefore, pediatric patients will need appropriate care, both physical and psychological. Pediatric patients have unique needs based on their anatomy and physiology, as well as their developmental levels. Each chapter will discuss the unique pediatric issues related to the topic being discussed. Examples of disaster responses requiring pediatric variations include decontamination, shelter management, and reunification, and, therefore, pediatric patients must be managed different from that of the adult population. Children are not small adults; nurses and other health care providers must be aware of the uniqueness of pediatric disaster victims.

The World Health Organization and the Pan American Health Organization define a *disaster* as "an event that occurs in most cases suddenly and unexpectedly, causing severe disturbances to people or objects affected by it, resulting in the loss of life and harm to the health of the population, the destruction or loss of community property, and/or severe damage to the environment. Such a situation leads to disruption in the normal pattern of life, resulting in misfortune, helplessness, and suffering, with adverse effects on the socioeconomic structure of a region or a country and/or modifications of the environment to such an extent that there is a need for assistance and immediate outside intervention" (Lynch and Berman 2009). When referring to disaster throughout the book, this is the definition that has been followed. In addition, the term MCI will be used to refer to both mass casualty incidents and mass casualty events (MCE). The term, "health care providers", will be used to address physicians, nurse practitioners, and physician assistants as they actually provide health care services (Code of Federal Regulations, 1995). This will differentiate health care providers from nurses caring for the patients.

Chapter 2 provides a thorough history of disaster nursing, beginning with Florence Nightingale's work caring for soldiers during the Crimean War. It emphasizes that nurses have been the consistent care providers deployed in a disaster and the largest group who care for patients in a disaster. It highlights that nurses need to have the competency and decision-making capacity to deal with issues including triage, trauma, mental health, and infection control. This chapter focuses on the role of nurses in many of the large disasters in the last two centuries. It is important to understand the history of disaster nursing in order to prepare for the role of nurses in disasters.

Chapter 3 provides a great overview of disaster planning and policy. It emphasizes the importance of nurses' understanding of the local, state, and federal laws that impact the "all-hazards approach". These laws address not only the oversight of the legal issues that occur during disasters but also the disaster response, which begins at the local level and then moves to the state and federal levels. It is important to be prepared at the local level as the federal response does not get deployed immediately and that nurses understand their roles in response at the local level. A significant change in disaster response began following the 9/11 attacks, following which the National Disaster Medical System was established in 2002. It was based on the National Incident Medical System (NIMS), which guides the disaster response of both governmental and nongovernmental agencies. This significantly changed the federal response to disasters and is very prescriptive on how the response should occur.

Chapter 4 provides a synopsis of the Incident Command System (ICS). Regardless of the type of event, ICS is a structured response used by government agencies and hospitals alike. The ICS was developed as a method to respond to domestic disasters by assimilating facilities, equipment, personnel, and communications under one operating structure (EMSI, 2019). It was developed in California following a large wildfire. During the response to this fire, there was a less than optimal response because of which it was determined during the after-action review that there were some key areas that required improvement: communications, common nomenclature, and a unified command between agencies. The ICS structure prescribes the same roles for each agency and each role has a job action sheet. Each role has a single supervisor, and the roles can be expanded as needed. Several other chapters cover the unique roles that can be added as needed, including those during decontamination and reunification. Several of the job action sheets are included as examples for the key roles.

Chapter 5 is a very detailed chapter covering the different types of disasters, both natural (forces of nature) and man-made (intentional). It begins with a thorough overview of the anatomical differences in children and the relevance of those differences in a disaster because of children's unique vulnerabilities. Included in this section are the behavioral differences in children as well as an in-depth review of disasters and the needs during a response, including the Strategic National Stockpile and the required supplies to care for children. Children are not just small adults; the equipments, supplies, and pharmaceuticals for children are unique. The remainder of the chapter is a comprehensive analysis of all the types of disasters.

Chapter 6 is a review of general disaster preparedness for families. This chapter emphasizes the role of nurses in educating patients and families to be prepared prior to and during disasters. Household preparedness has been low in the past, and it is important that families have a plan prior to disasters and that each member of the family is aware of the plan and his/her role in the response. It is important that families are aware of the plans of their community, local emergency management agency, and their local Red Cross. Nurses can educate families on these agencies.

Chapter 7 is an overview of the physical development and disaster preparedness in children. The focus is on the theories associated with physical development followed by the relevance of those theories and how they relate to disaster preparedness. The chapter details how knowledge of the developmental stage of the child will assist in disaster response.

Chapter 8 discusses the nuances of children with special health care needs (CSHCN) as well as the functional access needs, and how these needs are different than the usual needs of children. These needs can be both developmental and physical; federal definitions are included in this chapter. Throughout the book, CSHCN will also include children with functional and access needs. This chapter as others do, emphasizes the importance of preparedness in advance.

Chapter 9 addresses pediatric decontamination and the unique needs of children during decontamination. This chapter provides a general overview of decontamination during disasters and then focuses on the unique needs of children, especially small children, as they may not be able to understand what is going on and will not cooperate as much as adults do. It is important to have a plan for family decontamination when children are involved. It is also important to not contaminate the hospitals; therefore, decontamination training for nurses is an important competency.

Chapter 10 is a review of the unique needs of children in disaster shelters. This is a very important area of pediatric nursing and pediatric preparedness. Children are very vulnerable in shelters, and, therefore, should not be left alone with someone who is a volunteer that has not been fully vetted and known to the response team. The areas of shelters emphasized in this chapter include setting up mass care shelters, nursing care of displaced children, agency support for medically related issues, unaccompanied minors in shelters, and activities for children post disaster.

Chapter 11 describes the reunification process in disasters, which is a very important point in pediatric disaster preparedness. Whether the disasters happen while children are at school or child care, reunification becomes more complicated when the children are not with their families. Unfortunately, infants cannot tell you who their parents are, and, therefore, a reunification plan in place is very important to ensure that they are released to the appropriate family members. The National Center for Missing and Exploited Children is the agency that is designated responsible for reunification. This chapter also has recommendations for setting up reunification centers and holding areas for children until they can be reunified with their respective guardians.

Chapter 12 focuses on supporting children and families in the aftermath of disasters. The impact of disasters can be short- or long-term. The psychological impact of disasters can require long-term therapy by a qualified therapist. It is important that the primary first responders, including nurses, are able to identify those children that will need more than just immediate care. There is a detailed list of common symptoms of adjustment reactions in children after a disaster as well as post-traumatic stress issues with children. This chapter is filled with resources to help children who are impacted by disasters and may have post-disaster mental health issues.

Chapter 13 highlights hospital preparedness and the necessary plans that should be in place for hospitals prior to and during disasters. This chapter empasizes the importance of hospitals to conduct disaster drills with pediatric victims; this will ensure that hospital staff have the necessary training to care for pediatric victims and that hospitals have the necessary equipment and supplies to care for young victims. The importance of coordinating with the community is also covered in this chapter to ensure appropriate coordination during a disaster. It is important that these memorandums of understanding (MOUs) are in place in advance. The remainder of the chapter focuses on the response including triage and care for the patients and families.

Chapter 14 describes disaster preparedness in schools. The beginning of the chapter describes school emergencies and disaster preparedness. An addition to ICS is the School Emergency Operations Team which will be deployed as necessary if the incident happens to involve the school. There is a thorough description of school response in shootings and epidemics. The focus for schools should be for preparedness, response, and recovery. The remainder of the chapter covers the role of school nurses in disasters.

Chapter 15 focuses on child care center preparedness. This chapter provides the information on the history of emergency preparedness in child care centers. Federal regulations for child care centers requiring emergency preparedness plans and evacuation routes have only been required in the last 10 years. Numerous preparation and mitigation strategies are covered in this chapter. A step-by-step approach to preparedness in child care centers is also included in this chapter.

Chapter 16 addresses pediatric office preparedness. Numerous suggested practices by the American Academy of Pediatrics (AAP) are included in this chapter. Five components of office preparedness are described: office self-assessment, effective preparation for more commonplace pediatric emergencies, development of written emergency response and disaster protocols, practice using drills or mock codes, and knowledge and integration of greater local and regional disaster planning agencies and resources (Fuchs 2013; AAP 2015; Jones 2019). This chapter includes tables of supplies, equipments, and medications that are recommended in the event of a disaster.

Chapter 17 focuses on the importance of breastfeeding during disasters and offers information that breastfeeding is the cleanest way to provide nutrition during disasters. This chapter also dispels the myth that mothers are not able to breastfeed during a disaster. The benefits to mothers and infants as well as issues in the community are covered in this chapter. The chapter ends with recommendations to support mothers in order to allow them to breastfeed.

Chapter 18 is full of information on how nurses can volunteer during a disaster. In addition to material regarding volunteering and regulations, the actual information regarding the experience is addressed. Many nurses do not understand what they are getting into when they volunteer. There are numerous challenges including personal safety, rest, altered conditions, and tragic events that nurses may encounter. Most nurses are unaware of the conditions they may need to work in. The chapter provides the information on what nurses can expect when they volunteer.

This book is a great resource for nurses who would like to be better prepared for pediatric disaster nursing. It can be a reference for both pediatric and adult nurses. The book provides an overview of the care and treatment of pediatric patients during a disaster, and what nurses can do to prepare for disasters as well as educate patients and families on home preparedness and developing family preparedness plans. Disasters can happen when least expected, and it is important that nurses have pediatric disaster competencies and be prepared before they are needed.

References

American Academy of Pediatrics (AAP). Disaster preparedness advisory council and committee on pediatric emergency medicine. Ensuring the health of children in disasters. Pediatrics. 2015:2015–3112. https://doi.org/10.1542/peds.2015-3112.

Code of Federal Regulations. 1995. https://www.dol.gov/general/cfr. Accessed 1 Jan 2020.

EMSI. The history of ICS. 2019. http://www.emsics.com/history-of-ics/. Accessed 4 Dec 2019.

Fuchs S. Pediatric office emergencies. Pediatr Clin N Am. 2013;60:1153–61.

Jones M. Preparing an office practice for pediatric emergencies. 2019. https://www.uptodate.com/contents/preparing-an-office-practice-for-pediatric-emergencies?csi=b38cd7d1-9f98-4b1c-8536-59f8af49960a&source=contentShare.

Lynch JA, Berman S. Disasters and their effects on the population: key concepts. In: Berman S, editor. Pediatric education in disasters manual. Buenos Aires, Argentina: Service Point S.A; 2009.

History of Disaster Nursing

2

John S. Murray

2.1 Introduction

Nurses have played an important role in responding to a wide spectrum of disasters, from war and conflict to natural and man-made catastrophes globally, since the mid-1800s (Labrague et al. 2018). The responsibilities nurses have held in relation to disasters have also been broad in scope. These responsibilities range from minimizing the effects of disaster, planning for response, providing direct care, and helping communities to recover (Grochtdreis et al. 2017). Increasingly, it has become even more relevant to understand the contributions nurses make to disaster efforts as the world experiences an increasing number of catastrophic events (Achora and Kamanyire 2016).

2.2 Disaster Defined

It is important to understand the definition of disaster as it varies widely. In fact, disaster experts have identified the need to standardize a definition to further advance the state of the science as it relates to practice, education, policy, and research (Mayner and Arbon 2015). However, this is not a new phenomenon. Like disaster nursing, efforts to establish a uniform meaning have evolved for decades (Mayner and Arbon 2015; Al-Madhari and Keller 1997). It has been long believed that it may not be possible to establish a universally accepted definition across multiple disciplines and regions of the world. Instead, efforts should focus on doing so within professions (Mayner and Arbon 2015; Al-Madhari and Keller 1997). For the purpose of this chapter, the definition of disaster will reflect the principles of the World Health Organization (WHO). WHO created a definition based on the work of the

J. S. Murray (✉)
Bouvé College of Health Sciences, Northeastern University, Boston, MA, USA

© Springer Nature Switzerland AG 2020
C. J. Goodhue, N. Blake (eds.), *Nursing Management of Pediatric Disaster*,
https://doi.org/10.1007/978-3-030-43428-1_2

7

International Strategy for Disaster Risk Reduction (ISDR) as well as the Centre for Research on the Epidemiology of Disaster (CRED) (Labrague et al. 2018). Oversight of execution of the ISDR is provided by the United Nations Office for Disaster Risk Reduction as mandated by the United Nations General Assembly in Geneva, Switzerland (United Nations Office for Disaster Risk Reduction 2018). CRED promotes a variety of activities such as research, education, training, and technical expertise related to crises globally (Centre for Research on the Epidemiology of Disaster 2015). WHO defines disaster as any event which significantly impacts a considerable number of individuals in a community or country where physical and mental health, environment, and economy are negatively disrupted requiring national or international response (World Health Organization 2018). Consensus does exist when classifying disaster types which include natural and man-made or technological hazards (Grochtdreis et al. 2017). Natural disasters are considered physical events which are geophysical (e.g., earthquakes and landslides), hydrological (e.g., floods and tsunamis), climatological (e.g., temperature extremes, blizzards, droughts, and wildfires), meteorological (e.g., hurricanes and cyclones) or biological (e.g., toxin and bioactive substance exposure, disease epidemics, and vector-borne outbreaks) (World Health Organization 2018; The International Federation of Red Cross and Red Crescent Societies 2019). Technological, or man-made hazards, are disasters occurring as a result of human behavior frequently resulting in mass destruction, population displacement, and death (e.g., complex emergencies, war/conflict, bioterrorism, industrial fires, transport accidents, oil spills, and gas leaks) (Grochtdreis et al. 2017; United Nations Office for Disaster Risk Reduction 2018; World Health Organization 2018; The International Federation of Red Cross and Red Crescent Societies 2019). Please refer to Chap. 5 for more detailed information on types of disasters.

2.3 Nurses Responding to Disasters

Throughout history, nurses have frequently been the first health care professionals mobilized to respond to disasters (Achora and Kamanyire 2016). In fact, nurses practicing in various settings and roles have responded to disasters for as long as the profession has existed (Grochtdreis et al. 2017; Gebbie and Qureshi 2006; Edmonson et al. 2017; Hutchinson and Welch 2013). Experts note that nurses' *critical thinking, problem-solving,* and *communication skills* make them highly qualified to respond to the multifaceted and unique demands imposed by disasters (Edmonson et al. 2017; Hutchinson and Welch 2013). The high level of clinical competence and decision-making capacity possessed by nurses also makes them vastly adept in delivering a wide range of care (e.g., triage, trauma, life support, mental health, and infection control) across all phases of disasters from mitigation to recovery efforts (Noguchi et al. 2016). Nurses have responded to all types of disasters even when health care infrastructures have been taxed to maximum capacity or even destroyed (Achora and Kamanyire 2016; Global Alliance for Nursing and Midwifery 2015). A key contributor to the evolution of disaster nursing is taking note of lessons learned that might be useful for responding to future catastrophic events.

2.3.1   The Forerunner of Disaster Nursing

Many individuals can recall the significant role nurses played in responding to the terrorist attacks of September 11, 2001 (9/11). In addition to the nurses who responded directly, thousands more sought ways to volunteer their services to help victims in the days that followed (Stokowski 2015; Orr 2002; D'Antonio and Whelan 2004). However, long before this tragic day in United States (U.S.) history, nurses have been ready, willing, and able to respond to disasters. Florence Nightingale was one of the first nurses to make significant contributions to disaster nursing by addressing the disease outbreak during the Crimean War (1854–1856). During this military conflict, cholera and unsanitary conditions were responsible for more deaths of British soldiers than combat injuries.

While caring for troops in field hospitals, Nightingale significantly improved patient outcomes by implementing disease prevention and infection control measures (Hutchinson and Welch 2013; Gill and Gill 2005). Nightingale, considered the forerunner of contemporary nursing, continued to contribute to disaster nursing until her death in 1910 at the age of 90 (D'Antonio and Whelan 2004; Young et al. 2011; McDonald 2014). However, her greatest contribution to disaster nursing was establishing foundational principles related to infection control (Young et al. 2011; McDonald 2014). Her contributions would prove to be exceptionally helpful in the early 1900s.

2.3.2   Influenza Pandemic of 1918–1919

A short time following Nightingale's death, nurses rallied in large numbers to address one of the earliest, and largest, biological disasters in history—the Influenza Pandemic of 1918–1919, otherwise known as the Spanish flu (Fig. 2.1) (Library of Congress 1918). Millions of people became ill from the flu at the same time the U.S. was experiencing a shortage of health care professionals because of World War I. It is estimated that over 9000 nurses were deployed abroad, with an additional cadre assigned to stateside military hospitals, to support caring for wounded service members. This left many U.S. hospitals short of nurses (Keeling 2010). Further complicating this shortage was the failure of the U.S. to ask trained African-American nurses to assist with the response (Centers for Disease Control and Prevention 2018). Despite these challenges, nurses both paid and volunteer continued to play an enormous role in responding to this monumental disaster (Gebbie and Qureshi 2006; D'Antonio and Whelan 2004; Keeling 2010; Centers for Disease Control and Prevention 2018; Kolawole 2010; Robinson 1990). There was no prevention or treatment for the pandemic virus that was caused by an influenza A (H1N1) virus. What complicated the disaster exponentially was that the pandemic occurred in three waves (Keen-Payne 2000). It is believed that more than 30% of the world's population became ill with over 50 million succumbing to their illness (Centers for Disease Control and Prevention 2018). The role of nurses during the pandemic was enormous. Nurses worked tirelessly to provide interventions such as isolation, quarantine, and educating the public about handwashing and avoiding

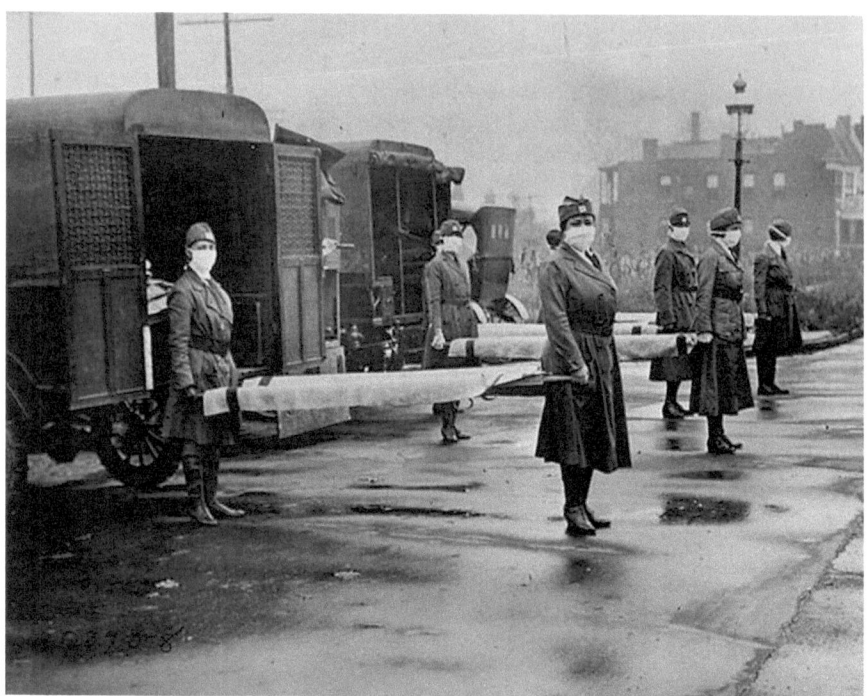

Fig. 2.1 St. Louis Red Cross Motor Corps on duty October 1918 Influenza epidemic. (Courtesy of the Prints and Photographs Division. Library of Congress)

gatherings to mitigate the transmission of disease (Centers for Disease Control and Prevention 2018; Robinson 1990). Again, one of the many lessons learned was the importance of nurses providing infection control measures given there were no effective therapeutic and/or prophylactic treatments available at the time (Robinson 1990; Keen-Payne 2000; Short et al. 2018).

2.3.3   Cocoanut Grove Fire

Just before the middle of the twentieth century, nurses played a critical role in responding to what continues to be Boston's most fatal disaster, and the nation's second-deadliest nightclub fire in history (Fig. 2.2) (Boston Public Library 1942). On the evening of November 28, 1942, over 1000 individuals crowded into the Cocoanut Grove, a trendy gathering place in Boston, Massachusetts to enjoy dinner and cocktails in the post-prohibition era. Occupancy guidelines restricted guests to 460 people. At approximately 10:15 p.m., a small fire spread very quickly. In less than 10 min, the fire fueled by establishment décor, completely engulfed the club killing 492 patrons (D'Antonio and Whelan 2004; Boston Public Library 1942; Connor-Ballard 2011). Most survivors of this man-made disaster suffered from respiratory distress and burn injuries. Boston City Hospital (now Boston Medical Center)

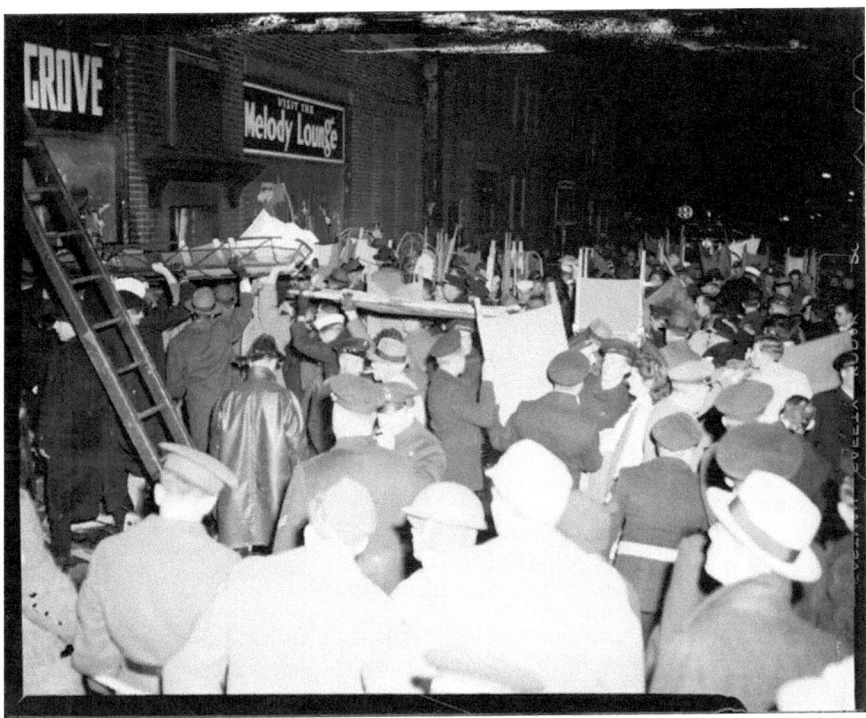

Fig. 2.2 Rescuers crowd entrance to Cocoanut Grove, November 1942. (Courtesy of Brearley Collection, Boston Public Library)

received most casualties. The majority of nurses employed at the hospital quickly mobilized to care for the injured. During the initial hours of the disaster, it is reported that one patient arrived at the hospital every 11 s rapidly exhausting resources (Connor-Ballard 2011). Nurses from surrounding hospitals quickly and willingly mobilized to support efforts to care for patients providing triage, fluid resuscitation, respiratory support, burn care, infection control, and pain management (D'Antonio and Whelan 2004; Connor-Ballard 2011). A significant lesson learned was the importance of the role of critical care nurses in disaster response that has been passed onto many generations of new nurses (Doona 2018). This became especially important with nurses responding to future man-made disasters related to terrorism.

2.3.4 Oklahoma City Bombing

Almost 25 years ago, on April 19, 1995, nurses were faced with responding to the largest terror attack in the U.S. at the time—the Oklahoma City Bombing (D'Antonio and Whelan 2004). Two American domestic terrorists, motivated by anti-government sentiment, devised and detonated a truck bomb carrying 4800 pounds of explosives that destroyed the Alfred P. Murrah Federal Building in Oklahoma City

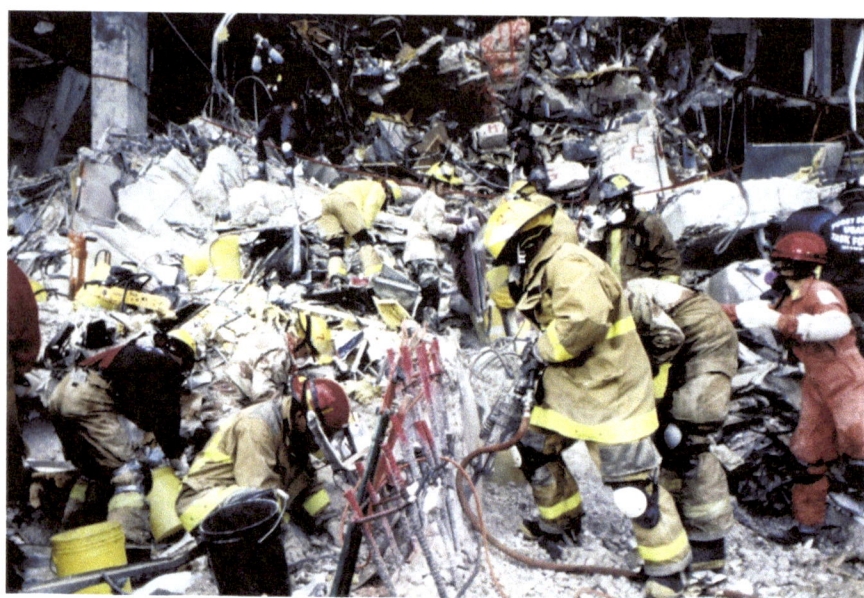

Fig. 2.3 Oklahoma City, OK, April 26, 1995. Search and rescue crews work to save those trapped beneath the debris, following the Oklahoma City Bombing. (Courtesy of the Federal Emergency Management Agency (FEMA))

(Fig. 2.3) (Federal Emergency Management Agency 1995). This large-scale technological disaster, that also destroyed hundreds of other structures within a 10-mile radius, killed 168 people mostly federal employees working at the building. Nineteen of the victims were infants and children attending the child care center at the Federal building. An additional 675 people were wounded (D'Antonio and Whelan 2004; Anteau and Williams 1997; Pfefferbaum 2001). Nurses throughout the community responded immediately to assist with care in the aftermath of the disaster. One nurse, 37-year-old Rebecca Needham Anderson, became the 168th casualty as a result of a head injury sustained while helping with rescue efforts (D'Antonio and Whelan 2004). Common injuries triaged and treated included, but not limited to, severe crush injuries, open fractures, multiple lacerations, traumatic amputations, head trauma, burns, and acute stress reaction (Anteau and Williams 1997; Buckner-Amundson and Burkle 1995). Critical lessons learned were the recognition of the need for nursing expertise in bomb disaster management and the importance of providing mental health care and support early on in the aftermath of catastrophes to patients, families, first responders, and hospital personnel (Anteau and Williams 1997; Buckner-Amundson and Burkle 1995). Additionally, this disaster highlighted the need for interagency coordination and cooperation (Anteau and Williams 1997). Experts have reported that response efforts could have been better. Response agencies did not have good visibility of each other's efforts. Lastly, it was noted that large metropolitan cities should have evacuation routes for civilians to leave disaster areas, especially in the event of bombings (Glenshaw et al. 2007). This would be acutely helpful with future man-made disasters related to terrorism.

2.3.5 Hurricane Katrina

On August 29, 2005, the U.S. experienced one of the deadliest and costliest natural disasters in the nation's history. At one point, Hurricane Katrina was a category five storm with maximum sustained winds above 170 miles per hour creating severe damage in South East Louisiana along the Gulf Coast spanning some 1400 miles. This natural disaster resulted in more than 1800 deaths and damages estimated at over $100 billion (Thomas 2018; Diamond 2015). Many challenges hampered rescue efforts. At least 80% of New Orleans was under water for weeks after the hurricane (Diamond 2015). Nine of 11 hospitals in the area were inoperable, and federal assistance did not arrive for several days after the disaster struck. Nurses were unable to provide even minimal standards of care, especially for critically ill patients. Without electricity, the use of mechanical ventilators, monitors, dialysis machines, etc., providing care was impossible. To the extent possible, nurses provided many of these functions manually and to the best of their ability (Thomas 2018; Franco et al. 2006). While some residents heeded early warnings and evacuated before the storm, over 250,000 others were left stranded. These residents remained in shelters, hospitals, long-term care facilities, and individual homes—all without potable water, electricity, or a means of communication as cell towers were decimated (Franco et al. 2006; Danna et al. 2010). The populations at greatest risk were the disabled, elderly, and poor. In the immediate aftermath of the disaster, nurses provided care in shelters in addition to the two functioning hospitals. However, the complete collapse of infrastructure in New Orleans ultimately required the mass evacuation of an entire city (Klein and Nagel 2007; Danna et al. 2010). The Louis Armstrong New Orleans International Airport served as the main evacuation site. At this location, nurses provided the mainstay of disaster response efforts such as triage, patient flow, and staging, as well as treatment (Klein and Nagel 2007). The scope of relief efforts was so great, additional nursing support was provided by DMAT (disaster medical assistance teams) from Washington state and Oregon. Other cadres of nurses were deployed from New Mexico, California, and Oklahoma to help with efforts to care for Hurricane Katrina survivors who had already been evacuated to shelter in Houston, Texas (Sanford et al. 2007) (Fig. 2.4) (Federal Emergency Management Agency 2005). One of the greatest lessons learned was the critical leadership role nurses play in managing care in disasters that helped shape subsequent relief efforts (Klein and Nagel 2007).

2.3.6 9/11

The 9/11 terrorist attacks on the U.S. are unquestionably the worst disaster of any kind the nation has experienced. On this day, 19 terrorists affiliated with al Qaeda highjacked four mid-to large-size jet airliners. Two jets struck the World Trade Center (WTC) in Lower Manhattan, New York City killing 2763 people and severely injuring 10,000 others (Fig. 2.5) (Library of Congress 2001). Another jet struck the Pentagon killing 189 people. The fourth flight killed 44 individuals when it crashed into a field in Shanksville, Pennsylvania. A total of 2996 people lost their lives as a

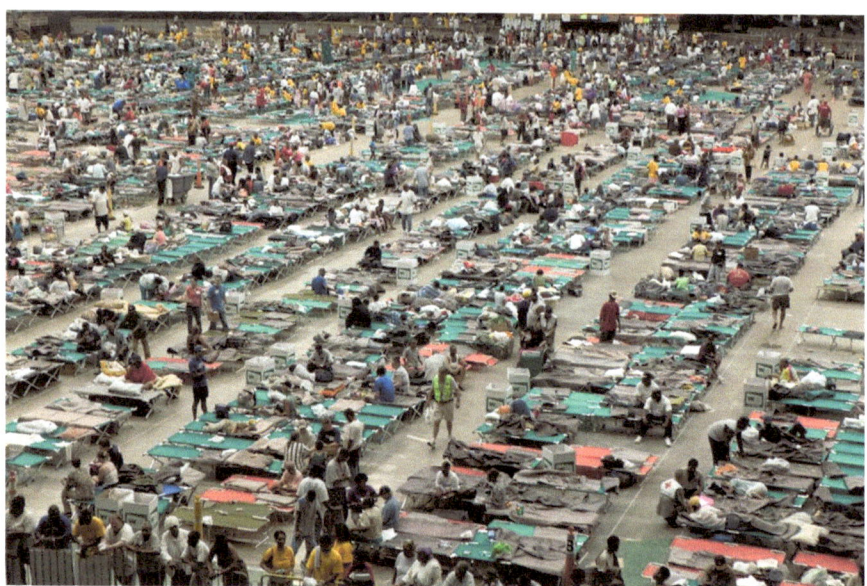

Fig. 2.4 New Orleans evacuees at the Astrodome in Texas. (Courtesy of FEMA)

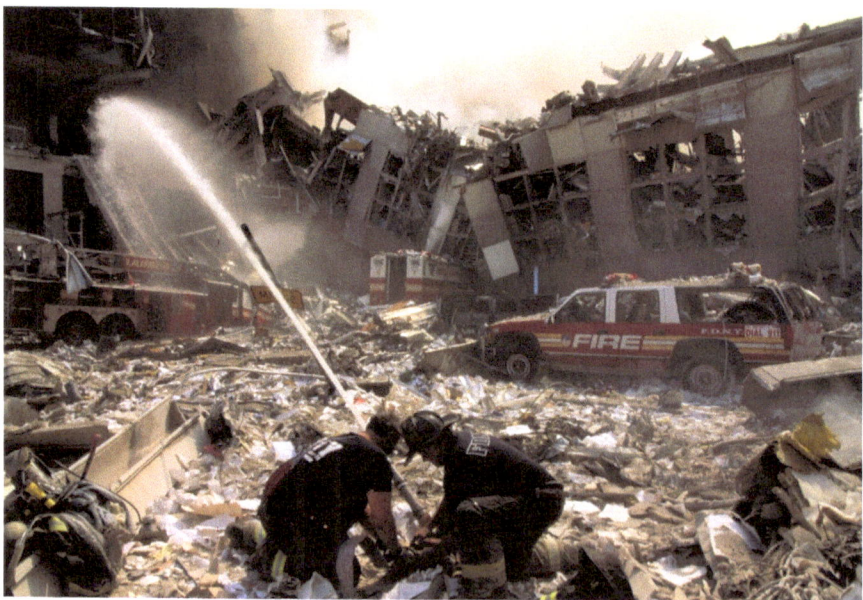

Fig. 2.5 Fire fighting in the aftermath of the September 11th terrorist attack. (Courtesy of the Prints and Photographs Division. Library of Congress)

result of this disaster (History.com 2019). The initial response by nurses to the WTC and Pentagon was swift and extensive. Nurses from around New York, Washington D.C., and beyond, including the U.S. Public Health Service, were quick to answer the call for help. Immediately following the attacks, nurses led efforts to set up makeshift triage areas and clinics both at the WTC and Pentagon (Knebel et al. 2010; Rosenfield et al. 2002). At the provisional sites, the injured (including first responders) were treated for burns, lacerations, fractures, psychological distress, etc. (Knebel et al. 2010; Rosenfield et al. 2002; Bills et al. 2008). Nurses in surrounding hospitals cared for patients admitted for injuries such as smoke inhalation, sustained burns, fractures, closed head trauma, and crush injuries (Centers for Disease Control and Prevention 2002). While there were many lessons learned from this disaster, some of the most important are the need for (1) disaster planning and training for health care professionals, (2) improved mechanisms to ensure efficient and appropriate coordination of resources, (3) better use of mental health professionals with the expertise and experience gained from responding to other terrorist attacks, and (4) recognizing early the critical role occupational nurses can play in ensuring responder safety and health (Rosenfield et al. 2002; Pak et al. 2008).

2.3.7 Boston Marathon Bombing

Unfortunately, responding to acts of terrorism have become commonplace for nurses. On April 15, 2013, 26,893 entrants and another 500,000 spectators gathered for the annual Boston Marathon (Naturale et al. 2017). Almost 3 h into the marathon, and after the winning runner crossed the finish line, two homemade improvised explosive devices were detonated seconds apart just 100 to 200 yards before the end of the race route (Gates et al. 2014). In a very short period of time, three spectators were killed and 281 injured at the scene. Initial triage and care were provided along the marathon route where the bombs were detonated (Fig. 2.6) (Wikimedia Commons 2013) in addition to medical aid stations that are routinely set up for the marathon each year. There is also a main medical tent at the finish line, staffed with upwards of 200 nurses and physicians, who are trained and equipped to provide a higher level of care. Finally, three DMATs are also available to support disaster care efforts (Nadworny et al. 2014). Almost half of those injured required transport and treatment at local trauma centers (Naturale et al. 2017; Gates et al. 2014). At trauma centers, nurses assisted in the care of victims with injuries reminiscent of those seen by military personnel deployed to Iraq (Bluman 2013). Almost 70% of the injured suffered from lower extremity soft tissue and skeletal injuries. Approximately 30% experienced exsanguinating hemorrhagic shock with 26 victims requiring the application of tourniquets at the scene of the disaster. Twelve patients eventually had to undergo lower extremity amputation (Bluman 2013). Many important lessons learned emerged from this disaster. The first is the importance of trauma center disaster response plans. The health care facilities receiving the injured had in place current marathon incident response plans that played a critical role in minimizing loss of life (Nadworny et al. 2014).

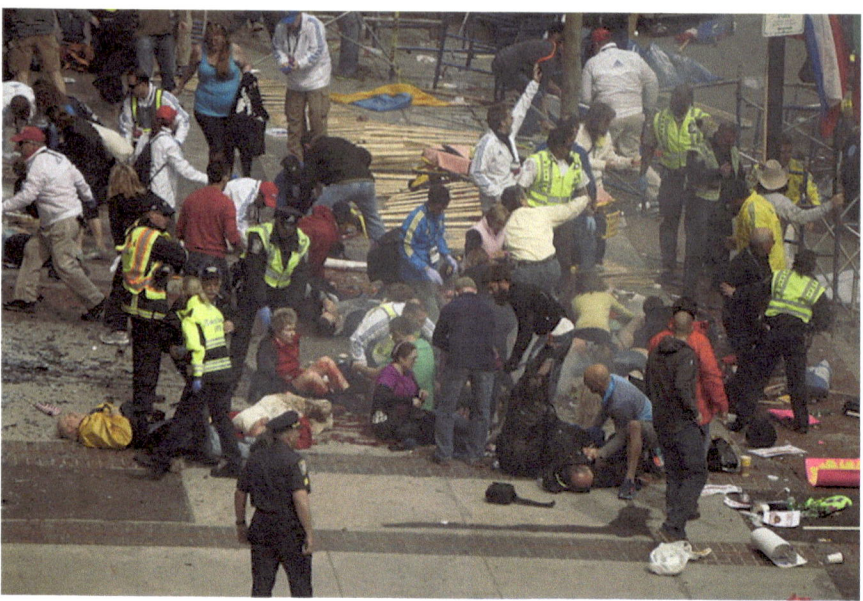

Fig. 2.6 Boston Marathon explosions. (Courtesy of Wikimedia Commons)

In disasters caused by terrorism, the safety of hospital personnel is critical. Four days following the Boston Marathon bombing, the suspects had not yet been apprehended. Many businesses, public institutions (including hospitals), and transit systems were on lock-down. Helicopters constantly circled communities in search of the suspects. Community members were told to shelter-in-place (Naturale et al. 2017; Gates et al. 2014; Bluman 2013). Law enforcement agencies were quick to provide additional protection for health care personnel caring for the injured (Nadworny et al. 2014). The lesson learned from the 9/11 attacks, regarding providing mental health support, was heeded early in the the aftermath of the bombing. At one major trauma center, psychiatric clinical nurse specialists were assigned to the Emergency Department (ED) waiting area to provide support to patients and families witnessing the arrival of mass casualties. Following the initial influx of patients, these nurses as well as social workers, psychologists, clergy, etc. provided ongoing support to staff involved in treating the injured throughout the hospital (Nadworny et al. 2014). The Massachusetts Office for Victim Assistance was also very instrumental in providing mental health support to victims of the disaster and their families (Naturale et al. 2017). One lesson learned, that was also experienced with the 9/11 attacks, and will be critical in future disasters, is to provide mental health support to children beyond the immediate location of the incident. With the Boston Marathon bombing, children beyond the immediate disaster zone were psychologically affected by what they observed in the media. The man-hunt related exposures (lock-down, sheltering-in-place, constant aerial surveillance, presence of large numbers of police and FBI agents patrolling neighborhoods and knocking on doors, etc.) created a lot of psychological stress among children spanning several communities. Future disaster planning should include a focus on addressing children's psychological well-being that is not limited to the immediate disaster area alone (Comer et al. 2014). Please see Chap. 12 for more information on post-disaster psychological effects. The Boston Marathon bombing was yet another reminder of the threat of man-made disasters involving terrorism that have become commonplace in the U.S. and around the world (Gates et al. 2014). As such, nurses need to be prepared even more than ever to respond to disasters of this scope and magnitude.

2.4   The Role of Military Nurses

As noted earlier in the chapter, Florence Nightingale was primarily responsible for the establishment of nursing disaster response. While not a military nurse, Nightingale made significant contributions to reducing mortality rates of British soldiers fighting in the Crimean War through infection control measures. Up until this time, infectious diseases such as typhoid, cholera, and dysentery were responsible for more soldier deaths than wounds sustained in combat. Nightingale's work would create the foundation upon which military nurses would practice in years to come (Hutchinson and Welch 2013; Gill and Gill 2005; Fee and Garofalo 2010).

Another nurse who made substantial contributions to the evolution of military nurses responding to disasters is Clara Barton. Like Nightingale, Barton started a long career in service to soldiers. In the early 1860s, she delivered much-needed supplies to Union soldiers serving on battlefields in Maryland, Virginia, and South Carolina which also led to her caring for the wounded. Barton would later go on to establish and lead the American Red Cross (ARC) answering the call for help during numerous disasters to come in the years that followed (e.g., Texas famine in 1887, Florida Yellow Fever Epidemic (1888), Johnstown, Pennsylvania flood (1889), etc.) (Rivers 2016; Strickler 2018). Barton, with a cadre of ARC nurses, also responded to the Spanish-American War. She initially offered her help to the U.S. Army War Department which declined her assistance. Recognizing the dramatic need of the Cuban people during this disaster, Barton subsequently offered her support to Cuban military forces which was readily accepted. The U.S. Army soon recognized the significant improvement in the health of Cubans occurring as a result of Barton's efforts. As such, they reversed their decision and asked Barton for her help. As a result of her contributions to the Spanish-American War, the U.S. Army Medical Department established a reserve corps of women nurses that was the genesis of the Army Nurse Corps (ANC) created in 1901 (Strickler 2018). Less than 10 years later, the Navy Nurse Corps would be formally established in 1908 (Navy Nurse Corps Association 2019). The Air Force Nurse Corps would emerge from the Army Nurse Corps later in 1949 (Smolenski et al. 2005).

The early 1920s is when military nurses began providing ongoing care during national and global disasters that would continue until today (Rivers 2016; Rivers and Gordon 2017). In 1923, two cadres of Army nurses deployed to Japan in response to the Great Kanto Earthquake which at the time was the worst natural disaster ever experienced by Japan. The effect of the initial disaster was exacerbated by an ensuing tsunami and several fires. Millions of people were trapped under falling debris and collapsed houses. All means of communication and transportation were disrupted. In the end, over 140,000 people lost their lives. Victims who survived were treated for inhalation and crush injuries, burns, and fractures (Smithsonian.com 2011). The extent of damage and number of injuries from the earthquake resulted in the U.S. Naval ships based in the Far East being deployed with medical personnel (Schencking 2013). This disaster reflected the critical role that the U.S. military nurses can play in disaster response (Rivers and Gordon 2017).

Throughout the next two to three decades, military nurses continued to provide disaster assistance both stateside and abroad. However, the U.S. still did not have a policy on providing disaster assistance to other countries. As such, in 1954, Congress passed the Agricultural and Trade Development and Assistance Act (Public Law [PL] 480) that granted the president authority to order support in response to international disasters. While intended to mainly provide surplus U.S. supplies, manpower was frequently also made available. This Act would evolve over time to improve disaster response efforts (Foster 1983). The establishment of PL 480 would be instrumental just six years later when a 9.5 magnitude earthquake (the largest ever instrumentally recorded) and ensuing tsunami struck Chile (National Oceanic and Atmospheric Administration National Centers for Environmental Information 2017). The magnitude of the disaster was so great that death and destruction resulted as far away as Japan, the Philippines, and Hawaii. Casualty data show that upward of 5000 Chileans died as well as 61 deaths and 43 injuries in Hawaii as a result of the tsunami (National Oceanic and Atmospheric Administration National Centers for Environmental Information 2017; Leifer and Glass 2008). Military nurses from Virginia and North Carolina were deployed to assist with disaster relief efforts (Foster 1983).

Another significant milestone for military nurses during the 1950s was the recognition that ANC personnel be properly prepared to respond to disasters. At the start of the Cold War era, when most Americans were acutely aware of the potential for nuclear disaster, Major Harriet H. Werley advocated for required disaster training for all Army nurses. An Army nurse herself, Werley felt strongly that disaster preparedness training be a routine aspect of continuing education. The significance of this recommendation was based on her knowledge of the casualties that could follow a nuclear disaster. Werley acquired this knowledge during the time she served as a consultant to the Department of Atomic Casualties Studies (Leifer and Glass 2008; River 2010). In the years to follow, Werley would develop a standardized disaster nursing exam in collaboration with the American Nurses Association (River 2010).

Throughout the 1960s and 70s military nurses continued to respond to calls for assistance when catastrophe struck such as natural disasters in Alaska, Chile, Iran, Nicaragua, and Yugoslavia (Rivers 2016). In more recent times, military nurses have responded to disasters such as the Pentagon Attack on 9/11, tsunami relief in Banda Aceh, Indonesia (2004), Hurricanes Katrina and Rita (2005), Haiti earthquake (2010), Japan earthquake and tsunami (2011), Hurricane Sandy (2013), Ebola epidemic in West Africa (2015), hurricane relief efforts in Puerto Rico (2017), Las Vegas shooting and mass casualty incident (2017), airlift of pediatric burn patients out of Guatemala (2018), etc. (Rivers 2016; Department of Defense 2017; Berry-Cabán et al. 2018). In addition, over 6326 military nurses have deployed to combat zones in Iraq and Afghanistan since 2001 (Berry-Cabán et al. 2018). During this period of time, disaster relief and emergency assistance legislation would also evolve (Federal Emergency Management Agency 2000) (refer to Chap. 3).

A guiding principle that military nurses live and practice by is mission readiness—being prepared to respond quickly and on short notice. At all times, military nurses are expected to be physically fit and in good health, have the required training to be clinically competent, and understand their responsibility to deploy as needed in the event of a disaster (Department of Defense 2017; Berry-Cabán et al. 2018; Federal Emergency Management Agency 2000). It is this value that has been key to the military contributing to the evolution of disaster care. Military nurses have a vast array of diverse clinical experiences serving in a multitude of different environments. They are encouraged to cross-train, pursue different clinical experiences (e.g., medicine, surgery, pediatrics, and women's health) so that care can be provided for patients with a wide array of medical conditions (e.g., traumatic amputations, penetrating trauma, blast injuries, gunshot wounds, and complex burns) in a range of setting from stateside clinics and medical centers to hospital ships, evacuation aircraft, field combat hospitals, etc. globally (Rivers 2016; Berry-Cabán et al. 2018; Murray 2015). For example, the Air Force's aeromedical evacuation capability has saved thousands of lives by evacuating injured service members from combat areas back to military bases in Europe or the U.S. within days of injury where more advanced care can be provided. Oftentimes this means that military nurses and medical technician crew members may be responsible for the care of up to 100 patients on one aircraft depending on patient acuity. This workload is further challenged by the difficult working conditions posed by the aircraft environment (e.g., poor lighting oftentimes to avoid gunfire and missile attacks during takeoff in hazardous areas, difficult regulation of environmental controls for heating or cooling, loud noise making use of stethoscopes impossible, tremendous amounts of vibration—the litters patients are transported on consist of a mere two-inch foam pad, etc.). However, the training military nurses receive helps in addressing these challenges as best possible. For example, patients with fractures and head injuries are situated in areas of the aircraft where there is less vibration. This training is provided through the Air Force's Critical Care Air Transport Team program where nurses train with the use of simulators that mirror the same challenges experienced in flight during missions (Fig. 2.7) (Hacinas 2012; Smith 2018; Wikimedia Commons 2015). Evolution of aeromedical evacuation capabilities since the 1940s has resulted in a present-day survival rate of 98% for injured troops compared to 75% during the Vietnam War (Bedi 2018).

Military nurses have an extensive amount of experience working in unique, and oftentimes hostile, environments. They provide care for large numbers of critically injured patients in locations where resources are oftentimes very limited, especially during the initial response phase (Murray 2015; Kenward and Kenward 2015). Increasingly, experts are recognizing the unique contributions the military offers to response efforts as a result of its long history of providing care in all types of

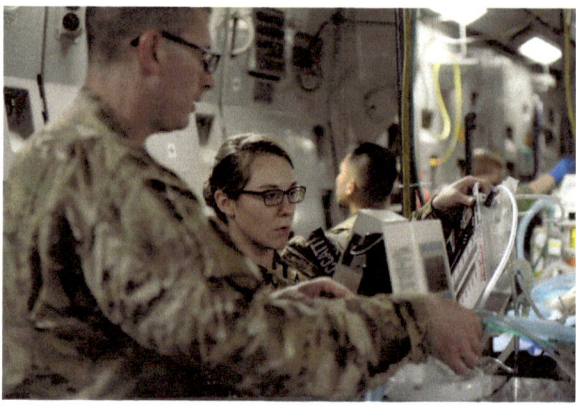

Fig. 2.7 U.S. Air Force Critical Care Air Transport Team members check on a patient prior to an aeromedical evacuation mission aboard a C-17 Globemaster III aircraft from Bagram Airfield, Afghanistan, to Ramstein Air Base, Germany, August 8, 2015. (Courtesy of the U.S. Air Force/Maj. Tony Wickman)

disasters. Several advancements, and lessons learned, in military health care are transferable to civilian disaster efforts: (1) response needs to be rapid and coordinated for the timely care of the injured, (2) patients must be stabilized and transferred to a higher level of care as soon as possible to improve outcomes, and (3) a system for collecting and critically analyzing lessons learned must be in place. It is imperative that data be collected as a fundamental aspect of disaster response. It is the ongoing assessment of these data that generate lessons learned that can be used to implement change as needed for future disaster response efforts. This process must be continuous and lessons shared with the international community to best prepare for future disasters (Zimlichman 2015).

2.5   Conclusion

Unfortunately, disasters of all types have become commonplace in the U.S. and around the world. It's not a matter of if another disaster will occur, but when, where, what type, and will the response be timely, appropriate, and effective. Nurses have consistently demonstrated being ready, willing, and able to respond to disasters. As a profession, we must ensure that we are prepared to respond to disasters utilizing the lessons learned from previous events.

Acknowledgments The author gratefully acknowledges Lauren Frost, Ada Genere, Marissa Grammar, Alina Mujukian, Stephanie Slater and Kathryn Teague, Nurse Anesthesia Program, Bouvé College of Health Sciences, and Northeastern University, Boston, MA for their help with reviewing the literature.

References

Achora S, Kamanyire JK. Disaster preparedness: need for inclusion in undergraduate nursing education. Sultan Qaboos Univ Med J. 2016;16(1):e15–9. https://doi.org/10.18295/squmj.2016.16.01.004.

Al-Madhari AF, Keller AZ. Review of disaster definitions. Prehosp Disaster Med. 1997;12(1):17–21. https://doi.org/10.1017/S1049023X0003716X.

Anteau CM, Williams LA. The Oklahoma bombing: lessons learned. Crit Care Nurs Clin North Am. 1997;9(2):231–6. https://doi.org/10.1016/S0899-5885(18)30282-X.

Bedi S. The evolution of aeromedical evacuation capabilities help deployed medicine take flight. 2018. https://www.airforcemedicine.af.mil/News/Display/Article/1466825/the-evolution-of-aeromedical-evacuation-capabilities-help-deployed-medicine-tak/. Accessed 11 Mar 2019.

Berry-Cabán C, Rivers F, Beltran T, Anderson L. Description of United States military nurses deployed to Afghanistan & Iraq, 2001-2015. Open J Nurs. 2018;8(1):93–101. https://doi.org/10.4236/ojn.2018.81008.

Bills CB, Levy N, Sharma V, Charney DS, Herbert R, Moline J, Katz CL. Mental health of workers and volunteers responding to events of 9/11: review of the literature. Mt Sinai J Med. 2008;75(2):115–27. https://doi.org/10.1002/msj.20026.

Bluman EM. Boston Marathon Bombing. Foot Ankle Int. 2013;34(8):1053–4. https://doi.org/10.1177/1071100713495811.

Boston Public Library. Rescuers crowd entrance to Cocoanut Grove. 1942. https://www.digitalcommonwealth.org/search/commonwealth:x346fh894. Accessed 12 Feb 2019.

Buckner-Amundson S, Burkle AM. Golden minutes: the Oklahoma nurses' stories. J Emerg Nurs. 1995;21(5):401–7. https://doi.org/10.1016/S0099-1767(05)80105-9.

Centers for Disease Control and Prevention. Rapid assessment of injuries among survivors of the terrorist attack on the World Trade Center—New York City, September 2001. 2002. https://www.cdc.gov/mmwr/preview/mmwrhtml/mm5101a1.htm. Accessed 19 Feb 2019.

Centers for Disease Control and Prevention. The 1918 flu pandemic: why it matters 100 years later. 2018. https://blogs.cdc.gov/publichealthmatters/2018/05/1918-flu/. Accessed 11 Feb 2019.

Centre for Research on the Epidemiology of Disaster. About us. 2015. https://www.cred.be/. Accessed 25 Jan 2019.

Comer JS, Dantowitz A, Chou T, Edson AL, Elkins RM, Kerns C, et al. Adjustment among area youth after the Boston Marathon Bombing and subsequent manhunt. Pediatrics. 2014;134(1):7–14. https://doi.org/10.1542/peds.2013-4115.

Connor-Ballard PA. The 1942 Cocoanut Grove Nightclub Fire: out of the ashes. In: Wall BM, Keeling AW, editors. Nurses on the front line: when disaster strikes, 1878-2010. New York: Springer; 2011. p. 167–93.

D'Antonio P, Whelan JC. Moments when time stood still: nursing in disaster. Am J Nurs. 2004;104(11):66–72.

Danna D, Bernard M, Schaubhut R, Mathews P. Experiences of nurse leaders surviving Hurricane Katrina, New Orleans, Louisiana, USA. Nurs Health Sci. 2010;12(1):9–13. https://doi.org/10.1111/j.1442-2018.2009.00497.x.

Department of Defense. The Defense Health Agency: 2017 stakeholder report. 2017. https://health.mil/Reference-Center/Reports/2018/05/01/Defense-Health-Agency-2017-Stakeholder-Report. Accessed 10 Mar 2019.

Diamond L. 10 years after Katrina: lessons learned, lessons to learn. 2015. http://www.rh.gatech.edu/features/10-years-after-katrina-lessons-learned-lessons-learn. Accessed 16 Feb 2019.

Doona ME. 75th anniversary memorial of the Cocoanut Grove Fire. 2018. https://d3ms3kxrsap50t.cloudfront.net/uploads/publication/pdf/1639/Massachusetts_3_18_WEB.pdf. Assessed 13 Feb 2019.

Edmonson C, McCarthy C, Trent-Adams S, McCain C, Marshall J. Emerging global health issues: a nurse's role. Online J Issues Nurs. 2017;22(1):1–17. https://doi.org/10.3912/OJIN.Vol22No01Man02.

Federal Emergency Management Agency. Oklahoma City, OK, April 26, 1995—search and rescue crews work to save those trapped beneath the debris, following the Oklahoma City bombing. 1995. https://commons.wikimedia.org/wiki/File:Oklahomacitybombing-fema-1567.jpg. Accessed 13 Feb 2019.

Federal Emergency Management Agency. Disaster Mitigation Act of 2000. 2000. https://www.fema.gov/media-library/assets/documents/4596. Accessed 11 Mar 2019.

Federal Emergency Management Agency. New Orleans evacuees at the Astrodome in Texas. 2005. https://www.fema.gov/media-library/assets/images/45219. Accessed 17 Feb 2019.

Fee E, Garofalo ME. Florence Nightingale and the Crimean war. Am J Public Health. 2010;100(9):1591. https://doi.org/10.2105/AJPH.2009.188607.

Foster GM. The demands of humanity: army medical disaster relief. 1983. https://history.army.mil/html/books/040/40-3/CMH_Pub_40-3.pdf. Accessed 2 Mar 2019.

Franco C, Toner E, Waldhorn R, Maldin B, O'Toole T, Inglesby TV. Systemic collapse: medical care in the aftermath of Hurricane Katrina. Biosecur Bioterror. 2006;4(2):135–46. https://doi.org/10.1089/bsp.2006.4.135.

Gates JD, Arabian S, Biddinger P, Blansfield J, Burke P, Chung S, et al. The initial response to the Boston Marathon bombing: lessons learned to prepare for the next disaster. Ann Surg. 2014;260(6):960–6. https://doi.org/10.1097/SLA.0000000000000914.

Gebbie K, Qureshi K. A historical challenge: nurses and emergencies. Online J Issues Nurs. 2006;11(3):1–11. https://doi.org/10.3912/OJIN.Vol11No03Man01.

Gill CJ, Gill GC. Nightingale in Scutari: her legacy reexamined. Clin Infect Dis. 2005;40(12):1799–805. https://doi.org/10.1086/430380.

Glenshaw MT, Vernick JS, Li G, Sorock GS, Brown S, Mallonee S. Preventing fatalities in building bombings: what can we learn from the Oklahoma City bombing? Disaster Med Public Health Prep. 2007;1(1):27–31. https://doi.org/10.1097/DMP.0b013e3180640cd7.

Global Alliance for Nursing and Midwifery. Strengthening a global nursing workforce: disaster preparedness & response. 2015. https://ganm.nursing.jhu.edu/strengthening-a-global-nursing-workforce-disaster-preparedness-response/. Accessed 1 Feb 2019.

Grochtdreis T, de Jong N, Harenberg N, Görres S, Schröder-Bäck P. Nurses' roles, knowledge and experience in national disaster preparedness and emergency response: a literature review. SEEJPH. 2017;7:1–19. https://doi.org/10.4119/unibi/seejph-2016-133.

Hacinas JD. The elements to succeed as a military nurse leader. Nurse Lead. 2012;10(4):48–9. https://doi.org/10.1016/j.mnl.2011.12.011.

History.com. 9/11 Attacks. 2019. https://www.history.com/topics/21st-century/9-11-attacks. Accessed 18 Feb 2019.

Hutchinson GB, Welch CA. Florence Nightingale: her legacy to humankind. Imprint. 2013;60(5):25–33.

Keeling AW. "Alert to the necessities of the emergency": U.S. Nursing during the 1918 Influenza Pandemic. Public Health Rep. 2010;125(2):105–12.

Keen-Payne R. We must have nurses: Spanish influenza in America 1918-1919. Nurs Hist Rev. 2000;8(1):143–56. https://doi.org/10.1891/1062-8061.8.1.143.

Kenward LJ, Kenward G. Experiences of military nurses in Iraq and Afghanistan. Nurs Stand. 2015;29(32):34–9. https://doi.org/10.7748/ns.29.32.34.e9248.

Klein KR, Nagel NE. Mass medical evacuation: Hurricane Katrina and nursing experiences at the New Orleans airport. Disaster Manag Response. 2007;5(2):56–61. https://doi.org/10.1016/j.dmr.2007.03.001.

Knebel AR, Martinelli AM, Orsega S, Doss TL, Balingit-Wines AM, Konchan CL. Ground Zero recollections of US Public Health Service nurses deployed to New York City in September 2001. Nurs Clin North Am. 2010;45(2):137–52. https://doi.org/10.1016/j.cnur.2010.02.010.

Kolawole B. Nursing and the 1918/1919 Spanish influenza pandemic. J Commun Nurs. 2010;24(6):30–4.

Labrague LJ, Hammad K, Gloe DS, Mcenroe-Petitte DM, Fronda DC, Obeidat AA, et al. Disaster preparedness among nurses: a systematic review of literature. Int Nurs Rev. 2018;65(1):41–52. https://doi.org/10.1111/inr.12369.

Leifer SL, Glass LK. Planning for mass disaster in the 1950s: Harriet H. Werley and nursing research. Nurs Res. 2008;57(4):237–44. https://doi.org/10.1097/01.NNR.0000313491.94906.8e.

Library of Congress. St. Louis Red Cross Motor Corps on duty Oct. 1918 Influenza epidemic. Available from: Library of Congress Prints & Photographs Online Catalog. http://www.loc.gov/pictures/item/2011661525/.

Library of Congress. Fire fighting in the aftermath of the September 11th terrorist attack. 2001. https://www.loc.gov/pictures/item/2012646014/. Accessed 18 Feb 2019.

Mayner L, Arbon P. Defining disaster: the need for harmonisation of terminology. Australas J Disaster Trauma Stud. 2015;19(Special Issue):19–23.

McDonald L. Florence Nightingale and Mary Seacole on nursing and health care. J Adv Nurs. 2014;70(6):1436–44. https://doi.org/10.1111/jan.12291.

Murray JS. The United States military and veterans administration health system: contemporary policy & political challenges. In: Mason DJ, Outlaw F, Gardener D, O'Grady E, editors. Policy & politics in nursing and health care. 7th ed. St. Louis: Elsevier; 2015. p. 326–35.

Nadworny D, Davis K, Miers C, Howrigan T, Broderick E, Boyd K, et al. Boston strong—one hospital's response to the 2013 Boston Marathon bombings. J Emerg Nurs. 2014;40(5):418–27. https://doi.org/10.1016/j.jen.2014.06.007.

National Oceanic and Atmospheric Administration National Centers for Environmental Information. On this day: 1960 Chilean earthquake and tsunami. 2017. https://www.ncei.noaa. gov/news/day-1960-chilean-earthquake-and-tsunami. Accessed 2 Mar 2019.

Naturale A, Lowney LT, Solè BC. Lessons learned from the Boston Marathon bombing victim services program. Clin Soc Work J. 2017;45(2):111–23. https://doi.org/10.1007/s10615-017-0624-7.

Navy Nurse Corps Association. History of the Navy Nurse Corps. 2019. https://nnca.org/nnca-history/about-navy-nurse-corps/. Accessed 2 Mar 2019.

Noguchi N, Inoue S, Shimanoe C, Shibayama K, Shinchi K. Factors associated with nursing activities in humanitarian aid and disaster relief. PLoS One. 2016;11(3):1–12. https://doi. org/10.1371/journal.pone.0151170.

Orr M. Ready or not, disasters happen. Online J Issues Nurs. 2002;7(3):1–8.

Pak VM, O'Hara ME, McCauley LA. Health effects following 9/11: implications for occupational health nurses. AAOHN J. 2008;56(4):159–65.

Pfefferbaum B. Lessons from the 1995 bombing of the Alfred P Murrah Federal Building in Oklahoma City. Lancet. 2001;358(9286):940. https://doi.org/10.1016/s0140-6736(01)06118-9.

River FM. Military nurses' experience in disaster response. 2010. https://apps.dtic.mil/dtic/tr/fulltext/u2/a630624.pdf. Accessed 9 Mar 2019.

Rivers FM. U.S. military nurses: serving within the chaos of disaster. Nurs Clin N Am. 2016;51(2016):613–23. https://doi.org/10.1016/j.cnur.2016.07.004.

Rivers FM, Gordon S. Military nurse deployments: similarities, differences, and resulting issues. Nurs Outlook. 2017;65(5S):S100–8. https://doi.org/10.1016/j.outlook.2017.07.006.

Robinson KB. The role of nursing in the influenza epidemic of 1918–1919. Nurs Forum. 1990;25(2):19–26. https://doi.org/10.1111/j.1744-6198.1990.tb00845.x.

Rosenfield A, Morse SS, Yanda K. September 11: the response and role of public health. Am J Public Health. 2002;92(1):10–1.

Sanford C, Jui J, Miller HC, Jobe KA. Medical treatment at Louis Armstrong New Orleans International Airport after Hurricane Katrina: the experience of disaster medical assistance teams WA-1 and OR-2. Travel Med Infect Dis. 2007;5(4):230–5. https://doi.org/10.1016/j. tmaid.2007.03.002.

Schencking JC. Aftermath: the ordeal of restoration and recovery. In: Schencking JC, editor. The Great Kanto Earthquake and the Chimera of National Reconstruction in Japan. New York: Columbia University Press; 2013. p. 47–77.

Short KR, Kedzierska K, van de Sandt CE. Back to the future: lessons learned from the 1918 Influenza Pandemic. Front Cell Infect Microbiol. 2018;8(343):1–19. https://doi.org/10.3389/fcimb.2018.00343.

Smith B. Bringing them home: U.S. Air Force aeromedical evacuation. 2018. https://www.emsworld.com/article/221142/bringing-them-home-us-air-force-aeromedical-evacuation. Accessed 10 Mar 2019.

Smithsonian.com. The Great Japan Earthquake of 1923. 2011. https://www.smithsonianmag.com/history/the-great-japan-earthquake-of-1923-1764539/. Accessed 2 Mar 2019.

Smolenski MC, Smith DG, Nanney JS. A fit, fighting force: the Air Force Nursing Services chronology. 2005. https://www.airforcemedicine.af.mil/Portals/1/Documents/History/A-Fit-Fighting-Force-The-AF-Nursing-Services-Chronology.pdf. Accessed 2 Mar 2019.

Stokowski LA. Ready, willing, and able: preparing nurses to respond to disasters. 2015. https://www.medscape.com/viewarticle/579888_2. Accessed 3 Feb 2019.

Strickler J. Clara Barton angel of the battlefield. Nursing. 2018;48(3):43–5. https://doi.org/10.1097/01.NURSE.0000529805.60418.26.

The International Federation of Red Cross and Red Crescent Societies. Types of disasters: definition of hazard. 2019. https://www.ifrc.org/en/what-we-do/disaster-management/about-disasters/definition-of-hazard/. Accessed 26 Jan 2019.

Thomas SL. Hurricane Katrina: a nurse practitioner's experience. J Am Assoc Nurse Pract. 2018;30(3):117–9. https://doi.org/10.1097/JXX.0000000000000026.

United Nations Office for Disaster Risk Reduction. What is the international strategy? 2018. https://www.unisdr.org/who-we-are/international-strategy-for-disaster-reduction. Accessed 25 Jan 2019.

Wikimedia Commons. Boston marathon explosions. 2013. https://commons.wikimedia.org/wiki/File:Boston_Marathon_explosions_(8652877581).jpg. Accessed 20 Feb 2019.

Wikimedia Commons. CCATT delivers critical care in the air. 2015. https://commons.wikimedia.org/wiki/File:CCATT_delivers_critical_care_in_the_air_150508-F-LH521-202.jpg. Accessed 10 Mar 2019.

World Health Organization. Humanitarian health action. 2018. https://www.who.int/hac/about/definitions/en/. Accessed 25 Jan 2019.

Young P, De Smith VH, Chambi MC, Finn BC. Florence Nightingale (1820-1910), 101 years after her death. Rev Med Chil 2011; 139(6): 807-813. https://doi.org/S0034-98872011000600017.

Zimlichman E. "Building the bridge": the launch of Disaster and Military Medicine journal. 2015. https://blogs.biomedcentral.com/on-medicine/2015/02/18/building-the-bridge-the-launch-of-disaster-and-military-medicine-journal/. Accessed 11 Mar 2019.

National Disaster Planning and Policy

Eileen K. Fry-Bowers

3.1 Introduction

Natural and man-made emergencies and disasters have been impacting communities, urban and rural, large and small, across the United States, with increasing regularity. All nurses and health care providers (HCPs) should be aware of the local, state, and national laws and regulations that govern the "all-hazards preparedness" (Federal Emergency Management Agency (FEMA) 2010). The readiness and resilience of communities requires a systems framework for preparedness across traditional and nontraditional medical and public health stakeholders, including community organizations, schools, and other partners in municipal planning. A proper understanding of the roles and responsibilities at each level of the government and the laws that direct governmental interface allows nurses and HCPs to better leverage resources to promote preparedness, response, and recovery. This chapter reviews the sources and scope of laws and regulations that govern national "all-hazards preparedness" policy and planning.

Public policy can be generally defined as "a system of laws, regulatory measures, courses of action, and funding priorities concerning a given topic, promulgated by a governmental entity or its representatives" (Kilpatrick 2000). A major aspect of emergency and disaster planning is law, which includes specific legislation. Over time, through law, regulation, and resource allocation, the local, state, tribal, and federal authorities have developed comprehensive strategies to address threats to public health and well-being.

E. K. Fry-Bowers (✉)

Hahn School of Nursing and Health Science, Betty and Bob Beyster Institute for Nursing Research, Advanced Practice, and Simulation, University of San Diego, San Diego, CA, USA

e-mail: efrybowers@sandiego.edu

C. J. Goodhue, N. Blake (eds.), *Nursing Management of Pediatric Disaster*,
https://doi.org/10.1007/978-3-030-43428-1_3

3.2   Sources of Law

The National Disaster Medical System Federal Partners Memorandum of Agreement defines a public health emergency as "[a]n emergency requirement for health care services to respond to a disaster, significant outbreak of an infectious disease, bio-terrorist attack, or other significant or catastrophic event" (Office of the Under Secretary of Defense for Personnel and Readiness 2016). Significant legal issues arise during these emergencies, such as the allocation of scarce health care resources and the establishment of crisis standards of care, which intersect nearly all levels of the public and private sectors involved in coordinating and providing emergency care during an event response (Committee on Guidance Establishing Crisis Standard of Care for Use in Disaster Situations 2012).

In the context of disasters and public health emergencies, understanding the interconnection among federal, state, and local laws begins with identifying the sources of law that govern behavior generally. *Law* may be defined as "[t]he system of rules which a particular country or community recognizes as regulating the actions of its members and which it may enforce by the imposition of penalties" (Oxford University Press 2019). There are four basic sources of law, all of which impact the national disaster policy preparedness, response, and recovery: (1) federal and state constitutions, which define and describe the role and authority of each branch of government, legislative, executive, and judicial; (2) statutes passed by the federal and state legislatures (laws passed by local officials are called ordinances); (3) case law; and (4) administrative law (which is derived from the executive branch). These sources of law address a number of issues relating to disasters and public health emergencies such as emergency declarations, quarantine and isolation, liability and licensure of nurses and HCPs, mutual aid, and others (Public Health Law Program 2017). Federal, state, and local authorities must work together during crises, but they may clash over who is in charge, who must expend resources, where those resources will be used, and so forth. The legal authority to act is centered at the distribution and allocation of powers enumerated in the U.S. Constitution (Hodge 2018).

Federalism is a system of government in which power is divided between a national (federal) government and various state governments. The U.S. Constitution, which is the primary source of all laws in the United States, enumerates the powers and limitations of the federal government, gives powers to the state governments, and in some cases, shares powers with the states. For example, the Constitution states that the federal government determines the foreign policy, with exclusive power to make treaties, declare war, and control imports and exports. Although the federal government has defined and limited powers, under the *doctrine of implied powers*, it has all authority "appropriate" to carry out such powers (*McCulloch v. Maryland*, 1819). As a result, the federal government can act broadly to address public health. Examples include the legislations on transportation safety, food safety, environmental protection, national security, and access to health services (Hodge 2018). Even so, through the Tenth Amendment, the states are reserved all powers "…not delegated to the United States by the Constitution, nor prohibited by it…" (National Archives 2019). These reserved powers give states the authority to regulate matters affecting the health and general welfare of the public and their citizens (Hodge 2018). In fact, provisions in *state* constitutions address public health emergency response. As such, state and local actors have substantial authority and responsibility for guiding response (Bjørnskov and Voigt 2017). If there is any conflict between the provisions of a state constitution and those of the federal Constitution, federal law takes precedence; this is known as federal supremacy.

In addition to the federal and state constitutions, the Congress and state legislatures provide a second source of law. Laws written by state legislatures, generally effective once signed by the state's governor, and laws drafted by Congress, effective once signed by the President, are called statutes. There are a substantial number of federal and state statutes that address issues pertinent to emergency preparedness, response, and recovery. A third and very important source of law, known as case law, results from judicial decisions made in settling disputes or "cases." Courts at the local, state, and federal levels provide a forum where facts of cases can be heard, the law applied, and the dispute resolved. Some court decisions serve as "precedent," establishing principles or rules that courts may adopt when deciding subsequent cases with similar issues or facts. For example, the seminal public health law case of *Jacobson v. Massachusetts* (1905) in which the U.S. Supreme Court upheld a board of health's authority to require vaccination against smallpox during a smallpox epidemic, serves as a precedent for courts when deciding how to balance the state authority with individual rights and interests, which are often implicated during disasters and other public health emergencies. Administrative rules and regulations are the fourth source of law. After a state legislature or Congress passes a law, it must be implemented by the administrative agencies under the state or federal executive branch. These agencies make rules and regulations for the enforcement of the statute. When conflicts arise regarding the application and interpretation of regulations, the administrative agency adjudicates the dispute through an administrative law process (by exercising "quasi-judicial" powers), with final decision subject to review by a court.

3.3 Federal Government Emergency Powers

As noted above, significant authority and responsibility for emergency preparedness, response, and recovery rest with the state and local officials and entities. The U.S. Constitution (Article 4, section 4), however, vests the supreme authority with the federal government to defend the nation and address matters of national security. Following the 9/11 terrorist attacks, officials strengthened the national disaster response policy through passage of a number of federal emergency preparedness laws, including:

- *Public Health Security and Bioterrorism Preparedness and Response Act of 2002*, which authorized the implementation of the National Disaster Medical System (NDMS), which coordinates the response of health and auxiliary services (e.g., Disaster Medical Response Teams (DMAT)) during public health emergencies, and established the Strategic National Stockpile (SNS) (see Table 3.1);

- *Project Bioshield Act of 2004*, which was a 10-year program (since reauthorized) to establish national requirements and acquisition strategies for pre- and postexposure countermeasures (e.g., vaccines) to be used in the event of chemical, biological, radiological, or nuclear (CBRN) emergencies;
- *Homeland Security Act of 2002*, which created and empowered the Department of Homeland Security to act as the focal point in securing the nation against terrorist attacks and coordinating planning and response to natural and man-made emergencies.

A number of other federal laws authorize the federal government to act in times of emergency. Examples of major emergency legal authorities, general laws as well as those specifically relating to public health emergencies are listed in Table 3.1.

In addition to statutes, the federal government can use its rule-making authority (administrative law) to direct and support emergency preparedness, response, and recovery. For example, on September 16, 2016, the Centers for Medicare and Medicaid Services (CMS), which is under the Department of Health and Human Services (HHS), issued a final rule entitled "Medicare and Medicaid Programs; Emergency Preparedness Requirements for Medicare and Medicaid Participating Providers and Suppliers," (42 CFR Parts 403, 416, 418, 441, 460, 482, 483, 484, 485, 486, 491, and 494), which "establishes national emergency preparedness requirements for Medicare- and Medicaid-participating providers and suppliers to plan adequately for both natural and man-made disasters, and coordinate with federal, state, tribal, regional, and local emergency preparedness systems." Specifically, the rule requires 17 provider types, including hospitals, long-term care facilities, home health agencies, community mental health centers, and rural health centers among others, to:

> • perform a risk assessment that uses an "all-hazards" approach prior to establishing an emergency plan;
> • develop and implement policies and procedures that support the successful execution of the emergency plan and risks identified during the risk assessment process;
> • develop and maintain an emergency preparedness communication plan that complies with both federal and state laws; and
> • develop and maintain an emergency preparedness training and testing program.
> (CFR, Vol. 81, No. 180, 63861-63862)

Just as the federal government can mandate certain activities by the entities participating in federal programs, it can also waive those requirements. For example, Section 1135 of the Social Security Act allows the HHS Secretary to waive or modify certain requirements of Medicare, Medicaid, Children's Health Insurance Program (CHIP), and Health Insurance Portability and Accountability Act (HIPAA), as well as the Emergency Medical Treatment and Active Labor Act (EMTALA) (known as "1135 waivers") to ensure that sufficient health care services are available to meet the needs of those enrolled in these programs during an emergency. HCPs who are unable to comply with certain requirements of these programs are

Table 3.1 Federal laws relating to public health emergencies

Federal statute	Key provisions
Robert T. Stafford Disaster Relief and Emergency Assistance Act of 1988 (Stafford Act); 42 U.S.C. §§ 5121-5207	• Authorizes the U.S. President to declare a "major disaster" or emergency in response to an event, most typically following the request of a state Governor; as of 2013, tribal leaders may also make a request • Directs Federal Emergency Management Agency (FEMA) to coordinate the administration of disaster relief to the states • Provides for a national system for all-hazards emergency preparedness, with authority at federal and state levels
National Emergencies Act; 50 U.S.C. §§ 1601-1651	• Authorizes the President to declare a "national emergency," which must be transmitted immediately to Congress and published in the Federal Register
Public Health Service Act (PHSA); 42 U.S.C. §§ 201 et seq.	• Section 319 of the PHSA provides the legal authority for the Department of Health and Human Services (HHS) to determine that a public health emergency exists; to respond to and lead federal public health and medical response to public health emergencies, and assist states in their response activities • Authorizes the HHS, in coordination with Homeland Security and the CDC, to maintain the Strategic National Stockpile (SNS), a stockpile of drugs, vaccines, biological products, medical devices and other medical supplies, to provide for the emergency health security of the United States and its territories to provide for the emergency health security of the United States and its territories
Pandemic and All-Hazards Preparedness Reauthorization Act (PAHPRA) of 2013; 42 U.S.C. §§ 201 et seq.	• Amends PHSA to reauthorize key portions of the *Project Bioshield Act of 2004* and the *Pandemic and All-Hazards Preparedness Act (PAHPA) of 2006* • Makes targeted improvements to preparedness and response programs and expands the role of the Assistant Secretary for Preparedness and Response (ASPR) • Emphasizes consideration of the unique needs of children and of persons with disabilities, including countermeasure-related needs for these populations • Creates the National Advisory Committee on Children and Disasters to advise, consult, and evaluate children's preparedness- and response-related needs • Expands Food and Drug Administration (FDA) authority to issue Emergency Use Authorizations (EUAs) that allow the use of unapproved medical products or unapproved use of approved products leading up to or during an emergency in the absence of adequate, available alternatives

(continued)

Table 3.1 (continued)

Federal statute	Key provisions
Volunteer Protection Act of 1997: 42 U.S.C. §§ 14501-14505	• Supports and promotes activities of organizations that rely on volunteers by providing volunteers with some protections from liability when acting for the organization
Emergency Medical Assistance Compact (EMAC) of 1996; ratified by U.S. Congress, PL 104-321	• An interstate mutual aid agreement that among states and territories of the United States facilitates sharing of resources during natural and man-made disasters, including terrorism • Requires a governor's declaration of emergency and request for assistance • Stipulates that a provider who is licensed or certified in one state will be considered licensed or certified in a receiving state, subject to limitations

Sources: Hodge JG Jr. *Public health law in a nutshell, 3rd ed.* St. Paul, MN: West Academic Publishing; 2018
Public Health Law Program, Centers for Disease Control and Prevention. Selected Legal Authorities Pertinent to Public Health Emergencies, 2017. Available at https://www.cdc.gov/phlp/docs/ph-emergencies.pdf

still reimbursed for the services they provide during the emergency and are exempted from sanctions for noncompliance absent fraud or abuse (Association of State and Territorial Health Officials 2019a). Section 1135 waivers require a declaration of a national emergency or disaster by the President under the National Emergencies Act or the Stafford Act and a public health emergency determination by the HHS Secretary under Section 319 of the Public Health Service Act (PHSA). Importantly, a 1135 waiver does not affect state laws or regulations, including those for licensure and conditions of participation (Association of State and Territorial Health Officials 2019a).

The federal government also uses its authority to promote the availability of resources during emergencies by limiting the legal liability of government employees and volunteers. Protection against liability serves an important public policy function by ensuring that sufficient numbers of medical, public health, and other individuals and institutions are willing to participate in emergency response efforts. Liability protections vary significantly and depend on who is protected (an individual, entity, or class), the law providing the protections, and the circumstances surrounding a particular emergency response (e.g., Volunteer Protection Act of 1997; Public Readiness and Emergency Preparedness (PREP) Act of 2005) (Association of State and Territorial Health Officials 2019b). For example, the HHS Secretary can issue a declaration that provides immunity from claims of harm to person or property resulting from the use of countermeasures (e.g., vaccines) against diseases or other threats of public health emergencies (Public Health Law Program 2017).

3.4   Local, State, and Tribal Government Emergency Powers

Under the Tenth Amendment of the U.S. Constitution, states have broad authority to act to protect the health of the public, which includes the times of emergency and disaster. Conversely, American-Indian tribal governments, which are sovereign nations, derive their power from the federal government through a series of federal laws. Previously, tribal governments were unable to directly request a presidential declaration of a major disaster in India; instead, tribes had to formally request their state governors to ask the President for federal assistance. However, the Sandy Recovery Improvement Act of 2013 amended the Stafford Act to provide federally recognized tribal governments the option of making an emergency declaration request directly to the President (Fugate 2017).

The dominant role of states, and by extension, local governments, in all-hazards preparedness, response, and recovery rests on the doctrines of "police powers" and "*parens patriae* powers" (Hodge 2018).

Police powers. Police powers refer to the authority of the states to enact laws and promulgate regulations for the promotion of public health, safety, morals, and welfare (Legarre 2007). Although this authority is broad, it remains subject to the restrictions of the Constitution's supremacy clause and must be balanced against the individual rights and private interests protected by Constitutional Amendments. The application of police powers has traditionally represented the state's capacity to: "(Federal Emergency Management Agency (FEMA) 2010) promote the public health, morals, or safety, and the general well-being of the community; (Kilpatrick 2000) enact and enforce laws for the promotion of the general welfare; (Office of the Under Secretary of Defense for Personnel and Readiness 2016) regulate private rights in the public interest; and (Committee on Guidance Establishing Crisis Standard of Care for Use in Disaster Situations 2012) extend measures to all great public needs" (Galva et al. 2005). States can delegate their police powers to local governments, either via the state Constitution or by a statute. Police powers support broad state action in regard to "health laws of every description," including those needed to manage public health emergencies like disasters (*Jacobson v. Massachusetts*, 1905: 25).

***Parens patriae* power.** The legal principle of *parens patriae*, "Latin for parent of the country," authorizes the state government to act in the interest of an individual's well-being as well as that of a community (Hodge 2018). Typically, *parens patriae* powers allow the state to look after the interests of minors, persons with mental disabilities, the elderly, prisoners, or other wards of the state, but they may also be used to support legal standing when states sue to support the well-being of a state's entire population (e.g., environmental concerns or natural disasters) (Hodge 2018).

Emergencies start and end locally; therefore, local officials must be empowered to act during times of crises. The authority of city, county, and other local officials to act during emergencies is derived from the state Constitution or state statute and is constrained by the federal and state laws. Specifically, the state may provide local governments with "home rule" over matters of local concern. The breadth of this "home rule" is limited to those powers expressly granted to the locality by the state (Hodge 2018). The scale and complexity of any emergency will dictate the level of response, local, state, or federal. Generally, the authority to declare an emergency is reserved with the chief executive officer (nationally, the President; at the state level, the governor) or their designee (other key governmental officials as determined by law). In some states, local officials may be able to declare local emergencies. Declaring an emergency triggers a number of actions, including suspension of routine governmental activity and implementation of emergency response, which includes making operational resources available. During catastrophic events, multiple jurisdictions, agencies, and levels of government are activated. Multiple emergency declarations and duplicative response efforts can create legal conflicts and impede action. Often times, the scope and scale of an emergency may exceed the capabilities of the jurisdictions impacted. Mutual aid agreements are an important legal tool that provides for the sharing of supplies, equipments, personnel, information, and other resources across jurisdictional boundaries. In 1996, the Congress ratified the Emergency Management Assistance Compact, creating the nation's all-hazards–all-disciplines state-to-state mutual aid system. Presently, all 50 states, the District of Columbia, Puerto Rico, Guam, and the U.S. Virgin Islands are members of the compact (Compact 2019).

3.5   Executive Branch Authority

Article II of the U.S. Constitution establishes the Executive Branch of the federal government and vests the roles of commander in chief, head of state, chief law enforcement officer, and head of the executive branch with the President. The President is obligated to "take care that the laws be faithfully executed" and is granted broad discretion over federal law enforcement decisions. One mechanism by which the President directs the actions of government officials and agencies is through the use of executive orders and presidential directives. An executive order can be used to execute a power the President already has under the Constitution or federal law, but it cannot be used to give the presidency new powers. Frequently, Presidents use executive orders and presidential directives to "establish policies, strategies, and frameworks, directing executive agency activities," including policies related to national security, disaster preparedness, response, and recovery (Association of State and Territorial Health Officials 2019c).

National Incident Management System (NIMS). Under Homeland Security Presidential Directive-5 (HSPD-5) (February 28, 2003), the federal government created the NIMS "[t]o enhance the ability of the United States to manage domestic incidents by establishing a single, comprehensive national incident management system." Now, in its third iteration, the NIMS guides all levels of government, nongovernmental organizations, and the private sector in the prevention and mitigation of, response to, and recovery from events and incidents of all sizes, regardless of the emergency declaration status (U.S. Department of Homeland Security, Federal Emergency Management Agency 2017). NIMS provides a common framework to integrate the diverse authorities, management structures, communication capabilities, and protocols of jurisdictions and organizations responding to emergencies, and specifically addresses the following: (Federal Emergency Management Agency (FEMA) 2010) resource management, (Kilpatrick 2000) command and coordination, and (Office of the Under Secretary of Defense for Personnel and Readiness 2016) communications and information management (U.S. Department of Homeland Security, Federal Emergency Management Agency 2017). NIMS specifically states, "[a]ll incident management efforts, regardless of the incident or location, should fully incorporate people with disabilities and other people who have access and functional needs," with functional needs defined as "individual circumstances requiring assistance, accommodation, or modification for mobility, communication, transportation, safety, health maintenance, etc., due to any temporary or permanent situation that limits an individual's ability to take action during an incident" (U.S. Department of Homeland Security, Federal Emergency Management Agency 2017).

National Preparedness System. The Homeland Security Presidential Directive-8 (HSPD-8) issued on December 17, 2003 and as a companion to HSPD-5 set forth policies to promote the coordination and implementation of all-hazards preparedness in the United States, including establishing mechanisms for the delivery of federal preparedness assistance to state and local governments. In 2011, HSPD-8 was superseded by the Presidential Policy Directive-8 (PPD-8), which focuses on augmenting and improving an "all-of-Nation, capabilities-based approach to preparedness" (U.S. Department of Homeland Security 2019). the Major elements of the PPD-8 include the following:

1. Developing a *National Preparedness Goal*, defining a series of national preparedness elements (called core capabilities) needed to achieve the goal, and emphasizing the need for individuals, families, communities, private and nonprofit sectors, faith-based organizations, and state, local, tribal, territorial, insular area, and federal government to work together in a variety of ways and make the best use of resources (U.S. Department of Homeland Security, Federal Emergency Management Agency 2019a).
2. Outlining the *National Preparedness System* that delineates the approach, resources, and tools for achieving the National Preparedness Goal (U.S. Department of Homeland Security, Federal Emergency Management Agency 2019b).
3. Producing an annual *National Preparedness Report* that summarizes progress toward achieving the National Preparedness Goal and is used to inform the President's budget (U.S. Department of Homeland Security, Federal Emergency Management Agency 2019c).
4. Preparing *National Planning Frameworks* addressing each of the five preparedness mission areas: prevention, protection, mitigation, response, and disaster recovery (U.S. Department of Homeland Security, Federal Emergency Management Agency 2019d).
5. Developing *Federal Interagency Operational Plans* to address how federal efforts can work together to support state and local plans, and describe critical tasks and responsibilities and specific provisions for rapidly integrating resources and personnel (U.S. Department of Homeland Security, Federal Emergency Management Agency 2019e).
6. Building and sustaining preparedness through a comprehensive campaign, including public outreach and community-based and private-sector programs; federal preparedness efforts; grants, technical assistance and other federal preparedness support; and research and development (U.S. Department of Homeland Security, Federal Emergency Management Agency 2019e).

Administrative Agency Action. Most federal agencies fall under the control of the executive branch. As a result, in addition to issuing executive orders and presidential directives, the President can direct policies through the activities of these agencies. A substantial number of federal agencies are implicated in disaster preparedness and response. The agency responsibility is generally divided into two broad areas of responsibility, general operational and medical (Table 3.2). Agencies work with the executive and legislative branches to create strategies and plans relating to national emergency planning and response activities. For example, the Department of Homeland Security drafted the *National Response Framework*, a policy document that serves to guide to how the Nation conducts all-hazards response and is built upon scalable, flexible, and adaptable coordinating structures to align key roles and responsibilities across the Nation, linking all levels of government, nongovernmental organizations (NGOs), and the private sector (U.S. Department of Homeland Security, Federal Emergency Management Agency 2016). The *National Response Framework* document uses the concepts identified in the NIMS to describe specific authorities and best practices for managing events

Table 3.2 Key federal agencies with responsibilities in public health emergencies

Federal agency/office	Responsibilities	Website
Centers for Disease Control and Prevention (CDC), Center for Preparedness and Response	Extensive capabilities in preparation for and response to a variety of public health threats, including biological threats, natural disasters, and chemical and radiological events	https://www.cdc.gov/cpr/index.htm
Department of Agriculture (USDA)	Responsible for protecting the safety of the nation's food supply; provides nutrition assistance to those most affected by emergencies and disasters	https://www.aphis.usda.gov/aphis/ourfocus/emergencyresponse
Department of Defense (DOD)	In addition to its traditional military role, the DOD supports the operations of other Federal Government agencies as well as state and local governments. Use of the military is subject to the Posse Comitatus Act, 18 U.S.C § 1385, which restricts the participation of the military in domestic law enforcement activities under many circumstances	https://www.defense.gov
Department of Energy (DOE), Office of Cybersecurity, Energy Security and Emergency Response	Responsible for coordinating the protection of critical energy assets and assisting federal, state, and local governments with disruption preparation, response, and mitigation	https://www.energy.gov/ceser/activities/energy-security/emergency-preparedness
Department of Health and Human Services (HHS), Office of the Assistant Secretary for Preparedness and Response	Leads medical and public health preparedness for, response to, and recovery from disasters and public health emergencies; collaborates with hospitals, health care coalitions, biotech firms, community members, state, local, tribal, and territorial governments, and other partners across the country to improve readiness and response capabilities	https://www.phe.gov
Department of Homeland Security (DHS)	General operational responsibility related to federal disaster response in the U.S.	https://www.dhs.gov/topic/disasters
Department of the Interior (DOI)	Prepares for and responds to incidents caused by natural or human effects that impact Federal lands, resources (including nationwide fish and wildlife resources, flood plains, wetlands, and cultural/historic resources), facilities, tenants, employees, visitors, and adjacent landowners	https://www.doi.gov/emergency

(continued)

Table 3.2 (continued)

Federal agency/office	Responsibilities	Website
Environmental Protection Agency (EPA)	Responds to oil spills, chemical, biological, radiological releases, and large-scale national emergencies; provides additional response assistance when state and local first responder capabilities have been exhausted or when additional support is requested.	https://www.epa.gov/emergency-response
FEMA	Coordinates disaster response to a disaster that overwhelms the resources of local or state authorities; operates as a regional group with regional response	https://www.fema.gov
Nuclear Regulatory Commission (NRC), Office of Nuclear Security and Incident Response (NSIR)	Integrates overall NRC capabilities for the response and recovery of radiological incidents and emergencies involving facilities and materials regulated by the NRC or an Agreement State.	https://www.nrc.gov/about-nrc/emerg-preparedness.html

Source: Disaster Information Management Research Center. U.S. Government Sources of Information, 2019 [Available from: https://disasterinfo.nlm.nih.gov/us-government-sources]

that range from local to large-scale terrorist attacks or catastrophic natural disasters (U.S. Department of Homeland Security 2019). Other relevant strategy documents for emergency response include the *National Health Security Strategy* (U.S. Department of Health and Human Services, Office of the Assistant Security of Preparedness and Response 2019), produced by the HHS, Office of the Assistant Secretary for Preparedness and Response, the *National Strategy for Pandemic Influenza (*U.S. Homeland Security Council 2005*)*, promulgated by the Centers for Disease Control and Prevention, and the *National Strategy for Homeland Security (*U.S. Homeland Security Council 2007*)*, administered by the Department of Homeland Security.

3.6 Conclusion

Understanding the legal structures that support the federal, state, and local interaction is an essential component of effective emergency preparedness and response. Although emergencies generally start locally, the scale and complexity of an emergency can necessitate a multijurisdictional response. Federal and state laws provide for the activation of emergency response activities, allocate resources, authorize the expenditure of funds, and enable powers such as implementation of quarantines, curfews, and evacuations. Although beneficial, the intersection of federal and state authorities adds complexity to response activities and intensifies the need for multijurisdictional and multiprofessional emergency management planning, exercises and training, and coordination.

References

Association of State and Territorial Health Officials. Emergency authority and immunity toolkit, Social Security Act, section 1135, waiver authority in national emergencies [Internet]. 2019a. http://www.astho.org/Programs/Preparedness/Public-Health-Emergency-Law/Emergency-Authority-and-Immunity-Toolkit/Social-Security-Act,-Section-1135-Waiver-Authority-in-National-Emergencies-Fact-Sheet/.

Association of State and Territorial Health Officials. Emergency authority and immunity toolkit, immunity issues in emergencies [Internet]. 2019b. http://www.astho.org/Programs/Preparedness/Public-Health-Emergency-Law/Emergency-Authority-and-Immunity-Toolkit/Immunity-Issues-in-Emergencies-Fact-Sheet/.

Association of State and Territorial Health Officials. Emergency authority and immunity toolkit, key federal laws and policies regarding emergency authority and immunity [Internet]. 2019c. http://www.astho.org/Programs/Preparedness/Public-Health-Emergency-Law/Emergency-Authority-and-Immunity-Toolkit/Key-Federal-Laws-and-Policies-Regarding-Emergency-Authority-and-Immunity/.

Bjørnskov C, Voigt S. Dealing with disaster: Analyzing emergency constitutions of the U.S. States. AZ State Law J. 2017;49(3 (Fall)):883–906.

Committee on Guidance Establishing Crisis Standard of Care for Use in Disaster Situations. Crisis standards of care for use in disaster situations. Washington, DC: National Academies Press; 2012. http://www.nationalacademies.org/hmd/Reports/2012/Crisis-Standards-of-Care-A-Systems-Framework-for-Catastrophic-Disaster-Response.aspx.

Compact EMA. Emergency management assistance compact [Internet]. 2019. https://www.emac-web.org/index.php.

Federal Emergency Management Agency (FEMA). Developing and maintaining emergency operations plans, version 2.0. Washington, DC: Department of Homeland Security; 2010. https://www.fema.gov/media-library-data/20130726-1828-25045-0014/cpg_101_comprehensive_preparedness_guide_developing_and_maintaining_emergency_operations_plans_2010.pdf.

Fugate C. FEMA Blog [Internet]. 2017. https://www.fema.gov/blog/2013-01-31/changing-laws-better-recognizing-tribal-sovereignty.

Galva JE, Atchinson C, Levey S. Public health strategy and police powers of the state. Public Health Rep. 2005;120(Suppl. 1):20–7.

Hodge J Jr. Public health law in a nutshell. 3rd ed. St. Paul, MN: West Academic Publishing; 2018.

Kilpatrick DG. Definitions of public policy and the law [Internet]. 2000. https://mainweb-v.musc.edu/vawprevention/policy/definition.shtml.

Legarre S. The historical background of the police power. J Constit Law. 2007;9(3):745–96.

National Archives. America's Founding Documents. The Constitution of the United States [Internet]. 2019. https://www.archives.gov/founding-docs/constitution.

Office of the Under Secretary of Defense for Personnel and Readiness. DoD Instruction 6010.22, National Disaster Medical System (NDMS). In: Department of Defense, editor [Internet]. 2016. https://www.esd.whs.mil/Portals/54/Documents/DD/issuances/dodi/601022p.pdf.

Oxford University Press. English Oxford Living Dictionary, Definition of law [Internet]. 2019. https://en.oxforddictionaries.com/definition/law.

Public Health Law Program. Centers for Disease Control and Prevention. Selected legal authorities pertinent to public health emergencies. Atlanta, GA: Centers for Disease Control and Prevention; 2017. https://www.cdc.gov/phlp/docs/ph-emergencies.pdf.

U.S. Department of Health and Human Services, Office of the Assistant Security of Preparedness and Response. National health security strategy, 2019-2022. Washington, DC: Department of Health and Human Services; 2019. https://www.phe.gov/Preparedness/planning/authority/nhss/Documents/NHSS-Strategy-508.pdf.

U.S. Department of Homeland Security. Presidential policy directive/PPD-8: National preparedness [Internet]. 2019. https://www.dhs.gov/presidential-policy-directive-8-national-preparedness#.

U.S. Department of Homeland Security, Federal Emergency Management Agency. National response framework. 3rd ed. Washington, DC: Department of Homeland Security; 2016. https://www.fema.gov/media-library-data/1466014682982-9bcf8245ba4c60c120aa915a-be74e15d/National_Response_Framework3rd.pdf.

U.S. Department of Homeland Security, Federal Emergency Management Agency. National incident management system. 3rd ed. Washington, DC: Department of Homeland Security; 2017. https://www.hsdl.org/?view&did=804929.

U.S. Department of Homeland Security, Federal Emergency Management Agency. National preparedness goal [Internet]. 2019a. https://www.fema.gov/national-preparedness-goal.

U.S. Department of Homeland Security, Federal Emergency Management Agency. National preparedness system [Internet]. 2019b. https://www.fema.gov/national-preparedness-system.

U.S. Department of Homeland Security, Federal Emergency Management Agency. National preparedness report [Internet]. 2019c. https://www.fema.gov/national-preparedness-report.

U.S. Department of Homeland Security, Federal Emergency Management Agency. National planning frameworks [Internet]. 2019d. https://www.fema.gov/national-planning-frameworks.

U.S. Department of Homeland Security, Federal Emergency Management Agency. Learn about presidential policy directive-8 [Internet]. 2019e. https://www.fema.gov/learn-about-presidential-policy-directive-8.

U.S. Homeland Security Council. National strategy for pandemic influenza. [Internet]. 2005. https://www.cdc.gov/flu/pandemic-resources/pdf/pandemic-influenza-strategy-2005.pdf.

U.S. Homeland Security Council. National strategy for homeland security [Internet]. 2007. https://www.dhs.gov/xlibrary/assets/nat_strat_homelandsecurity_2007.pdf.

Incident Command System

Nancy Blake

4.1 Introduction

The Incident Command System (ICS) originated in 1970 after a devastating wildfire in California (FEMA ICS Review 2018a). The fire in Southern California lasted 13 days, and 700 structures were destroyed, sixteen lives were lost, and it caused over $234M in damages. While responding agencies worked as well as they could together, there were multiple problems with communication and coordination resulting in a nonunified response. The issues discovered in the after action report were (1) at the field level, there was confusion based on the different agencies using different terminology, organizational structure, and operating procedures and (2) above the incident or field level, the mechanisms to coordinate and handle competing resource demands and to establish consistent resource priorities were inadequate (EMSI 2019).

Following the fire in 1971, Congress mandated that the U.S. Forest Service come together and design a system that would make "significant improvements" to coordinate efforts for response (Stambler and Barbera 2011). The group in Southern California that put the system together was the Firefighting Resources of Southern California Organized for Potential Emergencies (FIRESCOPE), and their tasks were to develop two systems: the Multiagency Coordination System (MACS) and the Incident Command System (ICS) (EMSI 2019).

The system grew in the late 1970s and 1980s and was used for fire response. ICS progressed beyond just a fire response to an all-hazards approach and was adopted nationally in the 1980s. FEMA recognized ICS as a model approach to hazard responses; interestingly, the organizational chart has not changed much over the

N. Blake (✉)
School of Nursing, University of California Los Angeles, Los Angeles, CA, USA

Harbor-UCLA Medical Center, University of California Los Angeles, Torrance, CA, USA
e-mail: nblake@dhs.lacounty.gov

© Springer Nature Switzerland AG 2020
C. J. Goodhue, N. Blake (eds.), *Nursing Management of Pediatric Disaster*,
https://doi.org/10.1007/978-3-030-43428-1_4

years. Following the 9/11 terrorist attacks, it was determined that a national approach was needed for incident response. As a result of this, President Bush issued a Homeland Security Presidential Directive—5 (HSPD-5) ordering the development of a single, national incident management system. As a result of this directive, ICS and MACS became the basis of the National Incident Management System (NIMS) command and management in 2004 (EMSI 2019).

4.2   NIMS

The most recent version of NIMS was released in 2017, and it has been adopted in all communities across the nation as an all-hazards approach. ICS is an approach to command and control under the NIMS system. The following characteristics are the foundation of incident command and coordination in the NIMS system and are the reasons for a successful approach:

- Common Terminology
- Modular Organization
- Management by Objectives
- Incident Action Planning
- Manageable Span of Control (1:5 is the guideline)
- Incident Facilities and Locations
- Comprehensive Resource Management
- Integrated Communications
- Establishment of Transfer and Command
- Unified Command
- Chain of Command and Unity of Command
- Accountability
- Dispatch/Deployment
- Information and Intelligence Management (ICS 100 2018b).

Some of the key features of NIMS, as listed above, will be covered in more detail. The common terminology includes organizational functions, resource descriptions, and facilities. The organizational functions and functional units, as well as the resource description, will be described further during the discussion on the organization structure and job action sheets in ICS. The incident facilities include the Incident Command Post (ICP), the incident base, staging areas, camps, mass casualty triage areas, points of distribution, and emergency shelters. Some of these facilities are defined below:

- Incident Command Post—The field location at which the primary tactical-level, on-scene incident command functions are performed.

- Staging Area—The location where resources can be placed while awaiting a tactical assignment.
- Incident Base—The location where primary logistics functions are coordinated. There is only one incident base per incident. The Incident Command Post may be collocated with the incident base.
- Camp—A location where food, water, rest, and sanitary services are provided to the incident personnel (ICS 100 2018b).

Integrated communications include a common plan for communication, interoperable communications process between agencies, and voice and data links. Without this common communication set of resources, the response agencies will not be able to have a unified response.

Establishment of command addresses the leadership, hand-off, and continual process addressing disasters. This process has common terminology and definitions that address who is responsible for the various locations. The term Unified Command is identified when there are multiple agencies and jurisdictions involved and there is not only one Incident Commander. A Unified Command results in jointly approved objectives and a unity of effort to allocate resources (Deal et al. 2010). The Transfer of Command results in a briefing that captures all of the important information at the time of transfer in command. The Chain of Command refers to the authority and levels of responsibility. More will be discussed later in this chapter when the organization structure of ICS is discussed. Unity of Command results in each individual only reporting to one person (FEMA ICS Review 2018a). This results in a clear understanding of accountability in each individual job.

4.3   Incident Command System (ICS)

The Incident Command System is a standardized approach to the command, control, and coordination of incident management for both governmental and nongovernmental (NGO) agencies. The concepts of ICS include a common hierarchy and standardized roles. The important features of ICS are that is integrates and coordinates procedures, personnel, equipment, facilities, communications, and, when necessary, intelligence and investigations. The five major functional areas that are staffed, as needed: Command, Operations, Planning, Logistics, and Finance Administration. The general ICS organizational chart is attached in Fig. 4.1.

The position titles (Table 4.1) for each of the roles change based on the role and the organizational element. While the organizational chart may expand in the larger incidents that occur over a longer time period, the system is modular and may not require expansion in short minor responses.

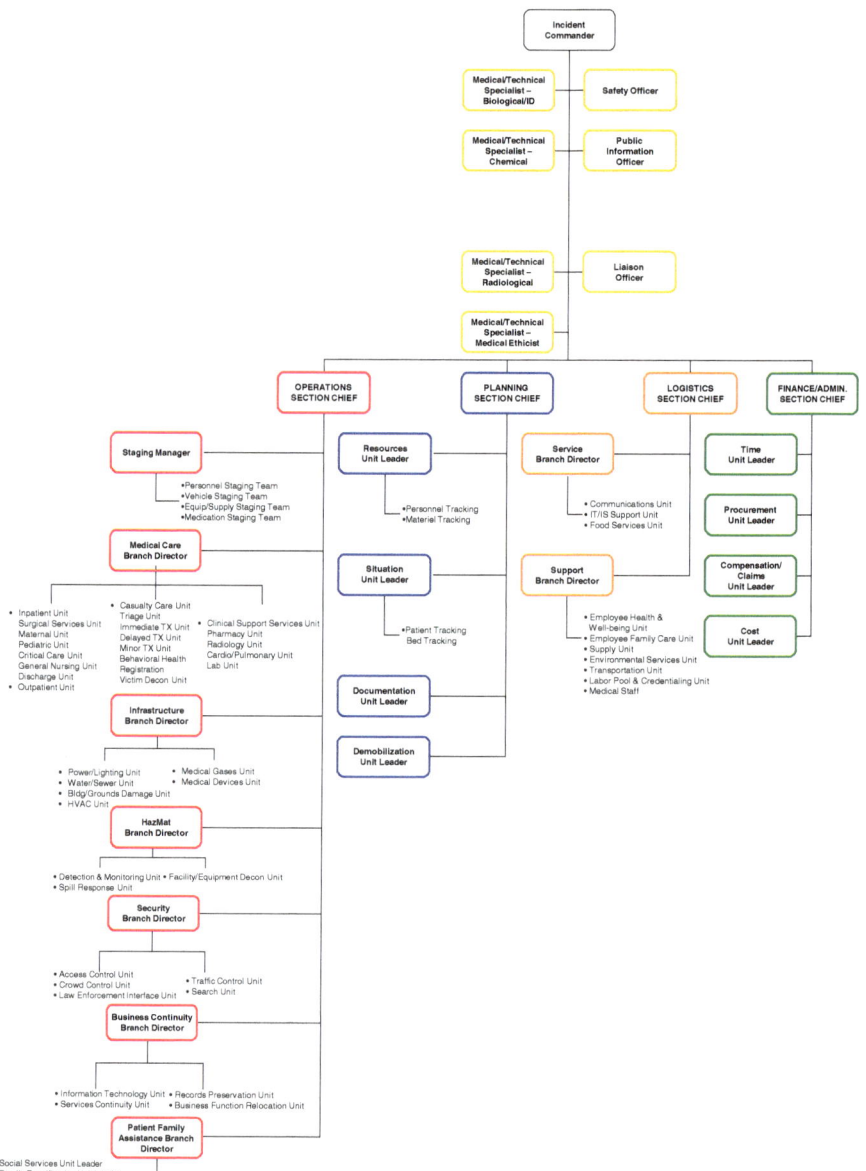

Fig. 4.1 HICS organization charts

HICS–Command Staff, Section Chiefs

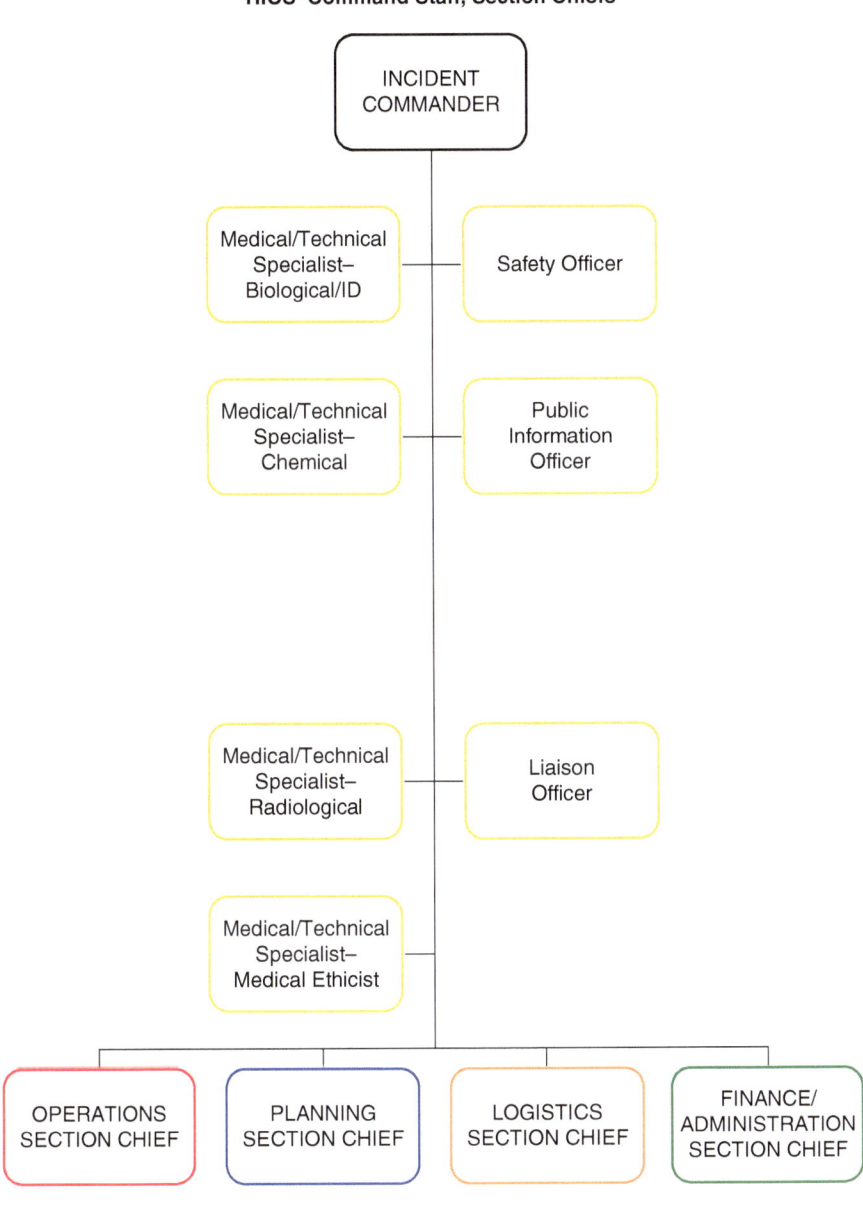

Fig. 4.1 (continued)

HICS–Command Staff, Section Chiefs, Branch Directors, Unit Leaders

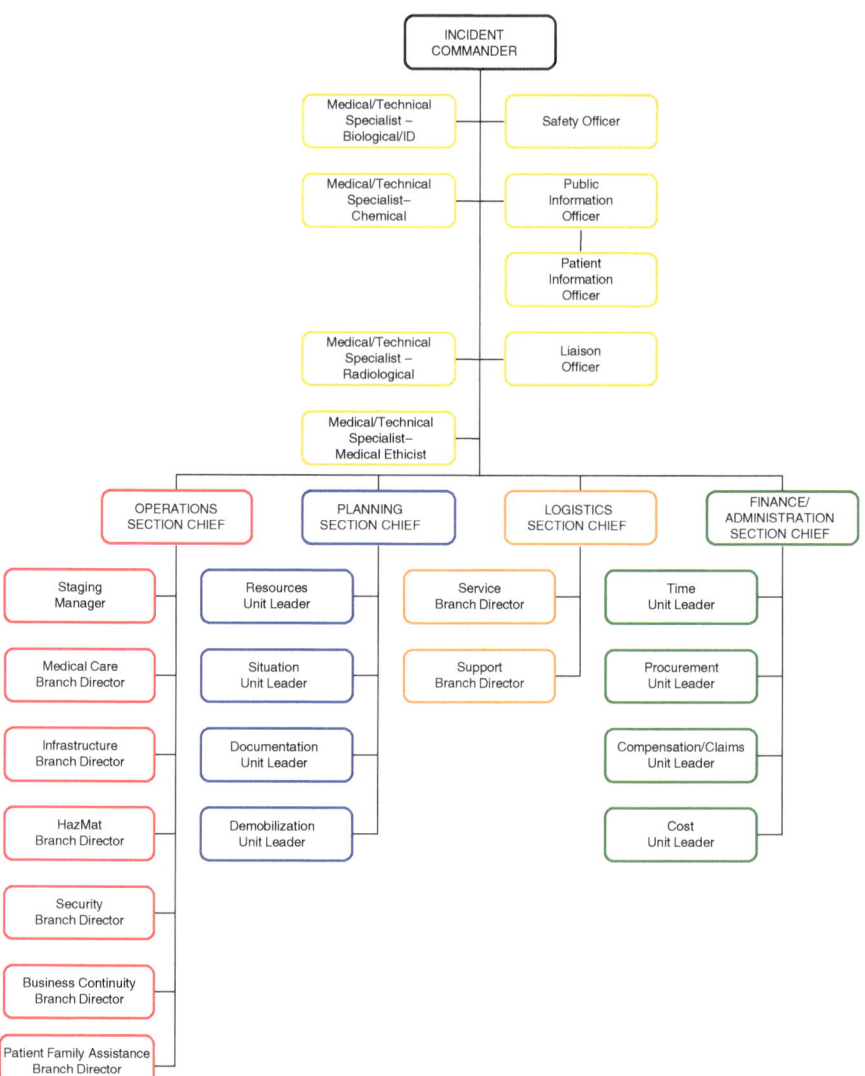

Fig. 4.1 (continued)

HICS–Finance/Administration

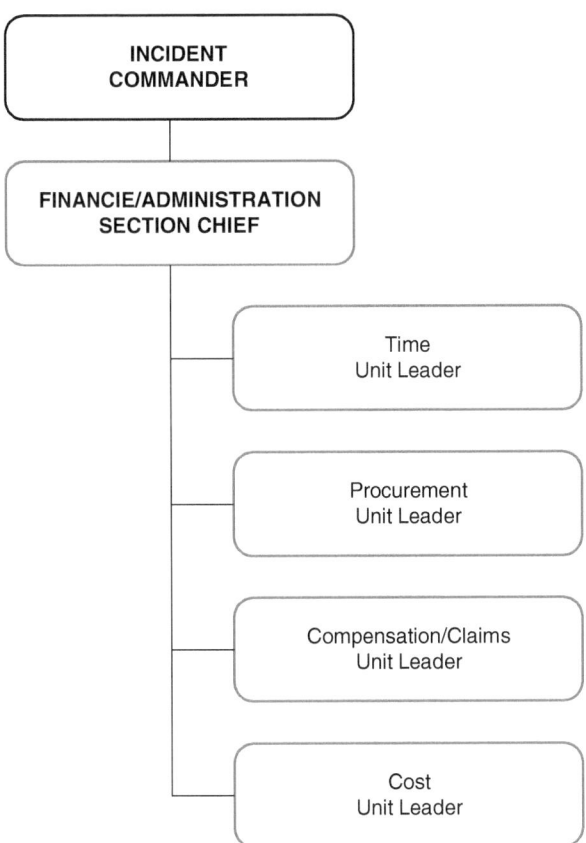

Fig. 4.1 (continued)

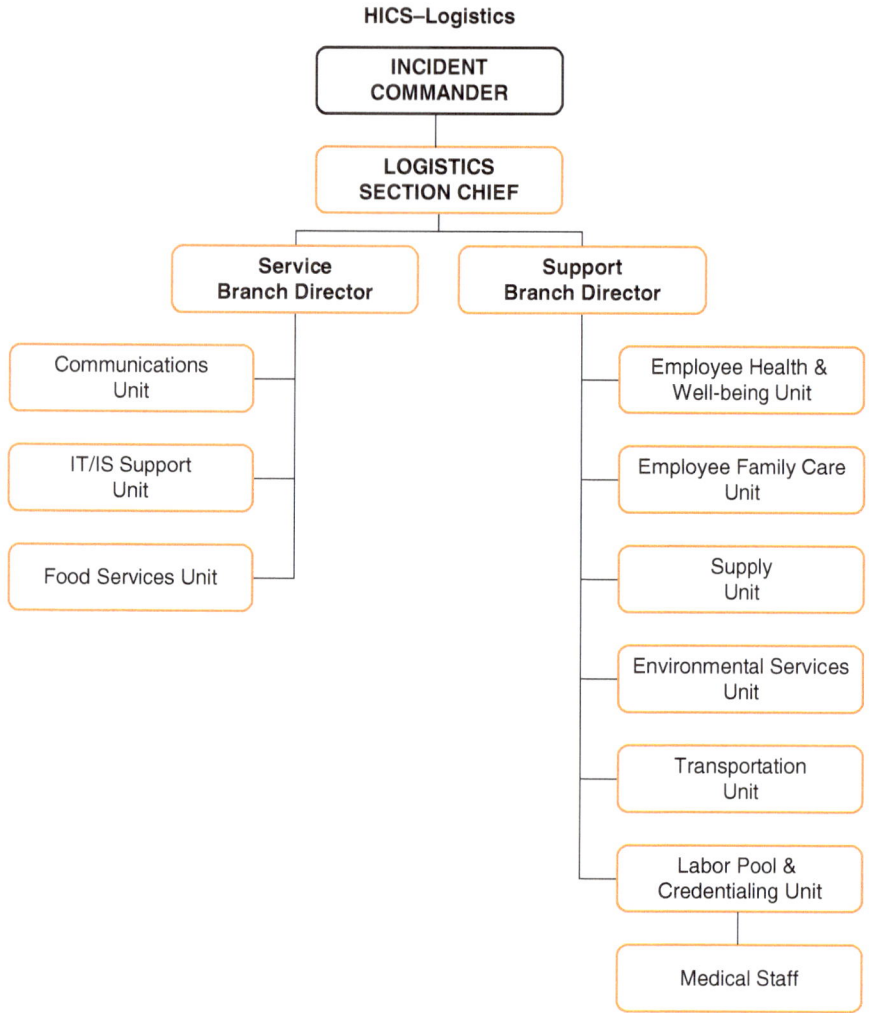

Fig. 4.1 (continued)

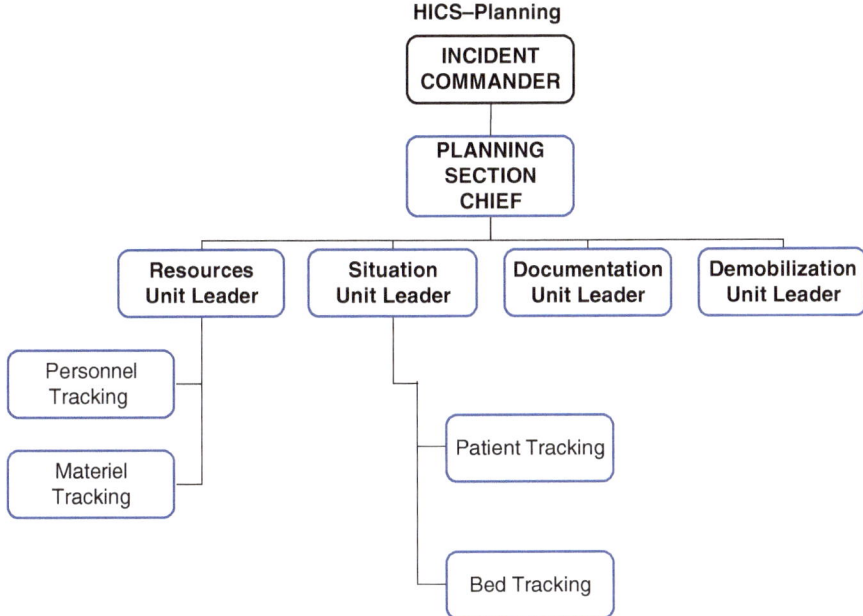

Fig. 4.1 (continued)

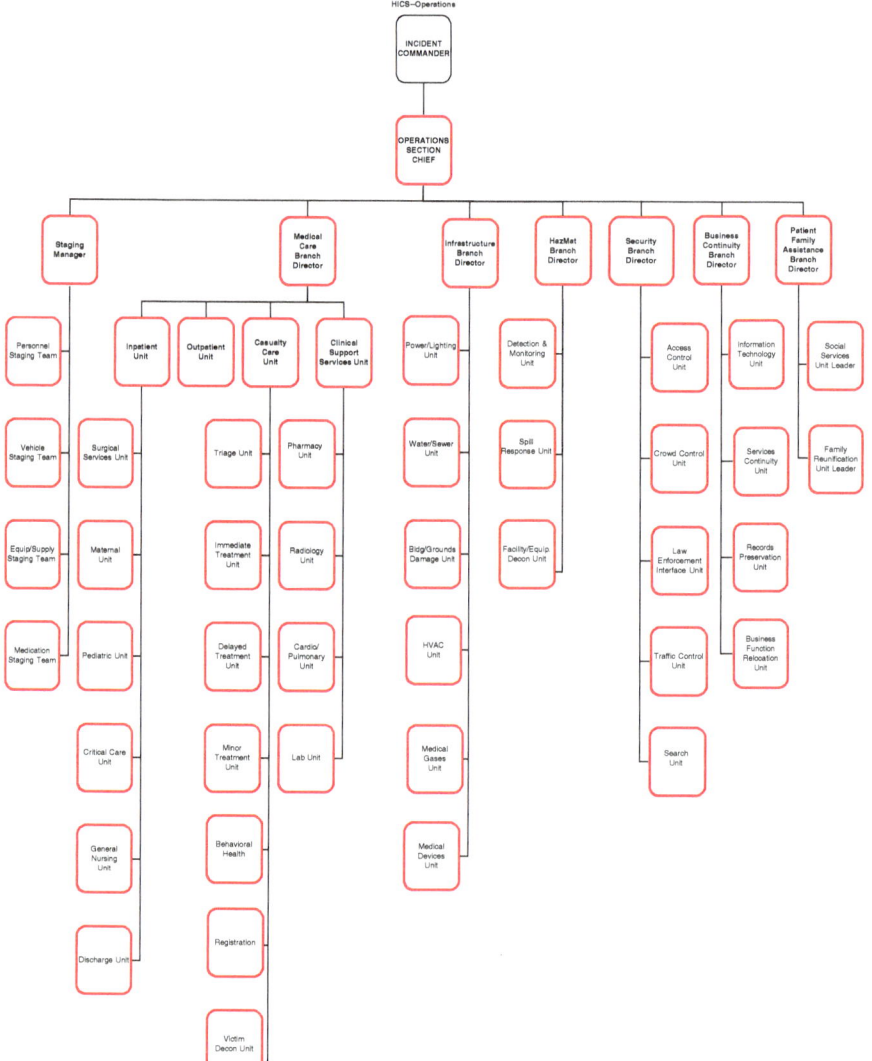

Fig. 4.1 (continued)

HICS–Operations, Staging

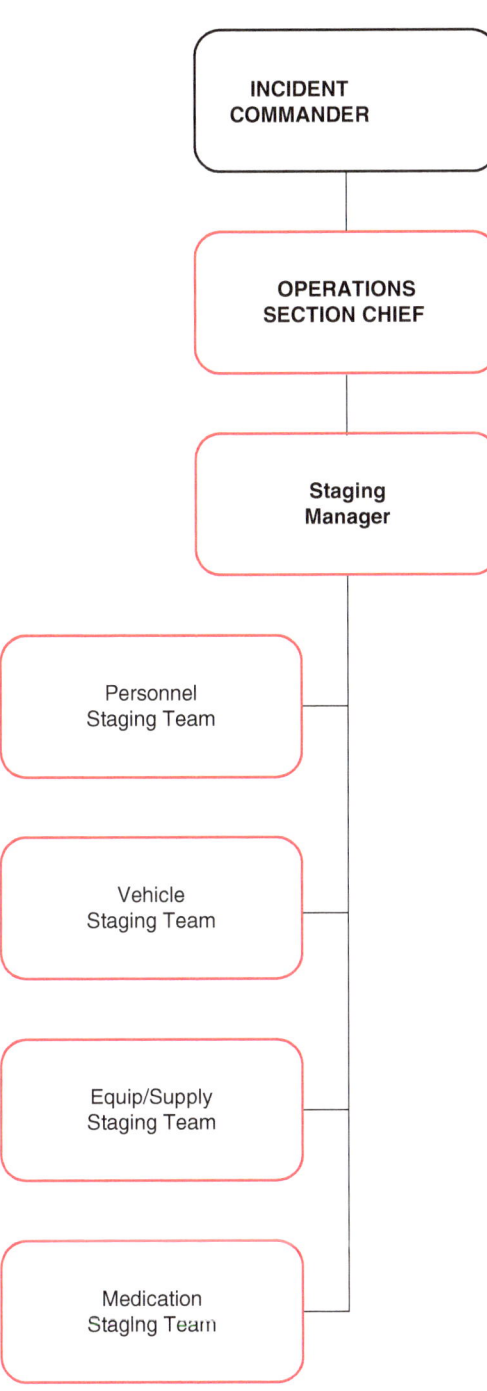

Fig. 4.1 (continued)

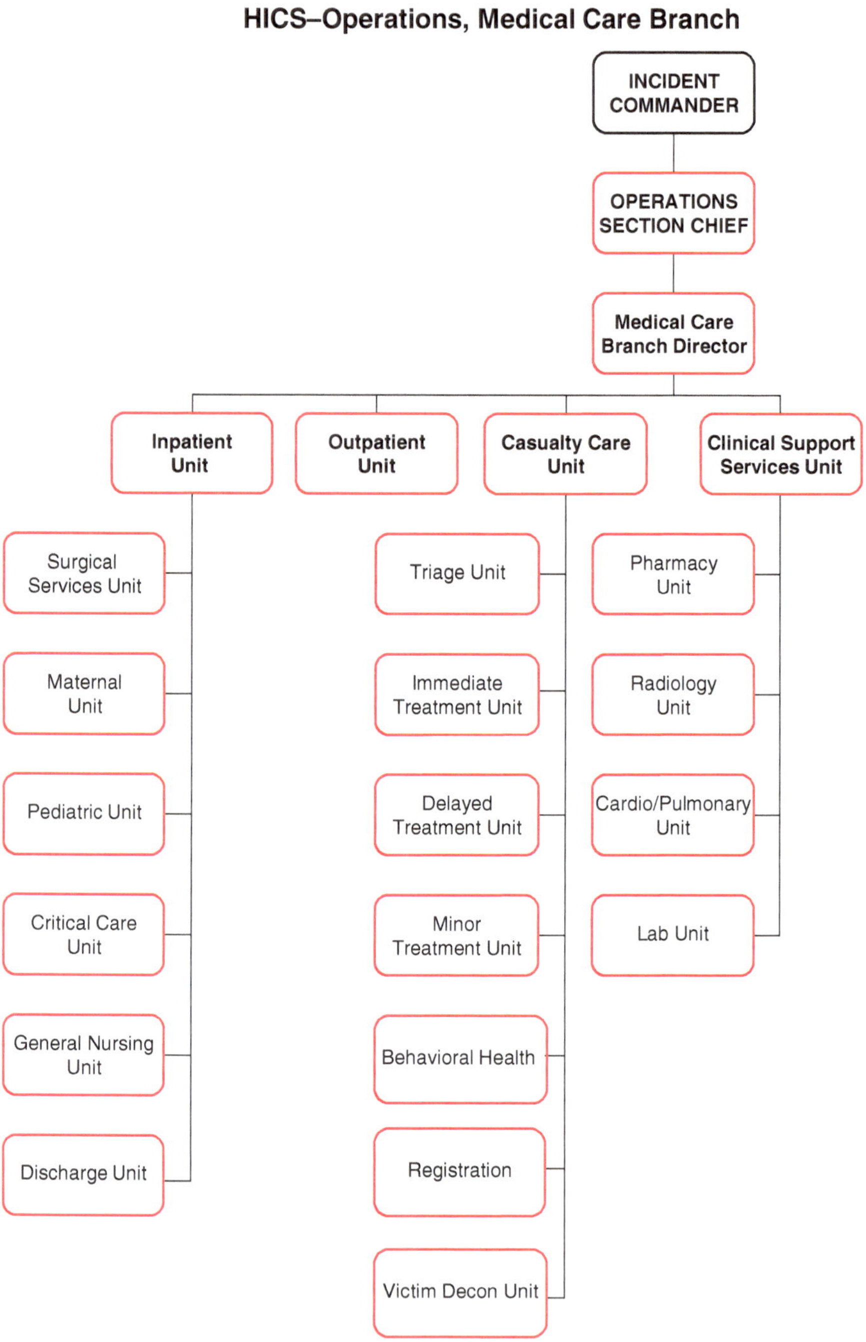

HICS–Operations, Medical Care Branch

INCIDENT COMMANDER

OPERATIONS SECTION CHIEF

Medical Care Branch Director

Inpatient Unit
- Surgical Services Unit
- Maternal Unit
- Pediatric Unit
- Critical Care Unit
- General Nursing Unit
- Discharge Unit

Outpatient Unit

Casualty Care Unit
- Triage Unit
- Immediate Treatment Unit
- Delayed Treatment Unit
- Minor Treatment Unit
- Behavioral Health
- Registration
- Victim Decon Unit

Clinical Support Services Unit
- Pharmacy Unit
- Radiology Unit
- Cardio/Pulmonary Unit
- Lab Unit

Fig. 4.1 (continued)

HICS–Operations, Infrastructure Branch

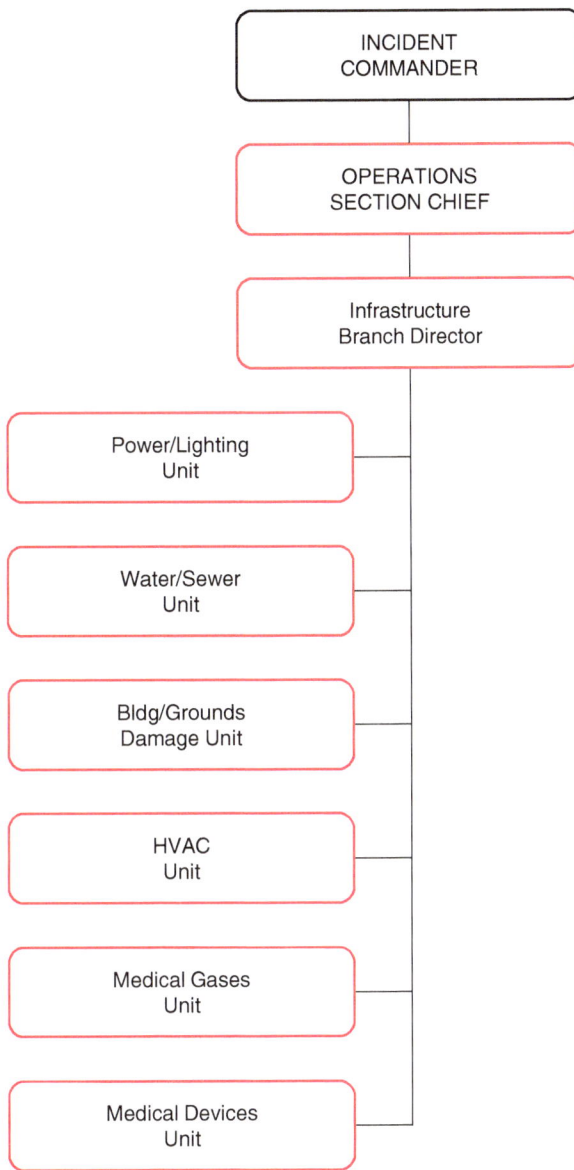

Fig. 4.1 (continued)

HICS–Operations, HazMat Branch

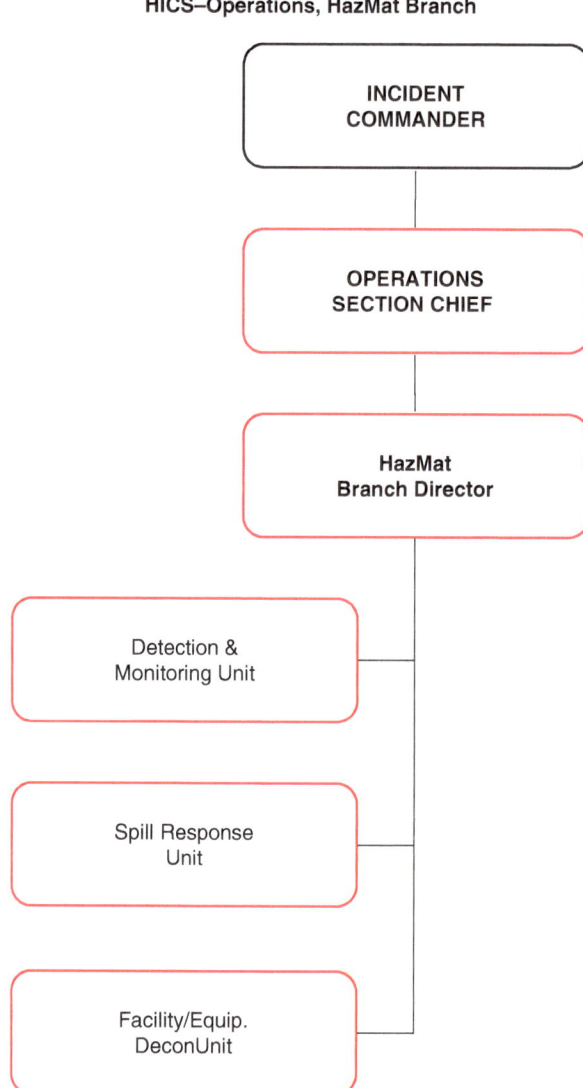

Fig. 4.1 (continued)

HICS–Operations, Security Branch

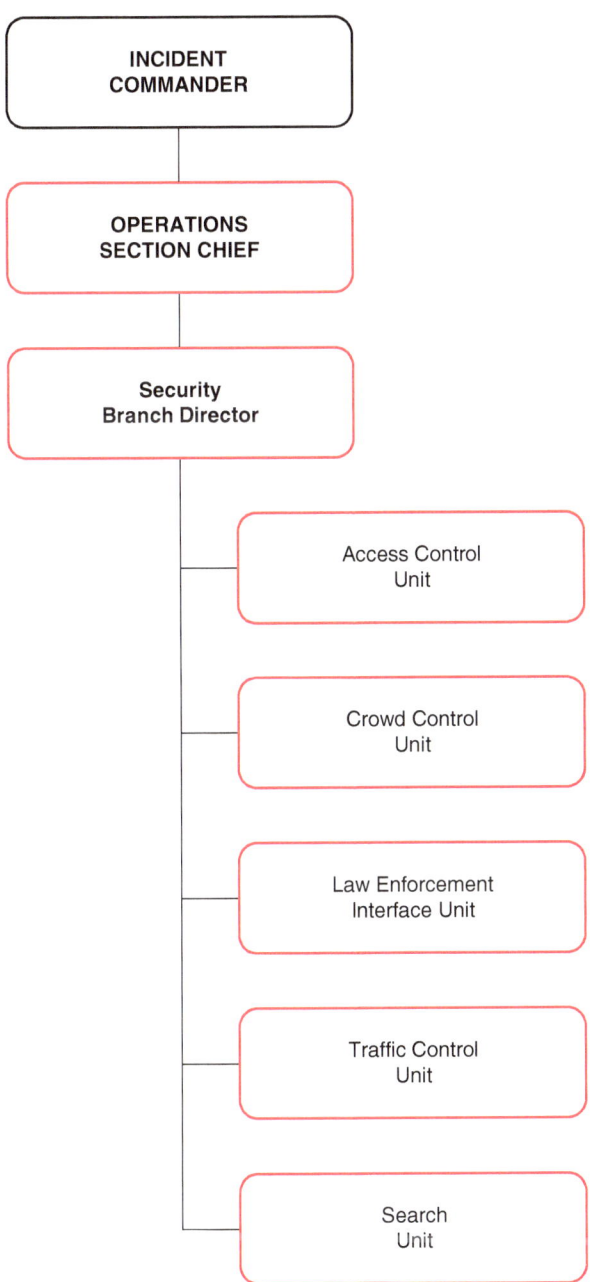

Fig. 4.1 (continued)

HICS–Operations, Business Continuity Branch

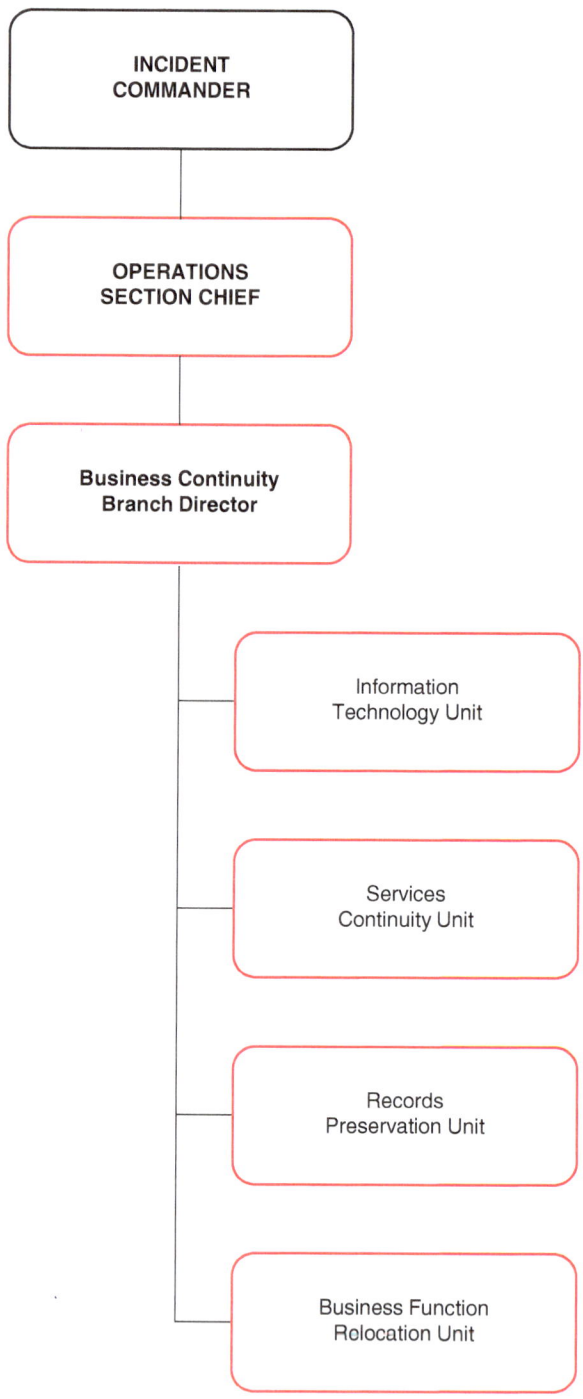

Fig. 4.1 (continued)

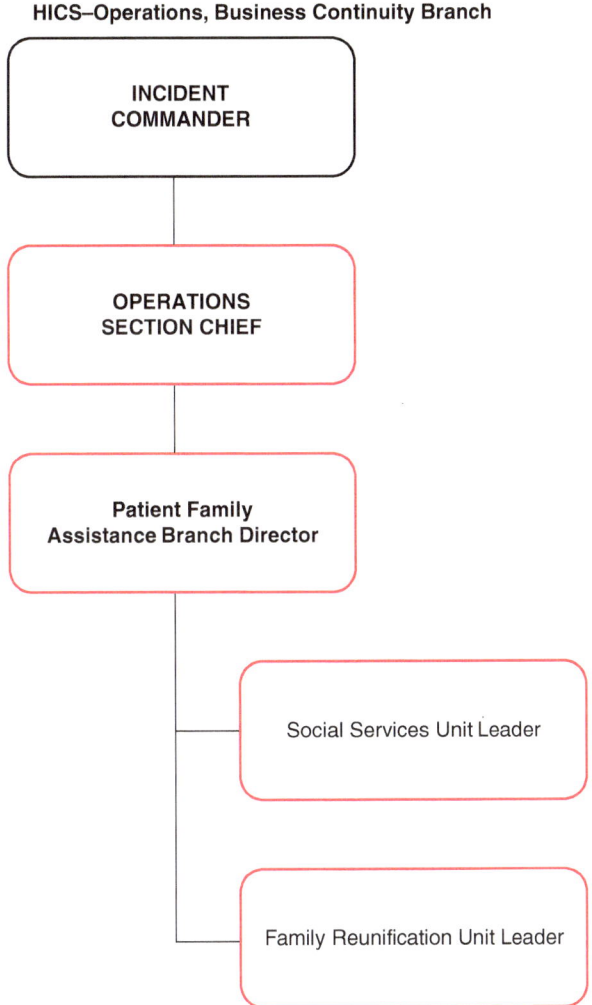

HICS–Operations, Business Continuity Branch

Fig. 4.1 (continued)

4.3.1   ICS Structure and Elements

The ICS roles and responsibilities are defined below. As mentioned earlier, not all of the roles may be deployed depending on the size and duration of the incident.

- Command Staff: The staff who report to the Incident Commander and include Public Information Officer (PIO), Safety Officer, Liaison Officer, and other positions as required.

Table 4.1 ICS position titles

Organizational element	Leadership position title	Support positions
Incident Command	Incident Commander	Deputy
Command Staff	Officer	Assistant
Section	Chief	Deputy, Assistant
Branch	Director	Deputy
Divisions/Groups	Supervisor	
Unit	Unit Leader	Manager, Coordinator
Strike Team/Resource Team/Task Force	Leader	Single Resource Boss
Single Resource	Boss, Leader	
Technical Specialist	Specialist	

- Section: The organizational level having responsibility for a major functional area (Operations, Planning, Logistics, Finance/Administration, and Intelligence/Investigations if established).
- Branch: The organization level having functional and/or geographical responsibility for major aspects of incident operations. A Branch is a level between the Section Chief and the Division or Group in the Operations, Section, and between the Section and Units in the Logistics Section.
- Division: The organizational level responsible for operations within a defined geographic area. The Division level is organizationally between the Strike Team and the Branch.
- Group: An organizational subdivision established to divide the incident into two functional areas of operation. Groups fall between Branches and Resources (personnel, equipment, teams, supplies, and facilities) in the Operations Section.
- Unit: The level with functional responsibility for a specific incident planning, logistics, or finance/administrative activity.
- Task Force: Any combination of resources set up to support a specific mission or operational need. A Task Force contains resources of different kinds and types. These resource elements will have common communications and a designated leader.
- Strike Team/Resource Team: A set number of resources of the same kind and type that have an established minimum number of personnel, common communications, and a designated leader. These are sometimes referred to Resource Teams.
- Single Resource: An individual or piece of equipment and its personnel, or a crew/team of individuals with an identified work supervisor that can be used on an incident. These resources will have a single resource boss.

4.3.2 ICS Functions

Figure 4.2 demonstrates the responsibilities of the Command and General staff leaders, including the Operations, Planning, Logistics, and Finance/Administration

ICS – Who Does What?

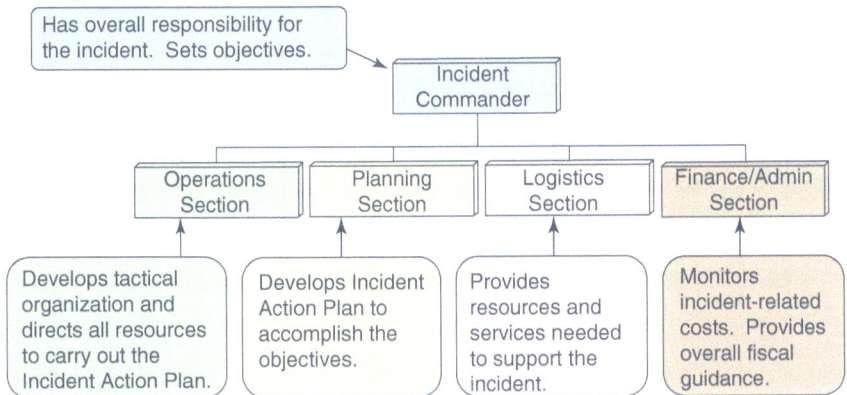

Fig. 4.2 Responsibilities in ICS

Sections. These five areas will be deployed no matter what the disaster or event. There will be a general discussion for each section and the leader titles that are in those sections. For more detailed information, it is recommended to take the FEMA ICS 100 online course found at www.training.fema.gov.

4.3.3   Incident Commander (IC)

The Incident Commander (IC) is in charge of all activities and the overall management of the incident. They are in charge of all functions until they delegate the duties to others, namely the section chiefs. The IC may not delegate any functions if the incident is very small scale and short in duration, but as time goes by and the incident gets bigger, the organizational chart expands. The IC is technically not part of the General or Command Staff. The Incident Commander is responsible for:

• Ensuring incident safety
• Establishing an Incident Command Post
• Providing information services to internal and external stakeholders
• Establishing incident priorities and determining the objectives and strategies to be followed
• Establishing and maintaining liaisons with other agencies
• Authorizing the release of information to the media
• Approving the Incident Action Plan (FEMA ICS Review 2018a).

See Appendix for the Job Actions Sheets.

4.3.4   Command Staff

The Command Staff that are mobilized in a disaster are the Safety Officer, the Public Information Officer (PIO), and the Liaison Officer. In an effort that requires an Intelligence or Investigations Officer that representative will work closely with the Command Staff. The Command Staff report directly to the Incident Commander and support functions needed to support the Incident Commander. The Incident Commander may designate one or more deputies that can assume the Incident Commander role if needed. Someone may be appointed as the Incident Commander but relinquish the role if someone more qualified arrives. When there is a hand-off to a new IC, a briefing must occur.

The Safety Officer is initiated when the incident response becomes larger and someone needs to focus on safety. A skilled safety professional is necessary when complex incidents require a higher degree of technical safety experience. It is a difficult position, and it is important that a professional trained in safety procedures can step in. The Safety Officer monitors incident operations, and they advise the IC on all things safety including the safety of the incident management personnel. The Safety Officer is responsible for:

- Identifying and mitigating hazardous situations
- Ensuring safety messages and briefings are made
- Stopping unsafe acts by exercising their authority
- Reviewing the Incident Action Plan for safety issues
- Assigning people who are qualified when there are special hazards, for example, radioactive exposure
- Primary accident investigations
- Reviewing and approving the Medical Plan
- Participating in planning meetings (FEMA ICS Review 2018a).

The Public Information Officer (PIO) has an important role because in any crisis the media is involved and the public wants information. Requests for information in disasters can be difficult to deal with because it is an overwhelming task. In large-scale disasters, the PIO is the one who briefs the media and the general public. This is one of the few roles in ICS that is primarily responsible for dealing with the public. In a larger incident, this role may interface with PIOs in other agencies, and there may be a Joint Information Center (JIC) opened to address issues together. The primary duties and responsibilities of the PIO are:

- Determining any limits on information release based on the incident
- Developing accurate, accessible, and timely information for press/media briefings
- Assisting the IC in developing the communication both internal and external to be shared and obtaining the IC's approval for release of information
- Monitoring media information about the incident
- Participating in planning meetings (FEMA ICS Review 2018a).

The last of the Command personnel is the Liaison Officer. This position is not as straightforward as the other two positions, but it is a very important position. It is helpful to have someone in that role who has relationships outside the facility with government agencies and elected officials. Their primary role is to deal with other Agency Representatives. To take on this role, individuals have to have good communication skills as they need to educate the elected officials on the incident and response. There are two primary functions including coordinating with other agencies to ensure the appropriate agencies are involved and to ensure the public's perception of the agencies working together as a team. The responsibilities of the Liaison Officer are:

- Acting as the point person for agency representatives
- Maintaining a current list of the assisting and cooperating agencies and agency representatives
- Assisting in setting up interagency contacts
- Participating in planning meetings, both with the IC and with other agencies (FEMA ICS Review 2018a).

See Appendix for the Job Actions Sheets

4.3.5   General Staff

The General Staff are responsible for the functional aspects of the response in the Incident Command Structure. The General Staff include the Operations, Planning, Logistics, Finance/Administrations, and, when necessary, the Intelligence/Investigations Function, which will not be discussed in this chapter. There is only one chief in every section. They may be filled with anyone knowledgeable of the organization, and they report to the IC. These chief positions should not be combined; it is best not filling one of them first. In a small-scale emergency, the section chiefs may be the only ones in that section that are deployed. Based on the need, the sections will be expanded as necessary.

The Operations Section Chief is primarily responsible for managing all tactical operations during an incident. In addition, it is the largest section once all roles are operationalized. It is important that whoever takes on this role has a strong knowledge of the Incident Command System as well as a working knowledge of the organization. The primary responsibilities of this role are:

- Managing tactical operations
- Ensuring tactical operations are implemented safely
- Developing the operations section of the Incident Action Plan (IAP)
- Supervising the operations portion of the IAP
- Approving the release of resources from their current active assignments
- Maintaining contact with the Incident Commander and responding to any requests from them (FEMA ICS 100 2018b).

The Planning Section Chief is responsible for providing planning services and procedures for the incident. This position can be challenging as the Planning Section is responsible for collection of situation and resource status information, evaluating it, and processing the information that will be used in developing action plans. These action plans can be disseminated via the Incident Action Plans, via formal briefings or through status boards (FEMA 300). The primary responsibilities of this role are:

- Managing the collection of all incident operational data
- Supervising the development of the Incident Action Plan and incorporating any additional plans within the system (Traffic, Medical, and Communication Plans)
- Providing current, accurate situational status and briefings for the Incident Command System, and keeping the Incident Commander informed
- Facilitating planning meetings
- Making recommendations for reassignment of personnel
- Developing and displaying all incident status information
- Identifying the need for specialized resources and assembling any Task Forces or Strike Teams not assigned to Operations
- Preparing and monitoring the preparation of the Demobilization Plan (FEMA ICS 100 2018b; Deal et al. 2010).

The Logistics Section Chief provides the incident support needs, and no incident can function long-term without this position. The only function that the Logistic Chief does not oversee is the logistics to air operations if that is necessary. The Logistics Chief is sometimes referred to as the "backbone" of a response (Deal et al. 2010). The duties the Logistics section is responsible for providing are:

- Facilities
- Transportation
- Communications
- Supplies
- Equipment maintenance and fueling
- Food services
- All off-incident resources (FEMA ICS 100 2018b).

The primary responsibilities for the Logistics Chief are:

- Providing facilities, transportation, communications, supplies, equipment maintenance and fueling, food and medical services for incident personnel, and all off-site resources as well as ensuring and overseeing of the action plans for these areas
- Managing all incident logistics
- Providing any logistical support and input to the Incident Action Plan
- Providing logistical briefings
- Requesting any additional support that may be needed (FEMA ICS 100 2018b).

The Logistics Section works closely together with all other areas as they are the major support unit to ensure these teams have what they need for disaster support.

The Finance/Administration Section Chief, as it sounds, is responsible for all financial aspects of an incident including purchasing and analysis of costs. This used to be an issue that people would not even think of until the response was complete. The expenses need to be addressed earlier during the response to minimize the risk to the organization. There needs to be financial management on-site in the Command Center to address any needs that may arise. This section will be activated when there is a financial need and may be the last to be mobilized. There are three reasons to mobilize this section: the financial response is complex; a Unified Command is established and there are multiple agencies involved; and there is a need for a number of tactical assets to be deployed (Deal et al. 2010). This position ensures finances that are expended as judiciously as possible and take the burden off the IC for such decisions.

The responsibilities for the Finance/Administration Section Chief are:

- Managing all financial aspects of an incident
- Providing any cost data for financial analysis that may be needed
- Ensuring any and all compensation and claims functions are addressed related to the incident, including contracting services, purchases, and payments
- Briefing the IC on any cost or budget issues
- Ensuring that personnel timekeeping is completed accurately and given to the appropriate agencies
- Determining the need and setting up an incident commissary if needed
- Ensuring at the close of the incident that all financial documents are in order, including purchasing, inventory, or funding requests
- Providing any input to the IAP
- Briefing the IC or any other agencies that need financial information (FEMA ICS Review 2018a).

When the Finance Section is mobilized, it is important that this team collects any expenses that may have taken place before their arrival. It is important that the Finance Section's documentation includes all finances and timekeeping for the entire incident.

It is important that the Incident Command System in the individual agencies is practiced in a drill on a regular basis. Although the Job Action Sheets make it easy to understand what to do in an incident, the relationships of the sections and the different roles and responsibilities are important to know in advance, so the responders are familiar with the process.

4.4 Conclusion

There is a lot more to know and understand about the Incident Command System, and it is recommended that if you want information that you take the online FEMA learning modules that have been referenced in this chapter. This chapter was an overview of the Incident Command System and focused on the highlights that should be known by leaders who would be responding. This system is meant to be used in whatever response unit there may be. It can be used in a hospital, in a local jurisdiction response, or even a school or child care center response as addressed in other chapters in this book. Some of the chapters include areas that may be deployed to address specific issues such as the decontamination unit covered in Chap. 9 and the reunification plan covered in Chap. 11. This information is part of all governmental and nongovernmental responses during an incident, and it is important that it is practiced regularly in order that the staff is prepared.

Appendix

HEICS Job Action Sheets—Incident Commander, Liaison Officer, Public Information Officer, Safety Officer, Operations Section Chief, Planning Chief, Logistics Chief, Finance Administration Chief. All reprinted with permission from California Emergency Medical Services Administration.

Finance Administration Section Chief

Mission: Monitor the utilization of financial assets and the accounting for financial expenditures. Supervise the documentation of expenditures and cost reimbursement activities.

Position Reports to: **Incident Commander**		Command Location: ———
Position Contact Information: Phone: ( )		Radio Channel: ———
Hospital Command Center (HCC): Phone: ( ) ———		Fax: ( ) ———
Position Assigned to:	Date: / /	Start: ___:___ hrs.
Signature:	Initials:	End: ___:___ hrs.
Position Assigned to:	Date: / /	Start: ___:___ hrs.
Signature:	Initials:	End: ___:___ hrs.
Position Assigned to:	Date: / /	Start: ___:___ hrs.
Signature:	Initials:	End: ___:___ hrs.

Immediate Response (0–2 h)	Time	Initial

Receive appointment
• Obtain briefing from the Incident Commander on:
  – Size and complexity of incident
  – Expectations of the Incident Commander
  – Incident objectives
  – Involvement of outside agencies, stakeholders, and organizations
  – The situation, incident activities, and any special concerns
• Assume the role of Finance/Administration Section Chief
• Review this Job Action Sheet
• Put on position identification (e.g., position vest)
• Notify your usual supervisor of your assignment		

Immediate Response (0–2 h)	Time	Initial

Assess the operational situation
• Obtain and ensure tracking of financial information and status
• Evaluate Finance/Administration Section needs and capacity to perform:
  – Time cost tracking
  – Procurement cost tracking and assistance
  – Compensation and claims cost tracking		

Determine the incident objectives, tactics, and assignments
• Determine which Finance/Administration Units need to be activated:
  – Time Unit
  – Procurement Unit
  – Compensation/Claims Unit
  – Cost Unit
• Document section objectives, tactics, and assignments on the HICS 204: Assignment List
• Make assignments and distribute corresponding Job Action Sheets and position identification
• Determine strategies and how the tactics will be accomplished
• Determine needed resources
• Brief section personnel on the situation, strategies, and tactics, and designate a time for the next briefing		

Activities
• Provide cost implications of incident objectives, activities, and resources
• Ensure that the Incident Action Plan (IAP) is within financial limits established by the Incident Commander
• Determine if any special contractual arrangements or agreements are needed
• Review existing contracts and Memoranda of Understanding (MOUs) to understand options and fiscal implications of implementation
• Obtain information and updates regularly from section units
• Provide status updates to the Incident Commander regularly, advising of accomplishments and issues encountered
• Provide regular updates to section personnel and inform them of strategy changes, as needed
• Communicate regularly with other Section Chiefs
  – Logistics Section for resource needs and activities
  – Inform Planning Section of activities that have occurred; keep updated with status and utilization of resources
  – Communicate with the Operations Section for personnel time records, potential compensation and claims, and canceled surgeries and procedures		

Documentation • HICS 204: Document assignments and operational period objectives on Assignment List • HICS 213: Document all communications on a General Message Form • HICS 214: Document all key activities, actions, and decisions in an Activity Log on a continual basis • HICS 252: Distribute Section Personnel Time Sheet to section personnel; ensure time is recorded appropriately, and submit it to the Time Unit Leader at the completion of a shift or end of each operational period • HICS 256: Initiate financial account tracking on Procurement Summary Report		

Immediate Response (0–2 h)	Time	Initial
Resources		
• Determine equipment and supply needs; request them from the Logistics Section Supply Unit Leader		
• Determine issues and needs in section areas; coordinate resource management		
• Make requests for external assistance, as needed, in coordination with the Liaison Officer		
Communication		
Hospital to complete: Insert communications technology, instructions for use, and protocols for interface with external partners		
Safety and security		
• Ensure that all section personnel comply with safety procedures and instructions		

Intermediate Response (2–12 h)	Time	Initial
Activities		
• Transfer the Finance/Administration Section Chief role, if appropriate		
– Conduct a transition meeting to brief your replacement on the current situation, response actions, available resources, and the role of external agencies in support of the hospital		
– Address any health, medical, and safety concerns		
– Address political sensitivities, when appropriate		
– Instruct your replacement to complete the appropriate documentation and ensure that appropriate personnel are properly briefed on response issues and objectives (see HICS Forms 203, 204, 214, and 215A)		
• Approve a cost-to-date incident financial status report to be submitted by the Cost Unit Leader at regular intervals (e.g., every 8 h) summarizing financial data relative to personnel, supplies, other expenditures, and expenses		
• Work with the Incident Commander and other Section Chiefs to identify short- and long-term issues with financial implications; establish needed policies and procedures		
• Brief the Incident Commander, Public Information Officer, and Liaison Officer regularly on the status of the Finance/Administration Section		
• Designate a time for briefing and updates with Finance/Administration Section leadership to update the Incident Action Plan (IAP)		
Documentation		
• HICS 204: Document assignments and operational period objectives on Assignment List		
• HICS 213: Document all communications on a General Message Form		
• HICS 214: Document actions, decisions, and information received on Activity Log		
Resources		
• Ensure equipment, supplies, and personal protective equipment (PPE) are replaced as needed, coordinating with Operations and Logistics Section Chiefs		

Intermediate Response (2–12 h)	Time	Initial
Communication *Hospital to complete: Insert communications technology, instructions for use, and protocols for interface with external partners*		
Safety and security • Ensure staff health and safety issues are being addressed; report issues to the Safety Officer and the Logistics Section Employee Health and Well-Being Unit		

Extended Response (greater than 12 h)	Time	Initial

Activities
• Transfer the Finance/Administration Section Chief role, if appropriate
  – Conduct a transition meeting to brief your replacement on the current situation, response actions, available resources, and the role of external agencies in support of the hospital
  – Address any health, medical, and safety concerns
  – Address political sensitivities, when appropriate
  – Instruct your replacement to complete the appropriate documentation and ensure that appropriate personnel are properly briefed on response issues and objectives (see HICS Forms 203, 204, 214, and 215A)
• Present financial updates to the Incident Commander and Command Staff at regular intervals (e.g., every 8 h) and as requested
• Ensure that routine nonincident-related administrative oversight of hospital financial operations is maintained
• Coordinate emergency procurement requests with the Logistics Section Supply Unit Leader
• Maintain cash on hand to ensure safe and efficient clinical and nonclinical operations
• Ensure automated teller machines (ATMs) located within the hospital are secured and maintained as appropriate
• Consult with local, state, and federal officials regarding reimbursement regulations and requirements; ensure required documentation is prepared according to guidance received
• Continue to monitor the ability of Finance/Administration Section personnel to meet workload demands, personnel health and safety, resource needs, and documentation practices
• Brief the Incident Commander, Public Information Officer, and Liaison Officer regularly on the status of the Finance/Administration Section
  – Designate a time for briefing and updates with Finance/Administration Section leadership to update the Incident Action Plan (IAP)		

Documentation • HICS 204: Document assignments and operational period objectives on Assignment List • HICS 213: Document all communications on a General Message Form • HICS 214: Document actions, decisions, and information received on Activity Log • HICS 257: Track equipment used during the response on the Resource Accounting Record		
Resources • Monitor levels of all supplies and equipment, and collaborate on needs with the Logistics Section Supply Unit Leader		

Extended Response (greater than 12 h)	Time	Initial
Communication *Hospital to complete: Insert communications technology, instructions for use, and protocols for interface with external partners*		
Safety and security • Coordinate Finance/Administration security needs with the Operations Section Security Branch • Observe all staff and volunteers for signs of stress and inappropriate behavior and report concerns to the Safety Officer and the Logistics Section Employee Health and Well-Being Unit Leader • Provide for personnel rest periods and relief • Ensure your physical readiness through proper nutrition, water intake, rest, and stress management techniques		

Demobilization/System Recovery	Time	Initial

Activities
 • Transfer the Finance/Administration Section Chief role, if appropriate
  – Conduct a transition meeting to brief your replacement on the current situation, demobilization actions, available resources, and the role of external agencies in support of the hospital
  – Address any health, medical, and safety concerns
  – Address political sensitivities, when appropriate
  – Instruct your replacement to complete the appropriate documentation and ensure that appropriate personnel are properly briefed on response issues and objectives (see HICS Forms 203, 204, 214, and 215A)
 • As objectives are met and needs decrease, return Finance/Administration Section personnel to their usual jobs and combine or deactivate positions in a phased manner, in coordination with the Planning Section Demobilization Unit Leader
 • Collect and analyze all financial-related data from Finance/Administration Section Units
 • Ensure processing and payment of invoiced costs
 • Submit required reimbursement documentation and track payments
 • Upon deactivation of your position, brief the Incident Commander on current problems, outstanding issues, and follow-up requirements
 • Participate in other briefings and meetings as required
 • Continue to become familiar with eligibility to apply for state and or federal reimbursement and assembly of needed materials including invoices, work orders, and pictures of items replaced and or hospital damage repaired
 • Participate in stress management and after action debriefings
 • Submit comments to the Planning Section for discussion and possible inclusion in an After Action Report and Corrective Action and Improvement Plan. Topics include:
  – Review of pertinent position descriptions and operational checklists
  – Recommendations for procedure changes
  – Accomplishments and issues		

Demobilization/System Recovery	Time	Initial
Documentation • HICS 221: Demobilization Check-Out • Ensure all documentation is submitted to the Planning Section Documentation Unit • Provide corporate reports as requested • Prepare with others as needed all invoices, overtime records, damage reports (including before and after pictures), and repair or replacement cost documentation for submission to state and federal authorities when requested • Work with risk management for submission of all insurance-related claims (personal injury, workmen's compensation, building damage, etc.)		

Documents/Tools
- HICS 203 - Organization Assignment List
- HICS 204 - Assignment List
- HICS 205A - Communications List
- HICS 213 - General Message Form
- HICS 214 - Activity Log
- HICS 215A - Incident Action Plan (IAP) Safety Analysis
- HICS 221 - Demobilization Check-Out
- HICS 252 - Section Personnel Time Sheet
- HICS 256 - Procurement Summary Report
- HICS 257 - Resource Accounting Record
- HICS 258 - Hospital Resource Directory
- Hospital financial data forms
- FEMA reimbursement guidance and forms
- State and Department of Homeland Security reimbursement forms
- Hospital Emergency Operations Plan
- Incident Specific Plans or Annexes
- Hospital organization chart
- Hospital telephone directory
- Telephone/cell phone/satellite phone/internet/amateur radio/2-way radio for communication

Logistics Section Chief

Mission: Organize and direct the service and support activities needed to ensure the material needs for the hospital's response to an incident are available when needed.

Position Reports to: **Incident Commander**		Command Location: ———————	
Position Contact Information: Phone: ( )		Radio Channel: ———————	
Hospital Command Center (HCC): Phone: ( ) ———————		Fax: ( ) ———————	
Position Assigned to:	Date: / /	Start: ____:____ hrs.	
Signature:	Initials:	End: ____:____ hrs.	
Position Assigned to:	Date: / /	Start: ____:____ hrs.	
Signature:	Initials:	End: ____:____ hrs.	
Position Assigned to:	Date: / /	Start: ____:____ hrs.	
Signature:	Initials:	End: ____:____ hrs.	

Immediate Response (0–2 h)	Time	Initial
Receive appointment		
• Obtain briefing from the Incident Commander on:		
– Size and complexity of incident		
– Expectations of Incident Commander		
– Incident objectives		
– Involvement of outside agencies, stakeholders, and organizations		
– The situation, incident activities, and any special concerns		
• Assume the role of Logistics Section Chief		
• Review this Job Action Sheet		
• Put on position identification (e.g., position vest)		
• Notify your usual supervisor of your assignment		
Assess the operational situation		
• Obtain information from the Operations Section Chief, Staging Manager, and the operational status of the Service and Support Branch Directors to assess critical issues and resource needs		
• Provide information to the Incident Commander on the Logistics Section operational situation including capabilities and limitations		
Determine the incident objectives, tactics, and assignments		
• Determine which Logistics Section functions need to be activated:		
– Service Branch		
– Support Branch		
• Document section objectives, tactics, and assignments on the HICS 204: Assignment List		
• Make assignments, distribute corresponding Job Action Sheets and position identification		
• Determine strategies and how the tactics will be accomplished		
• Determine needed resources		
• Brief section personnel on the situation, strategies, and tactics, and designate a time for the next briefing		
Activities		
• Ensure the Hospital Command Center (HCC) is set up and equipped with the necessary resources and services including communications and information technology		
• Appoint an assistant to manage the needs of the HCC, if needed		
• Establish and communicate the process for other sections to request personnel and additional resources		
• If relocation or additional care locations are necessary, coordinate with Operations and Planning Sections to determine the infrastructure requirements that are necessary to meet the operational needs, and conduct predeployment assessments		
• Establish Logistics Section work procedures (e.g., work hours, rotation schedule, contact list, need for, and monitoring of overtime hours)		
• Coordinate procurement and expense needs with Financial Section to determine proper authority and reimbursement ceilings		
• Participate in Incident Action Plan (IAP) preparation, briefings, and meetings as needed; assist in identifying strategies; determine tactics, work assignments, and resource requirements		

Immediate Response (0–2 h)	Time	Initial
Documentation		
• HICS 204: Document assignments and operational period objectives on Assignment List • HICS 205A: Distribute the Communications List appropriately • HICS 206: Ensure that a Staff Medical Plan is created and distributed • HICS 213: Document all communications on a General Message Form • HICS 214: Document all key activities, actions, and decisions in an Activity Log on a continual basis • HICS 252: Distribute Section Personnel Time Sheet to section personnel; ensure time is recorded appropriately, and submit it to the Finance/Administration Section Time Unit Leader at the completion of a shift or end of each operational period • HICS 256: Track requested equipment and services on a Procurement Summary Report • HICS 257: Track equipment used during the response on the Resource Accounting Record		
Resources		
• Determine equipment and supply needs; request them from the Supply Unit Leader • Assess issues and needs in section areas; coordinate resource management • Make requests for external assistance, as needed, in coordination with the Liaison Officer • Determine from all sections levels of personnel and additional resources needed for next operational period • Work with the Finance/Administration Chief on the preparation of additional service and equipment contracts • Maintain the current status of all areas in Logistics Section, inform Planning Section personnel of activities that have occurred; keep them updated with status and utilization of resources • Inform Finance/Administration Section of personnel time records and potential work-related claims		
Communication *Hospital to complete: Insert communications technology, instructions for use, and protocols for interface with external partners*		
Safety and security		
• Ensure that all section personnel comply with safety procedures and instructions • Ensure personal protective equipment (PPE) is available and utilized appropriately		

Intermediate Response (2–12 h)	Time	Initial
Activities		
• Transfer the Logistics Section Chief role, if appropriate		
– Conduct a transition meeting to brief your replacement on the current situation, response actions, available resources, and the role of external agencies in support of the hospital		
– Address any health, medical, and safety concerns		
– Address political sensitivities, when appropriate		
– Instruct your replacement to complete the appropriate documentation and ensure that appropriate personnel are properly briefed on response issues and objectives (see HICS Forms 203, 204, 214, and 215A)		
• Meet regularly with the Incident Commander and Hospital Incident Management Team (HIMT) staff to update the status of the response and relay important information on the capabilities and limitations of the Logistics Section		
• Designate a time for briefing and updates with the Logistics Section personnel to develop recommended updates to the Incident Action Plan (IAP) and to develop demobilization procedures		
• Ensure the following are being adequately supported with necessary resources:		
– Clinical areas, both inpatient and outpatient		
– Staging and Labor Pool including credentialing of staff and volunteers		
– Information technology and information systems network integrity		
– Food and water for patients, staff, and visitors		
– Employee health and well-being services		
– Clinical support services		
– Patient family care supply support		
– Hospital personnel family support		
– Environmental services		
– Transportation services		
• Coordinate and process requests for personnel and resources from other sections		
• Obtain needed materials and fulfill resource requests with the assistance of the Finance/Administration Section Chief and Liaison Officer		
• Communicate regularly with Hospital Incident Management Team (HIMT) staff		
• Ensure that the Logistics Section is adequately staffed and supplied		
Documentation		
• HICS 204: Document assignments and operational period objectives on Assignment List		
• HICS 213: Document all communications on a General Message Form		
• HICS 214: Document actions, decisions, and information received on Activity Log		
Resources		
• Ensure equipment, supplies, and personal protective equipment (PPE) are replaced as needed, coordinating with Operations Section Chief		
Communication		
Hospital to complete: Insert communications technology, instructions for use, and protocols for interface with external partners		
Safety and security		
• Ensure section personnel health and safety issues are being addressed; report issues to the Safety Officer and Employee Health and Well-Being Unit		

Extended Response (greater than 12 h)	Time	Initial
Activities		

• Transfer Logistics Section Chief role, if appropriate:
  – Conduct a transition meeting to brief your replacement on the current situation, response actions, available resources, and the role of external agencies in support of the hospital
  – Address any health, medical, and safety concerns
  – Address political sensitivities, when appropriate
  – Instruct your replacement to complete the appropriate documentation and ensure that appropriate personnel are properly briefed on response issues and objectives (see HICS Forms 203, 204, 214, and 215A)
• Continue to monitor the ability of Logistics Section personnel to meet workload demands, personnel health and safety, resource needs, and documentation practices
• Continue to maintain the HICS 257: Resource Accounting Record to track equipment used during the response
• Communicate regularly with the Hospital Incident Management Team (HIMT)
• Brief Incident Commander, Public Information Officer, and Liaison Officer regularly on the status of the Logistics Section
• Designate a time for briefing and updates with Logistics Section leadership to update the Incident Action Plan (IAP)		

Documentation		
• HICS 204: Document assignments and operational period objectives on Assignment List • HICS 213: Document all communications on a General Message Form • HICS 214: Document actions, decisions, and information received on Activity Log • HICS 257: Track equipment used during the response on the Resource Accounting Record		
Resources		
• Monitor levels of all supplies and equipment, and collaborate on needs with the Supply Unit Leader		
Communication		
Hospital to complete: Insert communications technology, instructions for use, and protocols for interface with external partners		
Safety and security		
• Observe section personnel for signs of stress and inappropriate behavior; report concerns to the Safety officer and the Employee Health and Well Being Unit • Provide for personnel rest periods and relief • Ensure your physical readiness through proper nutrition, water intake, rest, and stress management techniques		

Demobilization/System Recovery	Time	Initial
Activities		

• Transfer Logistics Section Chief role if appropriate
  – Conduct a transition meeting to brief your replacement on the current situation, demobilization actions, available resources, and the role of external agencies in support of the hospital
  – Address any health, medical, and safety concerns
  – Address political sensitivities, when appropriate
  – Instruct your replacement to complete the appropriate documentation and ensure that appropriate personnel are properly briefed on response issues and objectives (see HICS Forms 203, 204, 214, and 215A)
• Work with Planning and Finance/Administration Sections to complete cost data information
• Debrief section personnel on lessons learned and procedural or equipment changes needed
• Participate in other briefings and meetings as required
• Submit comments to the Planning Section for discussion and possible inclusion in an After Action Report and Corrective Improvement Plan. Topics include:
  – Review of pertinent position descriptions and operational checklists
  – Recommendations for procedure changes
  – Accomplishments and issues
• Participate in stress management and after action debriefings
• As objectives are met and needs decrease, return Logistics Section personnel to their usual jobs and combine or deactivate positions in a phased manner, in coordination with the Planning Section Demobilization Unit Leader
• Assist other Section Chiefs in restoring the hospital to normal operations		

Documentation		
• HICS 221: Demobilization Check-Out • Ensure all documentation is submitted to the Planning Section Documentation Unit		

Documents/Tools
• HICS 203 - Organization Assignment List • HICS 204 - Assignment List • HICS 205A - Communications List • HICS 206 - Staff Medical Plan • HICS 213 - General Message Form • HICS 214 - Activity Log • HICS 215A - Incident Action Plan (IAP) Safety Analysis • HICS 221 - Demobilization Check-Out • HICS 252 - Section Personnel Time Sheet • HICS 253 - Volunteer Registration • HICS 256 - Procurement Summary Report • HICS 257 - Resource Accounting Record • Hospital Emergency Operations Plan • Hospital Incident Specific Plans or Annexes • Hospital organization chart • Hospital telephone directory • Master Inventory Control lists • Telephone/cell phone/satellite phone/internet/amateur radio/2-way radio for communication

Operations Section Chief

Mission: Develop and implement strategies and tactics to carry out the objectives established by the Incident Commander. Organize, assign, and supervise the resources of the Staging Area, the Medical Care, Infrastructure, Security, Hazardous Materials (HazMat), Business Continuity, and Patient Family Assistance Branches.

Position Reports to: **Incident Commander**		Command Location: ———————	
Position Contact Information: Phone: ( )		Radio Channel: ———————	
Hospital Command Center (HCC): Phone: ( ) ————		Fax: ( ) ————	
Position Assigned to:	Date: / /	Start: ____:____ hrs.	
Signature:	Initials:	End: ____:____ hrs.	
Position Assigned to:	Date: / /	Start: ____:____ hrs.	
Signature:	Initials:	End: ____:____ hrs.	
Position Assigned to:	Date: / /	Start: ____:____ hrs.	
Signature:	Initials:	End: ____:____ hrs.	

Immediate Response (0–2 h)	Time	Initial
Receive appointment		
• Obtain a briefing from the Incident Commander on:		
– Size and complexity of the incident		
– Expectations of the Incident Commander		
– Incident objectives		
– Involvement of outside agencies, stakeholders, and organizations		
– The situation, incident activities, and any special concerns		
• Assume the role of Operations Section Chief		
• Review this Job Action Sheet		
• Put on position identification (e.g., position vest)		
• Notify your usual supervisor of your assignment		
Assess the operational situation		
• Obtain information and status from the Staging Manager, and the Medical Care, Infrastructure, Security, Hazardous Materials (HazMat), Business Continuity, and Patient Family Assistance Branch Directors		
• Provide information to the Incident Commander on the operational situation including capabilities and limitations		
Determine the incident objectives, tactics, and assignments		
• Determine which Operations Section functions need to be activated:		
– Staging Area		
– Medical Care Branch		
– Infrastructure Branch		
– Security Branch		
– HazMat Branch		
– Business Continuity Branch		
– Patient Family Assistance Branch		
• Document section objectives, tactics, and assignments on the HICS 204—Assignment List		
• Make assignments and distribute corresponding Job Action Sheets and position identification		
• Determine strategies and how the tactics will be accomplished		
• Determine needed resources		
• Brief section personnel on the situation, strategies, and tactics, and designate a time for the next briefing		

Immediate Response (0–2 h)	Time	Initial
Activities		
• Ensure the following are being addressed with the appropriate branch or unit:		
– Staff health and safety		
– Patient tracking		
– Patient care		
– Patient family support		
– Transfers into and from the hospital		
– Fatality management		
– Information sharing with other hospitals and local agencies (e.g., emergency medical services, fire, law, public health, and emergency management) in coordination with the Liaison Officer		
– Personnel and resource movement through the staging area		
– Documentation		
– Patient care treatment standards and case definitions with public health officials, as appropriate		
– Ensure coordination with any assisting or cooperating agency or corporate command center		
– Personnel needs with Logistics Section Labor Pool and Credentialing Unit Leader, supply and equipment needs with the Logistics Section Supply Unit Leader, projections and needs with the Planning Section, and financial matters with the Finance/Administration Section		
• Ensure that the Operations Section is adequately staffed and supplied		
• Communicate with Operations Section personnel to:		
– Obtain information and updates regularly from Operations Section Branch Directors and Staging Manager		
– Maintain the current status of all areas		
– Inform the Planning Section Situation Unit Leader of status information		
• Conduct an Operations Briefing to present the Incident Action Plan (IAP) to clarify staff responsibilities		
• Collaborate with appropriate Medical-Technical Specialists as needed		
• Communicate with other Section Chiefs:		
– Logistics Section for resource needs and activities		
– Planning Section for activities that have occurred; then keep updated with status and utilization of resources		
– Finance/Administration Section for personnel time records; potential compensation and claims and canceled surgeries and procedures		
Documentation		
• HICS 204: Document assignments and operational period objectives on Assignment List		
• HICS 205A: Distribute the Communications List appropriately		
• HICS 213: Document all communications on a General Message Form		
• HICS 214: Document all key activities, actions, and decisions in an Activity Log on a continual basis		
• HICS 251: As appropriate, complete a Facility System Status Report and report the results to the Incident Commander		
• HICS 252: Distribute a Section Personnel Time Sheet to section staff; ensure time is recorded appropriately, and submit to Finance/Administration Section Time Unit Leader at the completion of a shift or end of each operational period		
• HICS 257: Track the equipment used on the Resource Accounting Record		

Resources		
• Determine equipment and supply needs; request them from the Logistics Section Supply Unit Leader • Assess issues and needs in section areas; coordinate resource management • Make requests for external assistance, as needed, in coordination with the Liaison Officer		
Communication		
Hospital to complete: Insert communications technology, instructions for use, and protocols for interface with external partners		
Safety and security		
• Ensure that all section personnel comply with safety procedures and instructions • Determine if a communicable disease risk exists; implement appropriate response procedures collaborating with the appropriate Medical-Technical Specialist, if activated • Ensure personal protective equipment (PPE) is available and utilized appropriately		

Intermediate Response (2–12 h)	**Time**	**Initial**
Activities		

• Transfer the Operations Section Chief role, if appropriate
  – Conduct a transition meeting to brief your replacement on the current situation, response actions, available resources, and the role of external agencies in support of the hospital
  – Address any health, medical, and safety concerns
  – Address political sensitivities, when appropriate
  – Instruct your replacement to complete the appropriate documentation and ensure that appropriate personnel are properly briefed on response issues and objectives (see HICS Forms 203, 204, 214, and 215A)
• Ensure the following are being addressed with the appropriate section, branch, or unit:
  – Section personnel health and safety
  – Patient tracking
  – Patient care
  – Patient family support
  – Transfers into and from the hospital
  – Fatality management
  – Information sharing with other hospitals and local agencies (e.g., emergency medical services, fire, law, public health and emergency management) in coordination with the Liaison Officer
  – Personnel and resource movement through the staging area
  – Documentation
  – Patient care treatment standards and case definitions with public health officials, as appropriate
  – Ensure coordination with any assisting or cooperating agency
  – Personnel needs with Logistics Section Labor Pool and Credentialing Unit Leader, supply and equipment needs with the Logistics Section Supply Unit Leader, projections and needs with the Planning Section, and financial matters with the Finance/Administration Section
• Ensure that the Operations Section is adequately staffed and supplied
• Brief the Incident Commander, Public Information Officer, and Liaison Officer regularly on the status of the Operations Section
• Designate a time for a briefing and updates with Operations Section leadership to update the Incident Action Plan (IAP)
• Schedule meetings with the Branch Directors and Staging Manager to update the section plans and demobilization procedures		

Documentation
- HICS 204: Document assignments and operational period objectives on Assignment List
- HICS 213: Document all communications on a General Message Form
- HICS 214: Document actions, decisions, and information received on Activity Log

Resources
- Ensure equipment, supplies, and personal protective equipment (PPE) are replaced as needed, coordinating with Logistics Section Supply Unit Leader

Communication

Hospital to complete: Insert communications technology, instructions for use, and protocols for interface with external partners

Safety and security
- Review personnel protective equipment use; revise as needed
- Ensure staff health and safety issues are being addressed; report issues to the Safety Officer and Logistics Section Employee Health and Well-Being Unit
- Ensure patient safety issues are identified and addressed
- Ensure personal protective equipment (PPE) is available and utilized appropriately

Extended Response (greater than 12 h)	Time	Initial
Activities		
• Transfer the Operations Section Chief role, if appropriate		
– Conduct a transition meeting to brief your replacement on the current situation, response actions, available resources, and the role of external agencies in support of the hospital		
– Address any health, medical, and safety concerns		
– Address political sensitivities, when appropriate		
– Instruct your replacement to complete the appropriate documentation and ensure that appropriate personnel are properly briefed on response issues and objectives (see HICS Forms 203, 204, 214, and 215A)		
• Continue to monitor the ability of Operations Section personnel to meet workload demands, personnel health and safety, resource needs, and documentation practices		
• Address issues related to ongoing patient care including:		
– Ongoing patient arrival		
– Bed availability		
– Patient transfers		
– Patient tracking		
– Staff health and safety		
– Behavioral health for patients, families, staff, and incident management personnel		
– Fatality management		
– Staffing		
– Staff prophylaxis		
– Medications		
– Equipment and supplies		
– Personnel and resource movement through staging area		
– Coordination with other area hospitals		
– Documentation		
• Brief the Incident Commander, Public Information Officer, and Liaison Officer regularly on the status of the Operations Section		
• Designate a time for a briefing and updates with Operations Section leadership to update the Incident Action Plan (IAP)		

Extended Response (greater than 12 h)	Time	Initial
Documentation • HICS 204: Document assignments and operational period objectives on Assignment List • HICS 213: Document all communications on a General Message Form • HICS 214: Document actions, decisions, and information received on Activity Log • HICS 257: Track equipment used during the response on the Resource Accounting Record		
Resources • Monitor levels of all supplies and equipment, and collaborate on needs with the Logistics Section Supply Unit Leader		
Communication *Hospital to complete: Insert communications technology, instructions for use, and protocols for interface with external partners*		
Safety and security • Observe section personnel for signs of stress and inappropriate behavior; report issues to the Safety Officer and Logistics Section Employee Health and Well-Being Unit • Provide for personnel rest periods and relief • Ensure your physical readiness through proper nutrition, water intake, rest, and stress management techniques • Ensure personal protective equipment (PPE) is available and utilized appropriately		

Demobilization/System Recovery	Time	Initial

Activities
• Transfer the Operations Section Chief role, if appropriate
  – Conduct a transition meeting to brief your replacement on the current situation, demobilization actions, available resources, and the role of external agencies in support of the hospital
  – Address any health, medical, and safety concerns
  – Address political sensitivities, when appropriate
  – Instruct your replacement to complete the appropriate documentation and ensure that appropriate staff are properly briefed on response issues and objectives (see HICS Forms 203, 204, 214, and 215A)
• As objectives are met and needs decrease, return the Operations Section personnel to their usual jobs and combine or deactivate positions in a phased manner, in coordination with the Planning Section Demobilization Unit Leader
• Assist Section Chiefs in restoring the hospital to normal operations
• Through the Liaison Officer and Public Information Officer, share patient information with external agencies as needed and in accordance with patient privacy policies
• Work with the Planning and Finance/Administration Sections to complete cost data information collection
• Upon deactivation of your position, brief the Incident Commander on current problems, outstanding issues, and follow up requirements
• Debrief section personnel on lessons learned and procedural or equipment changes needed
• Participate in other briefings and meetings as required
• Submit comments to the Planning Section for discussion and possible inclusion in an After Action Report and Corrective Action and Improvement Plan. Topics include:
  – Review of pertinent position descriptions and operational checklists
  – Recommendations for procedure changes
  – Accomplishments and issues
• Participate in stress management and after action debriefings		

Demobilization/System Recovery	Time	Initial
Documentation • HICS 221: Demobilization Check-Out • Ensure all documentation is submitted to the Planning Section Documentation Unit		

Documents/Tools

- HICS 203 - Organization Assignment List
- HICS 204 - Assignment List
- HICS 205A - Communications List
- HICS 213 - General Message Form
- HICS 214 - Activity Log
- HICS 215A - Incident Action Plan (IAP) Safety Analysis
- HICS 221 - Demobilization Check-Out
- HICS 251 - Facility System Status Report
- HICS 252 - Section Personnel Time Sheet
- HICS 254 - Disaster Victim/Patient Tracking
- HICS 255 - Master Patient Evacuation Tracking
- HICS 257 - Resource Accounting Record
- HICS 259 - Hospital Casualty/Fatality Report
- HICS 260 - Patient Evacuation Tracking
- Hospital Emergency Operations Plan
- Incident Specific Plans or Annexes
- Hospital organization chart
- Hospital telephone directory
- Telephone/cell phone/satellite phone/internet/amateur radio/2-way radio for communication

Planning Section Chief

Mission: Oversee all incident-related data gathering and analysis regarding incident operations and resource management; develop alternatives for tactical operations; initiate long-range planning; conduct planning meetings; and prepare the Incident Action Plan (IAP) for each operational period.

Position Reports to: **Incident Commander**		Command Location: ———————	
Position Contact Information: Phone: ( )		Radio Channel: ———————	
Hospital Command Center (HCC): Phone: ( )———————		Fax: ( ) ———————	
Position Assigned to:	Date: / /	Start: ____:____ hrs.	
Signature:	Initials:	End: ____:____ hrs.	
Position Assigned to:	Date: / /	Start: ____:____ hrs.	
Signature:	Initials:	End: ____:____ hrs.	
Position Assigned to:	Date: / /	Start: ____:____ hrs.	
Signature:	Initials:	End: ____:____ hrs.	

Immediate Response (0–2 h)	Time	Initial
Receive appointment		
• Obtain briefing from the Incident Commander on:		
– Size and complexity of the incident		
– Expectations of the Incident Commander		
– Incident objectives		
– Involvement of outside agencies, stakeholders, and organizations		
– The situation, incident activities, and any special concerns		
• Assume the role of Planning Section Chief		
• Review this Job Action Sheet		
• Put on position identification (e.g., position vest)		
• Notify your usual supervisor of your assignment		
Assess the operational situation		
• Obtain information and status from the Operations and Logistics Section Chiefs to ensure the accurate tracking of personnel and resources by the Personnel Tracking and Materiel Tracking Managers, if appointed, or the respective Section Chiefs if not		
• Provide information to the Incident Commander on the Planning Section operational situation including capabilities and limitations		
Determine the incident objectives, tactics, and assignments		
• Determine which Planning Section Units need to be activated:		
– Resources Unit		
– Situation Unit		
– Documentation Unit		
– Demobilization Unit		
• Make assignments and distribute corresponding Job Action Sheets and position identification		
• Determine strategies and how the tactics will be accomplished		
• Determine needed resources		
• Brief section personnel on the situation, strategies, and tactics, and designate a time for the next briefing		
Activities		
• Ensure a bed report, staffing report, and current patient census and status are being prepared for the Incident Commander		
• Prepare and conduct a planning meeting to develop and validate the incident objectives for the next operational period		
• Coordinate the preparation, documentation, and approval of the Incident Action Plan (IAP) and distribute copies to the Incident Commander and Section Chiefs		
• Obtain and provide key information for operational and support activities, including the impact on affected departments		
• Gather additional information from the Liaison Officer		
• Collaborate with appropriate Medical-Technical Specialists as needed		
• Obtain information and updates regularly from Planning Section Unit Leaders		
• Maintain current status of all areas		
• Inform the Situation Unit Leader of status information		
• Communicate with the Operations and Logistics Sections for resource needs and projected activities		
• Inform Planning Section personnel of activities that have occurred; keep updates of status and utilization of resources		
• Communicate with the Finance/Administration Section for personnel time records, potential compensation and claims, and canceled surgeries and procedures		
• Activate Incident Specific Plans or Annexes as directed by the Incident Commander		

Immediate Response (0–2 h)	Time	Initial
Documentation		
• HICS 200: Consider use of the Incident Action Plan (IAP) Cover sheet		
• HICS 201: Draft Incident Briefing for Incident Commander as directed		
• HICS 202: Draft Incident Objectives for Incident Commander approval		
• HICS 203: Prepare Organization Assignment List as part of the IAP		
• HICS 204: Document assignments and operational period objectives on Assignment List		
• HICS 205A: Distribute the Communications List appropriately		
• HICS 213: Document all communications on a General Message Form		
• HICS 214: Document all key activities, actions, and decisions in an Activity Log on a continual basis		
• HICS 215A: Obtain completed Incident Action Plan (IAP) Safety Analysis from the Safety Officer for inclusion in the IAP		
• HICS 252: Distribute the Section Personnel Time Sheet to section personnel and ensure time is recorded appropriately		
• HICS 257: Track equipment used during the response on the Resource Accounting Record		
Resources		
• Determine equipment and supply needs; request them from the Logistics Section Supply Unit Leader		
• Assess issues and needs in section areas; coordinate for resource planning		
• Make requests for external assistance, as needed, in coordination with the Liaison Officer		
Communication		
Hospital to complete: Insert communications technology, instructions for use, and protocols for interface with external partners		
Safety and security		
• Ensure that all section personnel comply with safety procedures and instructions		

Intermediate Response (2–12 h)	Time	Initial
Activities		
• Transfer the Planning Section Chief role, if appropriate		
– Conduct a transition meeting to brief your replacement on the current situation, response actions, available resources, and the role of external agencies in support of the hospital		
– Address any health, medical, and safety concerns		
– Address political sensitivities, when appropriate		
– Instruct your replacement to complete the appropriate documentation and ensure that appropriate personnel are properly briefed on response issues and objectives (see HICS Forms 203, 204, 214, and 215A)		
• Ensure the following are being addressed:		
– Section personnel health and safety		
– Update the Incident Action Plan (IAP) with each operational period		
– Short- and long-term planning		
• Ensure that the Planning Section is adequately staffed and supplied		
• Work with the Incident Commander and other Section Chiefs to identify short- and long-term issues with financial implications; establish needed policies and procedures		
• Communicate regularly with Hospital Incident Management Team (HIMT) staff		
• Brief the Incident Commander, Public Information Officer, and Liaison Officer regularly on the status of the Planning Section		
• Designate a time for briefing and updates with Planning Section leadership to update the IAP		

Intermediate Response (2–12 h)	Time	Initial
Documentation • HICS 204: Document assignments and operational period objectives on Assignment List • HICS 213: Document all communications on a General Message Form • HICS 214: Document actions, decisions, and information received on Activity Log • HICS 257: Track equipment used during the response on the Resource Accounting Record		
Resources • Ensure equipment, supplies, and personal protective equipment (PPE) are replaced as needed, coordinating with the Operations and the Logistics Section Chiefs		
Communication *Hospital to complete: Insert communications technology, instructions for use, and protocols for interface with external partners*		
Safety and security • Review personnel protection practices; revise as needed • Ensure staff health and safety issues are being addressed; report issues to the Safety Officer and the Logistics Section Employee Health and Well-Being Unit		

Extended Response (greater than 12 h)	Time	Initial

Activities
 • Transfer the Planning Section Chief role, if appropriate
   – Conduct a transition meeting to brief your replacement on the current situation, response actions, available resources, and the role of external agencies in support of the hospital
   – Address any health, medical, and safety concerns
   – Address political sensitivities, when appropriate
   – Instruct your replacement to complete the appropriate documentation and ensure that appropriate personnel are properly briefed on response issues and objectives (see HICS Forms 203, 204, 214, and 215A)
 • Continue to monitor the ability of Planning Section personnel to meet workload demands, personnel health and safety, resource needs, and documentation practices
 • Continue to receive projected activity reports from Section Chiefs and Planning Section Unit Leaders at designated intervals to prepare status reports and update the Incident Action Plan (IAP)
 • Ensure the Demobilization Unit Leader assesses the ability to deactivate positions, as appropriate, in collaboration with Section Chiefs and develops and implements a Demobilization Plan
 • Ensure the Documentation Unit Leader is receiving and organizing all documentation, including HICS 214: Activity Logs and HICS 213: General Message Form
 • Communicate regularly with Hospital Incident Management Team (HIMT) staff
 • Brief the Incident Commander, Public Information Officer, and Liaison Officer regularly on the status of the Planning Section
 • Designate a time for a briefing and updates with the Planning Section leadership to update the IAP		

Extended Response (greater than 12 h)	Time	Initial
Documentation		
• HICS 204: Document assignments and operational period objectives on Assignment List • HICS 213: Document all communications on a General Message Form • HICS 214: Document actions, decisions, and information received on Activity Log • HICS 257: Track equipment used during the response on the Resource Accounting Record		
Resources		
• Monitor the levels of all supplies and equipment, and collaborate on needs with the Logistics Section Supply Unit Leader		
Communication		
Hospital to complete: Insert communications technology, instructions for use, and protocols for interface with external partners		
Safety and security		
• Observe all staff and volunteers for signs of stress and inappropriate behavior and report concerns to the Safety Officer and the Logistics Section Employee Health and Well-Being Unit Leader • Provide for personnel rest periods and relief • Ensure your physical readiness through proper nutrition, water intake, rest, and stress management techniques		

Demobilization/System Recovery	Time	Initial
Activities		

• Transfer the Planning Section Chief role, if appropriate
  – Conduct a transition meeting to brief your replacement on the current situation, demobilization actions, available resources, and the role of external agencies in support of the hospital
  – Address any health, medical, and safety concerns
  – Address political sensitivities, when appropriate
  – Instruct your replacement to complete the appropriate documentation and ensure that appropriate personnel are properly briefed on response issues and objectives (see HICS Forms 203, 204, 214, and 215A)
• As objectives are met and needs decrease, return Planning Section personnel to their usual jobs and combine or deactivate positions in a phased manner, in coordination with the Demobilization Unit Leader
• Assist Section Chiefs in restoring the hospital to normal operations
• Debrief section personnel on lessons learned and procedural or equipment changes needed
• Participate in other briefings and meetings as required
• Coordinate the final reporting of patient information with external agencies through the Liaison Officer and the Public Information Officer
• Work with Finance/Administration Section to complete cost data information
• Begin the development of the After Action Report and Corrective Action and Improvement Plan and assign staff to complete sections of the report. Topics include:
  – Review of pertinent position descriptions and operational checklists
  – Recommendations for procedure changes
  – Accomplishments and issues
• Participate in stress management and after action debriefings		

Demobilization/System Recovery	Time	Initial
Documentation • HICS 221: Collect and Distribute the Demobilization Check-Out form for Incident Commander approval • Ensure all documentation is submitted to the Documentation Unit		

Documents/Tools

- Incident Action Plan (IAP) Quick Start
- HICS 200 - Incident Action Plan (IAP) Cover Sheet
- HICS 201 - Incident Briefing
- HICS 202 - Incident Objectives
- HICS 203 - Organization Assignment List
- HICS 204 - Assignment List
- HICS 205A - Communications List
- HICS 213 - General Message Form
- HICS 214 - Activity Log
- HICS 215A - Incident Action Plan (IAP) Safety Analysis
- HICS 221 - Demobilization Check-Out
- HICS 252 - Section Personnel Time Sheet
- HICS 254 - Disaster Victim/Patient Tracking
- HICS 255 - Master Patient Evacuation Tracking
- HICS 256 - Procurement Summary Report
- HICS 257 - Resource Accounting Record
- Hospital Emergency Operations Plan
- Incident Specific Plans or Annexes
- Hospital organization chart
- Hospital telephone directory
- Telephone/cell phone/satellite phone/internet/amateur radio/2-way radio for communication

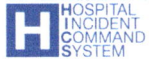

References

Deal T, de Bettencourt M, Deal V, Merrick G, Mills C. Beyond initial response: using the National Incident Management System's Incident Command System. Bloomington, IN: Author House; 2010.

Emergency Medical Services Agency (EMSA). Hospital Incident Command System. 2019. https://emsa.ca.gov/disaster-medical-services-division-hospital-incident-command-system-resources/. Accessed 24 Dec 2019.

EMSI. The history of ICS. 2019. http://www.emsics.com/history-of-ics/. Accessed 4 Dec 2019.

Federal Emergency Management Agency (FEMA). ICS review document. 2018a. https://training.fema.gov/emiweb/is/icsresource/assets/ics%20review%20document.pdf. Accessed 10 Dec 2019.

Federal Emergency Management Agency (FEMA). IS-0100.c: an introduction to the Incident Command System, ICS 100. 2018b. https://training.fema.gov/emiweb/is/is100c/student%20manual/is0100c_sm.pdf. Accessed 4 Dec 2019.

Stambler K, Barbera J. Engineering the incident command and multiagency coordination systems. J Homeland Secur Emerg Manag. 2011;8(1). https://doi.org/10.2202/1547-7355.1838. Accessed 26 Dec 2019.

Paul N. Severin and Phillip A. Jacobson

5.1 Unique Vulnerabilities of Children

Although pediatric patients are viewed as a unique population, they are the population: it has been estimated that more than 25% of the U.S. population fits within the pediatric age range. In all actuality, it is more appropriate to consider the pediatric patient as one with unique vulnerabilities. These vulnerabilities, especially with respect to disasters, are based on the following pediatric developmental differences: anatomy and physiology; behavior and development; and psychology and mental health (Hilmas et al. 2008; Jacobson and Severin 2012; Severin 2011).

5.1.1 Anatomy and Physiology

As depicted on pediatric burn assessment charts, the head accounts for a majority of the total body surface area, while the legs are much less. With growth, the head decreases in size to adult parameters by adolescence. The larger body surface area-to-mass ratio increases the risk of hypothermia. The decreased ability to shiver is another disadvantage to the pediatric patient as heat can be rapidly lost. Hypothermia can be a deadly combination with any trauma leading to coagulopathy and uncontrollable hemorrhage. When exposed to various toxins, the larger body surface area enhances the amount of absorption and end-organ toxicity. Their normally thin, delicate skin can add to absorption, especially in the presence of abrasions or burns. Orthopedic injuries are common in the pediatric patient due to pliability of the

P. N. Severin (✉) · P. A. Jacobson
Pediatric Critical Care Medicine, Rush Medical College and John H. Stroger,
Jr. Hospital of Cook County, Chicago, IL, USA
e-mail: Paul_N_Severin@rush.edu; pseverin@cookcountyhhs.org;
pjacobson@cookcountyhhs.org

© Springer Nature Switzerland AG 2020
C. J. Goodhue, N. Blake (eds.), *Nursing Management of Pediatric Disaster*,
https://doi.org/10.1007/978-3-030-43428-1_5

skeleton as a result of incomplete calcification and active bone growth centers. Protected organs, such as the lungs and heart, may be injured due to overlying fractures. Cervical spine injuries can also be pronounced, as in patients with head trauma. In fact, spinal cord injury may be present without any radiographic abnormalities of the spine. Finally, vital signs will vary based on the pediatric patient's age. This may be a pitfall during rapid evaluation by any nurse or HCP not accustomed to the care of children. Younger pediatric patients have higher metabolic rates and, therefore, higher respiratory rates and heart rates. This can be a distinct disadvantage versus older pediatric patients when encountering similar diseases. An example is inhaled toxins (e.g., nerve agents and lung-damaging agents). Infants and children will suffer greater toxicity since they inhale at a faster rate due to higher metabolic demands and thus, distribute the toxin more rapidly to various end-organs.

Understanding respiratory differences is essential to the management of the acutely ill pediatric patient. The most common etiology for cardiorespiratory arrest in children is respiratory pathology, typically of the upper airway. Most of the airway resistance in children occurs in the upper airway. Nasal obstruction can lead to severe respiratory distress due to infants being obligate nose breathers. Their relatively large tongue and small mouth can lead to airway obstruction quickly, especially when the neuromuscular tone is abnormal such as during sedation or encephalopathy. In infants, physiologic (i.e., copious secretions) and pathologic (i.e., edema, vomitus, blood, and foreign body) factors will exaggerate this obstruction. Securing the airway in such events can be quite challenging. Typically, the glottis is located more anterior and cephalad. Appropriate visualization during laryngoscopy can be further hampered by the prominent occiput that causes neck flexion and, therefore, reduces the alignment of visual axes. The omega or horseshoe-shaped epiglottis in young infants and children is quite susceptible to inflammation and swelling. As in epiglottitis, the glottis becomes strangulated in a circumferential manner leading to dangerous supraglottic obstruction. Children also have a natural tendency to laryngospasm and bronchospasm. Finally, due to weaker cartilage in infants, dynamic airway collapse can occur especially in states of increased resistance and high expiratory flow. Along with altered pulmonary compensation and compliance, a child may rapidly progress to respiratory failure and possibly arrest.

Cardiovascular differences are critical in the pediatric patient. Typical physiological responses tend to allow compensation with seemingly normal homeostasis. With tachycardia and elevated systemic vascular resistance, younger pediatric patients can maintain normal blood pressure despite decreased cardiac output and poor perfusion (compensated shock). Since children have less blood and volume reserve, they progress to this state quickly. In pediatric patients with multiorgan injury or severe gastrointestinal losses, these compensatory mechanisms are pushed to their limits. The unaccustomed HCP may be lulled into complacency since the blood pressure is normal. All the while, the pediatric patient's organs are being poorly perfused. Once these compensatory mechanisms are exhausted, the patient rapidly progresses to hypotension and, therefore, hypotensive shock. If not reversed expeditiously, this may lead to irreversible shock, ischemia, multiorgan dysfunction, and death.

Pediatric patients with altered mental status pose significant problems. The differential diagnosis will be very broad in the comatose patient based on development alone. For example, younger pediatric patients can present with nonconvulsive status epilepticus (NCSE) instead of generalized convulsive status epilepticus (GCSE). In fact, NCSE is more common among younger pediatric patients than GCSE, especially in those from 1 to 12 months of age. Furthermore, many of them are previously well without preexisting diseases such as epilepsy. Other disease states may include poisoning, inborn errors of metabolism, meningitis, and other etiologies of encephalopathy. Using the modified pediatric Glasgow Coma Scale (GCS) is the cornerstone when evaluating the young pediatric patient when they are preverbal. Pupillary response, external ocular movements, and gross motor response may be challenging to evaluate in a developmentally young or delayed pediatric patient.

Pediatric traumatic brain injury is extremely devastating. Whether considered accidental (motor vehicle crash) or nonaccidental (abusive head trauma), evaluation of the neurological status of the acutely injured pediatric patient can be problematic, especially the GCS. Some prefer to use the AVPU system (Alert, Responds to Verbal, Responds to Pain, and Unresponsive). Due to the disproportionately larger head and weaker neck muscles, there is more risk of acceleration–deceleration injuries (fall from a significant height, vehicular ejection, and abusive head trauma). Furthermore, the softer skull, dural structural differences, and vessel supply will place the pediatric patient at risk for brain injury and intracranial hemorrhage. Finally, due to pediatric brain composition, the risk of diffuse axonal injury and cerebral edema is much higher.

Although spinal cord injury is rare in young pediatric patients, morbidity and mortality are significant. In pediatric patients less than 9 years of age, the most commonly seen injuries are in the atlas, axis, and upper cervical vertebrae. In young pediatric patients, spinal injuries tend to be anatomically higher (cervical) versus adolescents (thoracolumbar). Furthermore, congenital abnormalities, such as atlantoaxial abnormalities (Trisomy 21), may exaggerate the process. The clinical presentation of spinal cord injury varies in young pediatric patients due to ongoing development. Laxity of ligaments, wedge-shaped vertebrae, and incomplete ossification centers contribute to specific patterns of injuries. Finally, Spinal Cord Injury without Radiographic Abnormality (SCIWORA) may result. Because of the disproportionately larger head, weaker neck muscles, and elasticity of the spine, significant distraction and flexion injury of the spinal cord may occur without apparent ligament or bony disruption (Hilmas et al. 2008; Jacobson and Severin 2012; Severin 2011).

5.1.2 Behavior and Development

Motor skills develop from birth. Gross and fine motor milestones are achieved in a predictable manner and must be assessed during each HCP encounter. Cognitive development will follow a similar pattern of maturation. The development of these skills can often predict injuries and their extent. For example, consider a house fire. A young infant, preschooler, and adolescent are sleeping upstairs in house when a fire breaks out in the middle of the night. The smoke detectors begin to alarm. Each child is awoken by the ensuing noise and chaos. Based on the development, the adolescent will most likely make it out of the house alive. He will comprehend the threat, run down the stairs, and exit the house without delay. Smoke inhalation may be minimal. If it is a middle adolescent, an attempt may be made to jump out of the window leading to multiple blunt trauma with or without traumatic brain injury. The preschooler most likely will be too scared and not understand how to escape. Tragically, he may hide under a bed or in a closet. When the firefighters arrive and search the house, the preschooler may remain silent because of fear, especially of strangers in the house. He will most likely succumb to thermal injuries along with the effects of carbon monoxide and die. As far as the infant, he cannot walk, climb, crawl, or run. Furthermore, he cannot scream for help or know how to escape. As the smoke engulfs the room, he will most likely suffer severe smoke inhalation injury including extensive carbon monoxide toxicity along with thermal injuries and die. This example also points out another important difference in pediatric patients: their dependence on caregivers. When considering neonates, for example, their entire existence depends on the caregiver, including feeding, changing of diapers, nurturing, and environmental safety. These dynamics are essential to the pediatric patient's health and survival, especially during a disaster.

Another aspect of development is the attainment of language skills. This, too, develops over time in a predictable fashion. One of the biggest challenges in pediatrics is the lack of the patient's ability to verbally convey complaints. As described above, verbal milestones vary among the different age ranges of the pediatric patient. HCPs are often faced with a caregiver's subjective assessment of the problem. Although it can be revealing and informative, this may not be available in an acute crisis situation. It will take the astute HCP to determine, for example, if an inconsolably crying infant is in pain from a corneal abrasion or something more life-threatening such as meningitis. This can also be a challenging task in a teenager, especially during middle adolescence. An HCP will have to determine, for example, if the seemingly lethargic middle adolescent is intoxicated with illicit drugs or has diabetic ketoacidosis.

Finally, the HCP will have to address developmental variances among their pediatric patients and any comorbid features. Young pediatric patients can regress developmentally during any illness or injury. This is especially seen in patients with chronic medical conditions (cancer) or during prolonged hospitalization with rehabilitation (multisystem trauma). Furthermore, those pediatric patients with developmental and intellectual disabilities, for example, will be difficult to evaluate based on the effects of their underlying pathology. These pediatric patients typically have unique variances in their physical exams (Jacobson and Severin 2012; Severin 2011). Please refer to Chap. 7 for more detailed information on pediatric development.

5.1.3 Psychology and Mental Health

Pediatric patients will often reflect the emotional state of their caregiver. They take verbal and physical cues from their caregiver. At times, this may also occur in the presence of a nurse or HCP. The psychological impact of illness will vary greatly with the child's development and experience. Children tend to have a greater vulnerability to post-traumatic stress disorder especially with disaster events. Furthermore, they are highly prone to becoming psychiatric casualties despite the absence of physical injury to themselves. And as any pediatric HCP can tell you, the younger pediatric patients tend to also have greater levels of anxiety, especially while preparing for invasive procedures such as phlebotomy and intravenous line placement (Hilmas et al. 2008; Jacobson and Severin 2012; Severin 2011). Please refer to Chap. 12 for more detailed content on mental health.

5.2   Pediatric Disaster Planning

The World Health Organization and the Pan American Health Organization define a *disaster* as "an event that occurs in most cases suddenly and unexpectedly, causing severe disturbances to people or objects affected by it, resulting in the loss of life and harm to the health of the population, the destruction or loss of community property, and/or severe damage to the environment. Such a situation leads to disruption in the normal pattern of life, resulting in misfortune, helplessness, and suffering, with adverse effects on the socioeconomic structure of a region or a country and/or modifications of the environment to such an extent that there is a need for assistance and immediate outside intervention" (Lynch and Berman 2009).

Types of disasters usually fall into two broad categories: natural and man-made. Natural disasters are generally associated with weather and geological events, including extremes of temperature, floods, hurricanes, earthquakes, tsunamis, volcanic eruptions, landslides, and drought. Naturally occurring epidemics, such as the 2009 H1N1, 2014 Ebola, and 2019 novel coronavirus (COVID-19) outbreaks, are often included in this category. Man-made disasters are usually associated with a criminal attack such as an active shooter incident, or a terrorist attack using weapons such as explosive, biological, or chemical agents. However, man-made disasters can also refer to human-based technological incidents, such as a building or bridge collapse, or events related to the manufacture, transportation, storage, and use of hazardous materials, such as the 1986 Chernobyl radiation leak and the 1984 Bhopal toxic gas leak. Even though disasters can be primarily placed into any of these two categories, they can often impact each other and compound the magnitude of any disaster incident (United States Department of Homeland Security, Office of Inspector General 2009). A prime example is the March 2011 Tohoku earthquake leading to a tsunami (natural) that triggered the Fukushima Daiichi nuclear disaster (man-made).

Disasters can also be characterized by the location of such an event. *Internal* disasters are those incidents that occur within the health care facility or system. Employees, physical plant, workflow and operations of the clinic, hospital, or system can be disrupted. *External* disasters are those incidents that occur outside of the health care facility or system. This impacts the community surrounding the facility, proximally or distally, but does not directly threaten the facility or its employees. As with natural and man-made disasters, internal and external disasters can impact each other. For example, an overflow of patients during a high census period may lead to the shutdown of the hospital to any new patients (internal disaster). This will place the hospital on bypass and possibly stress other hospitals in the community beyond their means (external disaster). A terrorist event, such as the release of sarin in a subway system during a busy morning commute, can lead to massive disruption in the community (external disaster). All the victims of the attack will seek medical care at nearby hospitals, possibly overwhelming the health care staff and depleting critical resources (internal disaster). Characterization of disasters by geography (local, state, national, and international) can also be used. Again, no matter the site of the incident, a disaster in one area could easily create a disaster in another geographical region. For example, a factory and its community could be ravaged by a hurricane (local disaster). If this is the only factory in the world to produce a certain medication, this could lead to critical shortages to hospitals all around the world (international disaster).

The term "disaster preparedness" has been used over the years as a way to describe efforts to manage any disaster event. However, preparedness is only one aspect of the process. The use of the term disaster planning is more appropriate. It considers all aspects needed for an effective effort and is dependent on additional phases, not just preparedness. National preparedness efforts, including planning, are now informed by the Presidential Policy Directive (PPD) 8 that was signed by the president in March 2011 and describes the nation's approach to preparedness (United States Department of Education, Office of Elementary and Secondary Education, Office of Safe and Healthy Students 2013; United States Department of Homeland Security 2018b). A recommended method for disaster preparedness efforts is the utilization of an "all-hazards" model of emergency management (Adini et al. 2012; Waugh 2000). The four overlapping phases of the model include mitigation, preparedness, response, and recovery. The *mitigation* phase involves "activities designed to prevent or reduce losses from a disaster" (Waugh 2000). Examples include land use planning in flood plains, structural integrity measures in earthquake zones, and deployment of security cameras. The *preparedness* phase includes the "planning of how to respond in an emergency or a disaster, and developing capabilities for more effective response" (Waugh 2000). Examples include training programs for emergency responders, drills and exercises, early warning systems, contingency planning, and development of equipment and supply caches. Up to this point, all planning efforts are proactive and not reactive. Often times, a hazard analysis is conducted to delineate areas of strengths and identify potential risks. It helps in "the identification of hazards, assessment of the probability of a disaster, and the probable intensity and location; assessment of its potential impact on a community; the property, persons, and geographic areas that may be at risk; and the determination of agency priorities based on the probability level of a disaster and the potential losses" (Waugh 2000). After a disaster or emergency incident occurs, the *response* phase, or "immediate reaction to a disaster",(Waugh 2000) begins. Examples include mass evacuations, sandbagging buildings and other structures, providing emergency medical services, firefighting, and restoration of public order. In some situations, the response period may be a short (e.g., house fire), intermediate (e.g., bomb detonation), or extended (e.g., pandemic influenza) duration. After a period of time, the *recovery* phase follows. These are "activities that continue beyond the emergency period to restore lifelines" (Waugh 2000). Examples include the provision of temporary shelter, restoration of utilities such as power, critical stress debriefing for responders, and victims, job assistance and small business loans, and debris clearance. Recovery always seems to be the most unpredictable; it may take days to months to years. As demonstrated with recent hurricanes Harvey, Irma, and Maria in 2017, the most affected regions are still in the phase of recovery and may be along a prolonged track as Hurricane Katrina in 2005.

As mentioned, the early phases of planning (mitigation and preparedness) truly hinge upon the environment or community surrounding the health care site (e.g., clinic, hospital, or long-term care facility). Identification of potential hazards and risks is a key step in disaster planning. Using a Hazard Vulnerability Assessment (HVA) or a Threat and Hazard Identification and Risk Assessment (THIRA) can provide a basis for mitigation and prevention tasks. An HVA/THIRA emphasizes which types of natural or man-made disasters are likely to occur in a community (e.g., tornado, flood, chemical release, or terrorist event). They further highlight the impact those disasters may have on the community and any capabilities that are in place that may lessen the effects of the disaster (Illinois Emergency Medical Services for Children 2018).

A basic principle of the HVA methodology is to determine the risk of such an event or attack occurring at a given hospital or hospital system. Simply, the risk is a product of the probability of an event and the severity of such an event if it occurs (risk = probability × severity). However, there are many complexities in quantifying terrorism risk (Waugh 2005; Woo 2002). It is important to note that in some circumstances, exposure may need to be included in the equation (risk = probability × severity × exposure), but usually for operational risk management applications (Mitchell and Decker 2004). At any rate, issues to consider for the probability of an event occurring include, but are not limited to, geographic location and topography, proximity to hazards, degree of accessibility, known risks, historical data, and statistics of various manufacturer/vendor products. Severity, on the other hand, is dependent on the gap between the magnitude of an event and mitigation for the given event (severity = magnitude – mitigation). Magnitude varies upon the impact of the event to humans, property, and/or business. Mitigation varies upon the development of internal and external readiness before a disaster strikes. As one can surmise, if the magnitude of the event outstrips the mitigation, the event is considered a threatening hazard. Once the HVA is completed, the health care site should immediately prioritize planning efforts for the top 5–10 hazards and develop plans accordingly. All other identified hazards must also be addressed to ensure a broad and robust disaster plan. It is important to realize that local and regional entities also perform comprehensive HVAs. A concerted analysis among a hospital and key community stakeholders is optimal for a coordinated plan.

An HVA/THIRA contains both quantitative and qualitative components. Specific tools have been developed through private and public organizations (e.g, FEMA) that can help in the analysis (United States Department of Homeland Security, Federal Emergency Management Agency 2001). Using these tools as a guide, the entity can determine what types of hazards have a high, medium, or low probability of occurring within specific geographic boundaries. Typically, these tools do not have components specific to children or other at-risk populations. However, the tools can be adapted either directly by adding children to specific hazards or ensuring considerations specific to children are incorporated into the HVA/THIRA calculations. The HVA/THIRA should be reviewed and updated minimally on an annual basis to identify changing or external circumstances. This includes conducting a pediatric-specific disaster risk assessment to identify where children congregate and their risks (e.g., schools, popular field trip designations, summer camps, houses of worship, and juvenile justice facilities) (Illinois Emergency Medical Services for Children 2018).

Of note, HVA techniques have been utilized for pediatric-specific disaster plans. Having a separate pediatric HVA (PHVA) is crucial to a well-rounded and robust health care disaster plan. First, it demonstrates the extent of the pediatric population in the community. It is estimated that 25% of the population fits within the age range of pediatric patients. In some situations, it may be more. During the performance of a PHVA, it was demonstrated that 29% of the community was less than 19 years of age (Jacobson and Severin 2012). Second, a PHVA increases the situational awareness of those tasked to plan for disasters that involve children and adolescents. Often times, children and adolescents are excluded from local and regional disaster plans. The unique vulnerabilities of pediatric patients will demand appropriate drills, exercises, equipment, medications, and expertise. Thirdly, identifying pediatric risks in a community will help prioritize efforts of planning, especially in those hospitals not accustomed to caring for pediatric patients. Finally, a PHVA helps to develop a framework for global pediatric disaster planning. This can extend beyond a local community and actually advance city, state, regional, and national disaster planning efforts. There has been a development of web-based tools to simplify and enhance the PHVA process (Jacobson and Severin 2012).

After an HVA/THIRA has been completed, the results should be used to help direct and plan drills/exercises based on high impact and high probability threats. It is advised to conduct an HVA/THIRA on an annual basis to assess specific threats unique to your organization's physical structure as well as the surrounding geographic environment. It will also provide insight into whether there is an improvement in previous planning efforts. Completion of a population assessment that provides a demographic overview of the community with a breakdown of the childhood population is strongly recommended in conjunction with the HVA/THIRA. Collaborating with other community partners, such as local health departments and emergency management agencies, can assist an organization with the conduction of a comprehensive HVA/THIRA (Illinois Emergency Medical Services for Children 2018). Please see Chap. 13 for further information on hospital planning.

5.3 General Resuscitation, Equipment, Supplies, and Medications

Pediatric supplies, equipment, and medications will be scarce during a disaster. It will become more of an issue if the health care facility is not accustomed to caring for acutely ill pediatric patients. This will be further exacerbated by a massive surge of acutely ill pediatric patients, a widespread or prolonged disaster, and supply line disruptions. To protect the health security of children and families during a public health emergency, the Assistant Secretary for Preparedness and Response (ASPR) manages and maintains the Strategic National Stockpile (SNS), a cache of medical countermeasures for rapid deployment and use in response to a public health emergency or disaster (Fagbuyi et al. 2016). Various pediatric-specific supplies and countermeasures are included in the SNS. Maintaining a supply of medications and medical supplies for specific health threats allows the stockpile to respond with the right product when a specific disease or agent is known. If a community experiences a large-scale public health incident in which the disease or agent is unknown, the first line of support from the stockpile is to send a broad-range of pharmaceuticals and medical supplies. The majority of stockpile assets are held in storage and kept as managed inventory. Each package contains 50 tons of emergency medical resources. The SNS is deployed along with a Federal Medical Station Strike Team who have in-depth knowledge of the stockpile and supply operations (Assistant Secretary for Preparedness and Response, United States Department of Health and Human Services 2018). The SNS, depending upon the threat, is intended to only supplement state and local supplies used for immediate care during the initial response. Contents are prepacked and configured in transport-ready containers for rapid delivery anywhere in the U.S. within 12 h of the federal decision to deploy (Assistant Secretary for Preparedness and Response, United States Department of Health and Human Services 2018). However, the federal recommendation is to always maintain a local stockpile of supplies to support patients, families, and staff independently for at least 96 h (Illinois Emergency Medical Services for Children 2018).

There are hospital guidelines for pediatric-specific medications, equipment, and supplies for pediatric emergency preparedness (American Academy of Pediatrics, Committee on Pediatric Emergency Medicine, American College of Emergency Physicians, Pediatric Committee, and Emergency Nurses Association Pediatric Committee 2009) (Tables 5.1 and 5.2). Much of the equipment is already recommended for ambulance services responding to pediatric emergencies (American College of Surgeons Committee on Trauma, American College of Emergency Physicians, National Association of EMS Physicians, Pediatric Equipment Guidelines Committee Emergency Medical Services for Children (EMSC) Partnership for Children Stakeholder Group, American Academy of Pediatrics 2009) and health care centers tasked with receiving acutely ill pediatric patients (American Academy of Pediatrics, Committee on Pediatric Emergency Medicine, American College of Emergency Physicians, Pediatric Committee, and Emergency Nurses Association Pediatric Committee 2009; Place and Martin 2012). The emergency equipment and supply lists can easily be adapted for any pediatric disaster emergency (Place and Martin 2012) or incident requiring pediatric mass critical care (Desmond et al. 2011). Age-appropriate nutrition, hygiene, bedding, and toys/distraction devices should also be available (Illinois Emergency Medical Services for Children 2013) (Tables 5.3 and 5.4).

Table 5.1 Potentially useful medications in pediatric emergencies[a]

Adenosine	Diphenhydramine	Glucagon	Lorazepam	Phenytoin
Albuterol	Dobutamine	Glucose	Magnesium sulfate	Prednisone/Prednisolone
Alprostadil (PGE1)	Dopamine	Hydrocortisone	Mannitol	Procainamide
Amiodarone	Epinephrine	Ipratropium bromide	Methylprednisolone	Propranolol
Atropine	Epinephrine, racemic	Kayexalate™ (sodium polystyrene sulfonate)	Midazolam	Rocuronium
Bicarbonate, sodium	Fentanyl		Milrinone	Succinylcholine
Calcium chloride	Flumazenil	Ketamine	Morphine	Vecuronium
Charcoal, activated	Fosphenytoin	Levalbuterol	Naloxone	
Dexamethasone	Furosemide	Lidocaine	Nitroprusside	
Diazepam			Norepinephrine	
			Phenobarbital	

[a]References: (American Academy of Pediatrics and American College of Emergency Physicians et al. 2012; American Academy of Pediatrics, Committee on Pediatric Emergency Medicine, American College of Emergency Physicians, Pediatric Committee, and Emergency Nurses Association Pediatric Committee 2009; Hegenbarth 2008)

Table 5.2 Guidelines for pediatric-specific equipment and supplies[a]

General equipment	Patient warming device (infant warmer)
	Restraint device for children
	Weight scale for infants and children
	Length-based resuscitation tape
	Pain-scale assessment tools appropriate for age
Monitoring equipment	Blood pressure cuffs (neonatal, infant, child, adult)
	Doppler ultrasound devices
	ECG monitor/defibrillator with pediatric and adult capabilities, including pediatric-sized pads/paddles
	Invasive thermometer
	Pulse oximeter with pediatric and adult probes
	Continuous end-tidal carbon dioxide monitoring device
Respiratory	Endotracheal tubes
	• Uncuffed: 2.5 and 3.0 mm
	• Cuffed or uncuffed: 3.5, 4.0, 4.5, 5.0, and 5.5 mm
	• Cuffed: 6.0, 6.5, 7.0, 7.5, and 8.0 mm
	Feeding tubes (5F and 8F)
	Laryngoscope blades curved: 2 and 3; straight: 0, 1, 2, and 3
	Laryngoscope handle
	Magill forceps (pediatric and adult)
	Nasopharyngeal airways (infant, child, and adult)
	Oropharyngeal airways (sizes 0–5)
	Stylets for endotracheal tubes (pediatric and adult)
	Suction catheters (infant, child, and adult)
	Tracheostomy tubes (sizes 2.5, 3.0, 3.5, 4.0, 4.5, 5.0, and 5.5 mm)
	Yankauer suction tip
	Bag-mask device (manual resuscitator), self-inflating (infant size: 450 mL; adult size: 1000 mL)
	Clear oxygen masks (standard and nonrebreathing) for an infant, child, and adult
	Masks to fit bag-mask device adaptor (neonatal, infant, child, and adult sizes)
	Nasal cannulas (infant, child, and adult)
	Nasogastric tubes (sump tubes): infant (8F), child (10F), and adult (14F–18F)
	Laryngeal mask airway[a]
Vascular access	Arm boards (infant, child, and adult sizes)
	Catheter over-the-needle device (14–24 gauge)
	Intraosseous needles or device (pediatric and adult sizes)
	Intravenous catheter–administration sets with calibrated chambers and extension tubing and/or infusion devices with ability to regulate rate and volume of infusate
	Umbilical vein catheters (3.5F and 5.0F)[b]
	Central venous catheters (4.0F–7.0F)
	Intravenous solutions to include normal saline, dextrose 5% in normal saline, and dextrose 10% in water
Fracture-management devices	Extremity splints, including femur splints (pediatric and adult sizes)
	Spine-stabilization method/devices appropriate for children of all ages[c]

(continued)

Table 5.2 (continued)

Pediatric trays or kits	Lumbar puncture tray, including infant (22-gauge), pediatric (22-gauge), and adult (18- to 21-gauge)
	Lumbar puncture needles
	Supplies/kit for patients with difficult airway conditions (to include but not limited to supraglottic airways of all sizes, such as the laryngeal mask airway, two-needle cricothyrotomy supplies, and surgical cricothyrotomy kit)
	Tube thoracostomy tray
	Chest tubes to include infant, child, and adult sizes (infant: 10F–12F; child, 16F–24F; adult, 28F– 40F)
	Newborn delivery kit (including equipment for initial resuscitation of a newborn infant: umbilical clamp, scissors, bulb syringe, and towel)
	Urinary catheterization kits and urinary (indwelling) catheter (6F–22F)

References: (American Academy of Pediatrics and American College of Emergency Physicians et al. 2012; American Academy of Pediatrics, Committee on Pediatric Emergency Medicine, American College of Emergency Physicians, Pediatric Committee, and Emergency Nurses Association Pediatric Committee 2009; American College of Surgeons Committee on Trauma, American College of Emergency Physicians, National Association of EMS Physicians, Pediatric Equipment Guidelines Committee Emergency Medical Services for Children (EMSC) Partnership for Children Stakeholder Group, American Academy of Pediatrics 2009; Desmond et al. 2011)
[a]Laryngeal mask airways could be shared with anesthesia but must be immediately accessible to the ED
[b]Feeding tubes (size 5F) may be used as umbilical venous catheters but are not ideal. A method for securing the umbilical catheter, such as an umbilical tie, should also be available
[c]A spinal stabilization device is one that can stabilize the neck of an infant, child, or adolescent in a neutral position

Table 5.3 Useful general care items for managing the needs of children[a]

Nutrition, hygiene, and sleeping supplies			
Nutrition	Nutrition supplies	Hygiene	Sleeping supplies
Baby formula Baby food/cereal Oral electrolyte solutions, age-appropriate	Baby bottles and nipples for bottles Plastic bowls Sippy cups Toddler feeding spoons/forks Manual breast pumps with bottles Small towels for spit up Pacifiers	Hand sanitizer Washcloths/towels Diapers (sizes 1–6) Pull ups (sizes 4 T–5 T) Diaper wipes Container for soiled diapers Diaper rash ointment Disposable changing pads Toddler toilet seat (potty chairs) Cloth diapers Infant wash (soap) Infant bathing bins Baby laundry detergent (dye and fragrance free)	Portable cribs, bassinets, play pens Laundry baskets (can be used for infant bed) Bed sheets Lightweight hypoallergenic blankets

[a]Reference: (Illinois Emergency Medical Services for Children 2013)

Table 5.4 Age-appropriate Toys/Distraction Devices[a]

For safety and infection control reasons, only stock toys for children that are washable, nontoxic, difficult to break, and without small pieces (NOTE: Toys with small parts may present a potential choking hazard). Consider including some toys/objects that could be given to the child to keep (small new stuffed animals, cars, stickers, coloring books/crayons, etc.).			
Infants/toddlers	Preschool/school age	Adolescents	General
Musical/light toys	Plastic animals, action figures, cars	Teen rated games	Bubbles
Pop-up toys	action figures, cars	Video/electronic games	Balls
Mirrors	Building blocks	games	Coloring books and supplies
Shape sorters	Books	Journal and writing supplies	supplies
Stacking rings	Dolls	supplies	Arts and craft supplies
Activity blocks	Elementary school rated games	Books and magazines	Music
Teething rings	rated games	Activity sets	Stickers
Board books	Foam balls	Music	Sculpting clay
Beginner toy cars			

[a]Reference: (Illinois Emergency Medical Services for Children 2013)

When a pediatric disaster victim presents acutely ill to the hospital, various emergency interventions will be needed to stabilize the patient. Evaluation of the pediatric patient should include a primary survey (ABCDE), secondary survey (focused SAMPLE history and focused physical examination), and diagnostic assessments (laboratory, radiological, and other advanced tests). This will guide further therapeutic interventions. Particular attention should be given to the identification of respiratory and/or circulatory derangements of the child, including airway obstruction, respiratory failure, shock, and cardiopulmonary failure. Interventions will be based on physiologic derangements of the pediatric patient and determined by the scope of practice and protocols, such as standard resuscitation algorithms for neonatal (American Academy of Pediatrics and American Heart Association et al. 2016) and pediatric (American Heart Association 2016) victims.

The HCP must be knowledgeable of various emergency medications (Table 5.1) used for children, the appropriate dosages and their mechanism of action, any potential side effects, and drug/drug interactions. Other medications, such as antibiotics, antidotes, or countermeasures, may be needed as well. Pharmacologic therapy should be initiated immediately based on clinical suspicion and not delayed due to pending laboratory tests (e.g., antibiotics for presumed infection/sepsis or antidotes for suspected nerve agents). Dosages should be based on the patient's weight or a length-based weight system. Utilizing current resuscitation references, such as *Handbook of Emergency Cardiovascular Care for Healthcare Providers*, (American Heart Association 2015) *Neonatal Resuscitation Program*, (American Academy of Pediatrics and American Heart Association et al. 2016) *Pediatric Advanced Life Support*, (American Heart Association 2016) or *Advanced Pediatric Life Support*, (American Academy of Pediatrics and American College of Emergency Physicians 2012) is highly recommended (American Academy of Pediatrics, Committee on Pediatric Emergency Medicine, American College of Emergency Physicians, Pediatric Committee, and Emergency Nurses Association Pediatric Committee

2009; Hegenbarth 2008). Pediatric countermeasure dosing recommendations for various chemical, biological, and radiological/nuclear exposures can be found online through the U.S. Department of Health and Human Services (United States Department of Health and Human Services, Office of the Assistant Secretary for Preparedness and Response, National Library of Medicine 2019; United States Department of Health and Human Services, Chemical Hazards Emergency Medical Management (CHEMM) 2019) or Centers for Disease Control and Prevention (Centers for Disease Control and Prevention 2018a). Pediatric antidote dosing cards (Montello et al. 2006) or hard copy countermeasure manuals may be more practical, especially during a disaster incident when computer service or internet access may be unreliable.

5.4   Natural Disasters

In 1988, the Centre for Research on the Epidemiology of Disasters (CRED) launched the Emergency Events Database (EM-DAT). EM-DAT was created with the initial support of the World Health Organization (WHO) and the Belgian Government. The main objective of the database is to serve the purposes of humanitarian action at national and international levels. The initiative aims to rationalize decision-making for disaster preparedness as well as provide an objective base for vulnerability assessment and priority setting. EM-DAT contains essential core data on the occurrence and effects of over 22,000 mass disasters in the world from 1900 to the present day. The database is compiled from various sources, including United Nation agencies, nongovernmental organizations (NGOs), insurance companies, research institutes, and press agencies (CRED 2019). As described in the CRED report entitled *Natural disasters 2017: lower mortality, higher cost*, a disaster is entered into the database if at least one of the following criteria is fulfilled: 10 or more people reported killed; 100 or more people reported affected; declaration of a state of emergency; and/or call for international assistance (CRED 2018).

In *Economic losses, poverty and disasters 1998–2017: CRED/UNISDR Report*, the CRED defines a disaster as "a situation or event which overwhelms local capacity, necessitating a request at national or international level for external assistance; an unforeseen and often sudden event that causes great damage, destruction and human suffering" (CRED 2018). The CRED EM-DAT classifies disasters according to the type of hazard that triggers them. The two main disaster groups are natural and technological disasters.

There are six natural disaster subgroups. *Geophysical* disasters originate from the solid earth and include earthquake (ground movement and tsunami), dry mass movement (rock fall and landslides), and volcanic activity (ash fall, lahar, pyroclastic flow, and lava flow). Lahar is a hot or cold mixture of earthen material flowing on the slope of a volcano either during or between volcanic eruptions. *Meteorological* disasters are caused by short-lived, micro- to meso-scale extreme weather and atmospheric conditions that last from minutes to days and include extreme temperatures (cold wave, heat wave, and severe winter conditions such as snow/ice or frost/freeze), fog, and storms. Storms can be extra-tropical, tropical, or convective. Convective storms include derecho, hail, lightning/thunderstorm, rain, tornado, sand/dust storm, winter storm/blizzard, storm/surge, and wind. Derecho is a widespread and usually fast-moving windstorm associated with convection/convective storm and includes downburst and straight-line winds. *Hydrological* disasters are caused by the occurrence, movement, and distribution of surface/subsurface freshwater and saltwater and include floods, landslides (an avalanche of snow, debris, mudflow, and rockfall), and wave action (rogue wave and seiche). Flood types can be coastal, riverine, flash, or ice jam. *Climatological* disasters are caused by long-lived, meso- to macro-scale atmospheric processes ranging from intraseasonal to multidecadal climate variability and include drought, glacial lake outburst, and wildfire (forest fire, land fire: brush, bush, or pasture). *Biological* disasters are caused by the exposure to living organisms and their toxic substances or vector-borne diseases that they may carry and include epidemics (viral, bacterial, parasitic, fungal, and prion), insect infestation (grasshopper and locust), and animal accidents. *Extraterrestrial* disasters are caused by asteroids, meteoroids, and comets as they pass near-earth, enter Earth's atmosphere, and/or strike the earth, and by changes in the interplanetary conditions that affect the Earth's magnetosphere, ionosphere, and thermosphere. Types include impact (airbursts) and space weather (energetic particles, geomagnetic storm, and shockwave) events (CRED 2019).

There are three technological disaster subgroups. *Industrial* accidents include chemical spills, collapse, explosion, fire, gas leak, poisoning, radiation, and oil spills. A chemical spill is an accidental release occurring during the production, transportation, or handling of hazardous chemical substances. *Transport* accidents include disasters in the air (airplanes, helicopters, airships, and balloons), on the road (moving vehicles on roads or tracks), on the rail system (train), and on the water (sailing boats, ferries, cruise ships, and other boats). *Miscellaneous* accidents vary from collapse to explosions to fires. Collapse is an accident involving the collapse of a building or structure and can either involve industrial structures or domestic/nonindustrial structures (CRED 2019). Technological disasters are considered man-made, but as suggested by their subgroup, they are accidental and not intentional.

The United Nations Office for Disaster Risk Reduction (UNISDR) and CRED report, *Economic losses, poverty, and disasters 1998–2017*, reviews global natural disasters during that time period, their economic impact, and the relationship with poverty. Between 1998 and 2017, climate-related and geophysical disasters killed 1.3 million people and left a further 4.4 billion injured, homeless, displaced, or in need of emergency assistance. Although the majority of fatalities were due to geophysical events, mostly earthquakes and tsunamis, 91% of all disasters was caused by floods, storms, droughts, heatwaves, and other extreme weather events. The financial impact was staggering. In 1998–2017, disaster-hit countries reported direct economic losses valued at US$ 2908 billion, of which climate-related disasters caused US$ 2245 billion or 77% of the total. This was up from 68% (US$ 895 billion) of losses (US$ 1313 billion) reported between 1978 and 1997. Overall, reported losses from extreme weather events rose by 151% between these two 20-year periods. In absolute monetary terms, over the last 20-years, the USA recorded the biggest losses (US$ 945 billion), reflecting high asset values as well as frequent events. China, by comparison, suffered a significantly higher number of disasters than the USA (577 vs. 482) but lower total losses (US$ 492 billion) (CRED 2018) (Figs. 5.1, 5.2, 5.3, 5.4, 5.5, 5.6, 5.7, 5.8 and 5.9).

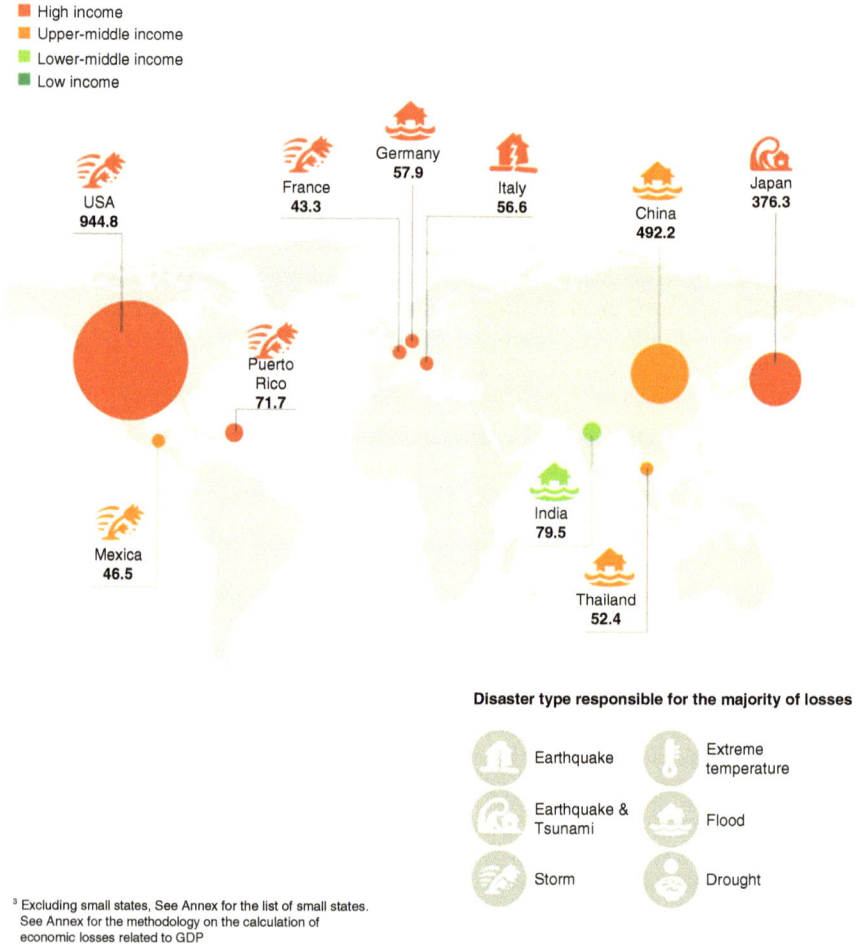

³ Excluding small states, See Annex for the list of small states.
See Annex for the methodology on the calculation of
economic losses related to GDP

Fig. 5.1 Top 10 countries/territories in terms of absolute losses*. *Used with permission from CRED (2018)

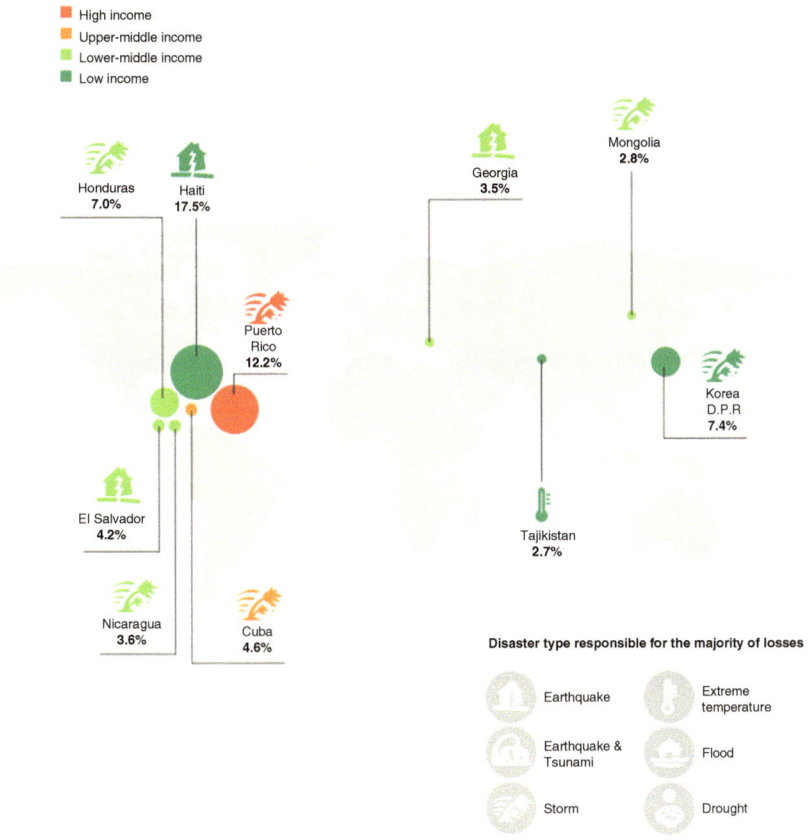

Fig. 5.2 Top 10 countries/territories in terms of average annual percentage losses relative to GDP*. *Used with permission from CRED (2018)

In 2018, 281 climate-related and geophysical incidents in the world were estimated with 10,733 deaths and over 60 million people impacted. Indonesia recorded approximately half of the deaths with India accounting for half of those impacted by disasters. Notable features of 2018 were intense seismic activity in Indonesia, a series of disasters in Japan, floods in India, and an eventful year for both volcanic activity and wildfires. However, an ongoing trend of lower death tolls from previous years continued into 2018 (Centre for Research on the Epidemiology of Disasters (CRED) and United Nations Office for Disaster Risk Reduction (UNISDR) 2019) (Tables 5.5, 5.6, 5.7, 5.8, 5.9, 5.10 and 5.11).

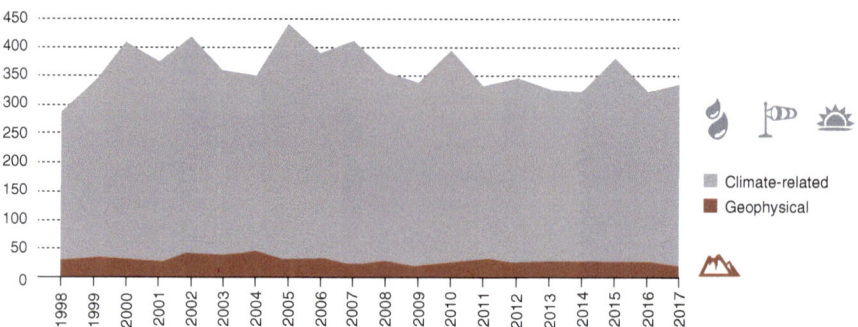

Fig. 5.3 Number of disasters by major category per year 1998–2017*. *Used with permission from CRED (2018)

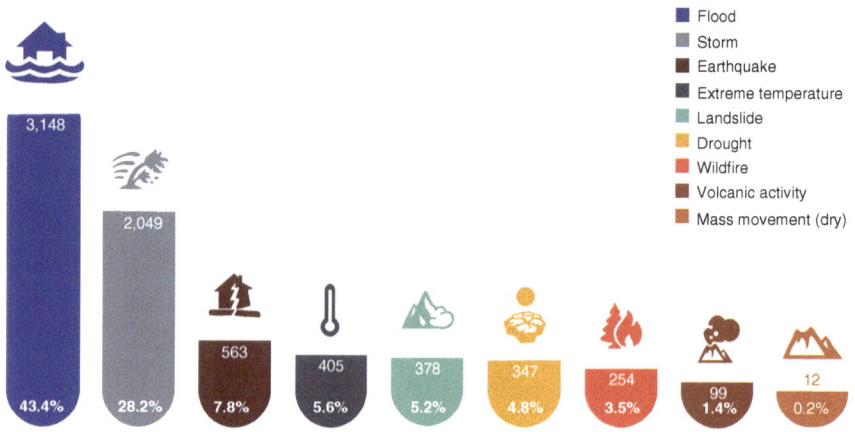

Fig. 5.4 Numbers of disasters per type 1998–2017*. *Used with permission from CRED (2018)

There are no specific deviations when medically managing children after a natural disaster. According to Sirbaugh and DiRocco (2012) "Small-scale mass casualty incidents occur daily in the United States. Few present unusual challenges to the local medical systems other than in the number of patients that must be treated at one time. Except in earthquakes, explosions, building collapses, and some types of terrorist attacks, the same holds true for large-scale disasters. Sudden violent disaster mechanisms can produce major trauma cases, including patients needing field amputations or management of crush syndrome. For the most part, medicine after a disaster is much the same as it was before the disaster, with more minor injuries, more people with exacerbations of their chronic illnesses, and number of patients

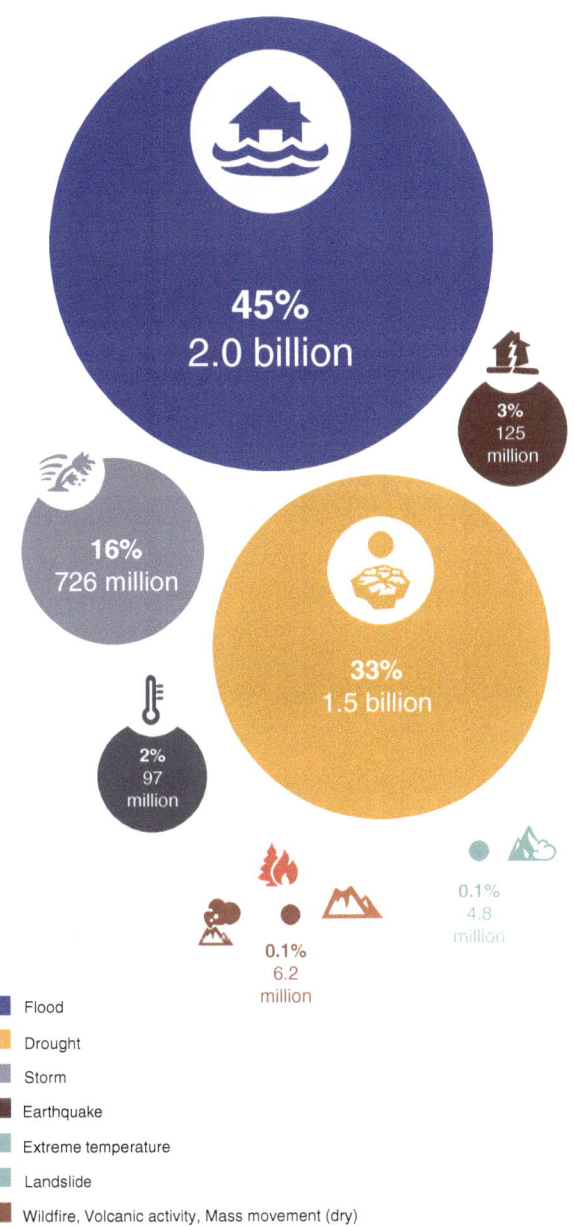

45%
2.0 billion

3%
125
million

16%
726 million

33%
1.5 billion

2%
97
million

0.1%
4.8
million

0.1%
6.2
million

- ■ Flood
- ■ Drought
- ■ Storm
- ■ Earthquake
- ■ Extreme temperature
- ■ Landslide
- ■ Wildfire, Volcanic activity, Mass movement (dry)

Fig. 5.5 Number of people affected per disaster type 1998–2017*. *Used with permission from CRED (2018)

Fig. 5.6 Number of deaths per disaster type 1998–2017*. *Used with permission from CRED (2018)

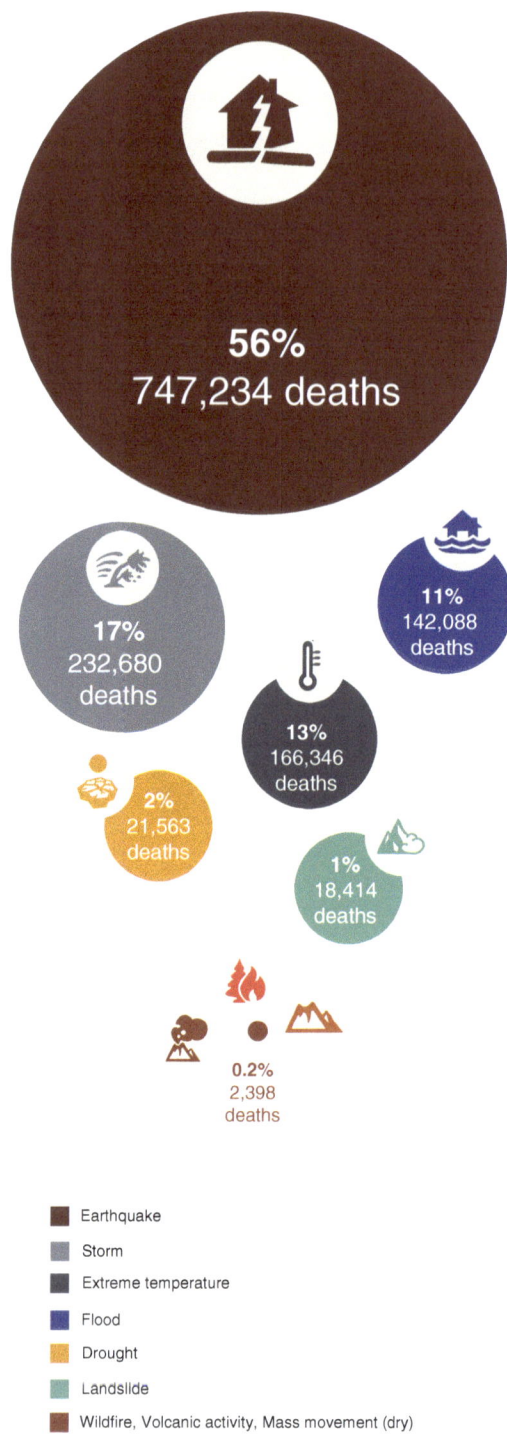

56%
747,234 deaths

17%
232,680
deaths

11%
142,088
deaths

13%
166,346
deaths

2%
21,563
deaths

1%
18,414
deaths

0.2%
2,398
deaths

Earthquake
Storm
Extreme temperature
Flood
Drought
Landslide
Wildfire, Volcanic activity, Mass movement (dry)

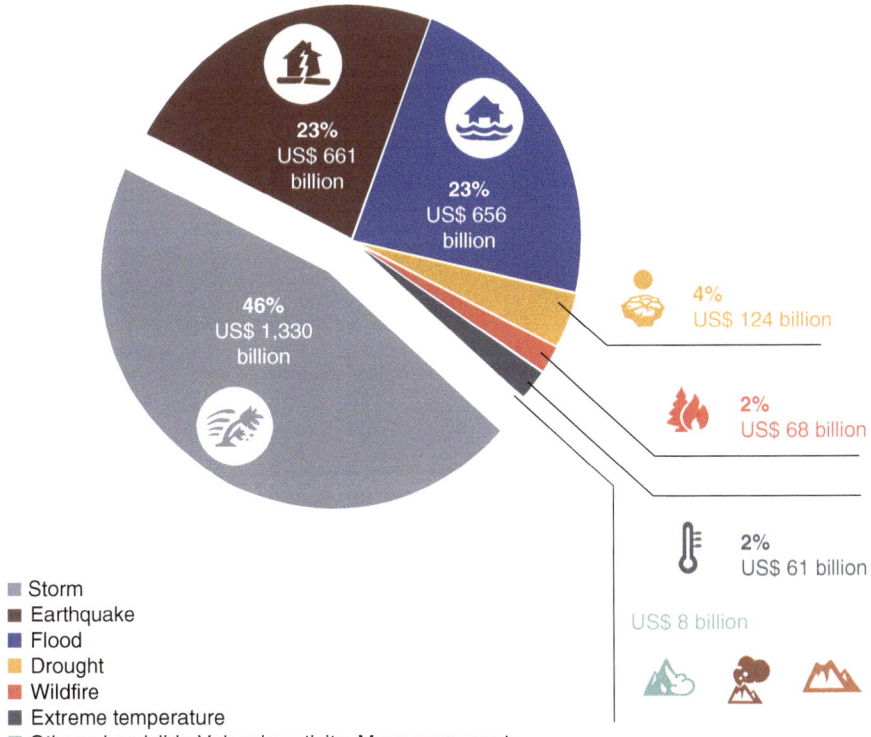

Fig. 5.7 Breakdown of recorder economic losses (US$) per disaster type 1998–2017. *Used with permission from CRED (2018)

seeking what is ordinarily considered primary care. This is true for children and adults." It should be noted, however, that children have a predisposition to illness and injury after natural disasters. The HCP must be able to identify any health problems and treat the child effectively and efficiently while utilizing standard resuscitation protocols as indicated.

Traumatic injuries may be seen after any natural disaster. The injuries can range from minor scrapes and bruises to major blunt trauma or traumatic brain injury. Children are at increased risk for injury since adults are distracted by recovery efforts and may not be able to supervise them closely. The environment may not be safe due to environmental hazards, such as collapsed buildings, sinkholes, and high water levels. Dangerous equipment used during relief efforts may be present, such as heavy earth moving equipment, chainsaws, and power generators. Hazardous chemicals, such as gasoline and other volatile hydrocarbons, may be readily accessible or taint the environment. Without suitable shelter, children are also exposed to weather, animals, and insects (Sirbaugh and DiRocco 2012).

Infectious diseases may also pose a problem to children after a natural disaster. Infectious patterns will persist during a disaster based on the season and time of

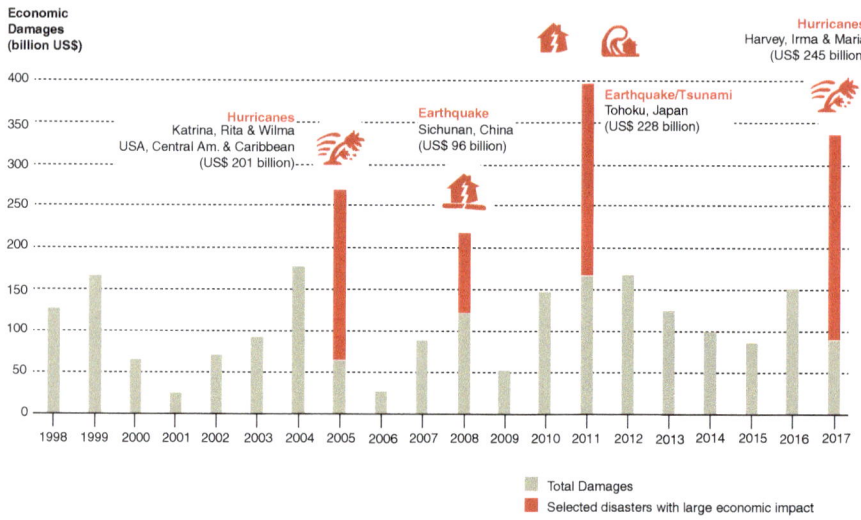

Fig. 5.8 Total reported economic losses per year with major events highlighted 1998–2017. *Used with permission from CRED (2018)

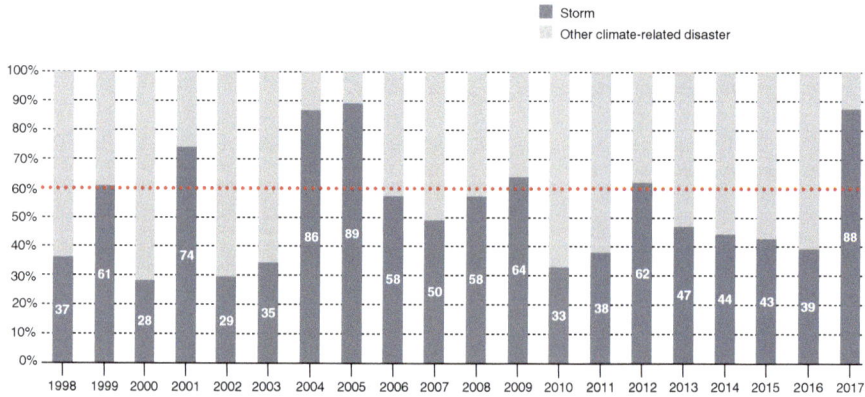

Fig. 5.9 Share of losses due to storms as a percentage of annual climate-related disaster losses 1998–2017. *Used with permission from CRED (2018)

year. There may be outbreaks or epidemics of highly contagious infections (e.g., influenza, respiratory syncytial virus, *Streptococcus pyogenes*) due to mass sheltering of children and families. Poor nutrition or decreased availability of food may lower their resistance against infections. Various water-borne or food-borne diseases may cause illnesses in children. Poor hygiene and mass shelter environments may exacerbate these illnesses. Immunized children should be protected against

Table 5.5 Summary of disaster events in 2018[a]

Natural disaster category	Events	Key details
Droughts and extreme temperature	39	Kenya: three million people affected Afghanistan: 2.2 million people affected Central America: 2.5 million affected Europe
Earthquakes and Tsunamis	20	Papua New Guinea: 181 killed, over half million affected Island of Lombok, Indonesia: 564 killed Island of Sulawesi, Indonesia: 3400 killed
Floods	108	Somalia: 700,000 affected Nigeria: 300 killed, four million affected Japan: 230 killed Kerala, India: 504 killed, over 23 million affected
Storms	84	United States: Hurricanes Florence and Michael Japan: Typhoon Jebi Asia China India Philippines
Volcanic activity	7	Volcan de Fuego, Guatemala: 400 killed, 1.7 million affected Anak Krakatau, Indonesia: resulting tsunami resulted in 400 killed on the islands of Sumatra and Java
Wildfires	9	Attica Fires, Greece: 126 killed Camp Fire, California, US: 88 killed

[a]Used with permission from CRED, 2019 (Centre for Research on the Epidemiology of Disasters (CRED) and United Nations Office for Disaster Risk Reduction (UNISDR) 2019)

Table 5.6 Top 10 countries by number of people affected (2018)[a]

Rank	Country	Total number of people affected
1	India	23,900,348
2	Philippines	6,490,216
3	China	6,415,024
4	Nigeria	3,938,204
5	Guatemala	3,291,359
6	Kenya	3,211,188
7	Afghanistan	2,206,750
8	USA	1,762,103
9	Japan	1,599,497
10	Madagascar	1,472,190

[a]Used with permission from CRED, 2019 (Centre for Research on the Epidemiology of Disasters (CRED) and United Nations Office for Disaster Risk Reduction (UNISDR) 2019)

Table 5.7 Top 10 countries by total death toll (2018)[a]

Rank	Country	Total death toll
1	Indonesia	4535
2	India	1388
3	Guatemala	427
4	Japan	419
5	China	341
6	Nigeria	300
7	USA	298
8	Pakistan	240
9	Korea DPR	237
10	Philippines	221

[a]Used with permission from CRED, 2019 (Centre for Research on the Epidemiology of Disasters (CRED) and United Nations Office for Disaster Risk Reduction (UNISDR) 2019)

Table 5.8 Top 10 deadliest disaster events (2018)[a]

Rank	Event	Country	Death toll
1	Earthquake/Tsunami	Indonesia	3400
2	Earthquake, August	Indonesia	564
3	Flood, August	India	504
4	Volcanic Activity/Tsunami, December	Indonesia	453
5	Volcanic Activity, June	Guatemala	425
6	Flood, June	Japan	220
7	Flood, September	Nigeria	199
8	Heatwave, May	Pakistan	180
9	Flood, August	Korea DPR	151
10	Earthquake, February	Papua New Guinea	145

[a]Used with permission from CRED, 2019 (Centre for Research on the Epidemiology of Disasters (CRED) and United Nations Office for Disaster Risk Reduction (UNISDR) 2019)

common preventable diseases after a natural disaster but still could be a problem in mass groups that are not completely or appropriately immunized. After the 2010 Haiti earthquake, there were increased cases of diarrhea, cholera, measles, and tetanus in children months after the earthquake despite some level of vaccination (Sirbaugh and DiRocco 2012).

Children are at risk for various environmental emergencies. Austere environments will impact children greatly. Heat exposure coupled with minimal access to drinkable water may lead to severe dehydration. Exposure to the cold may lead to frostbite or hypothermia. Children are at risk for carbon monoxide toxicity due to generator use or natural gas poisoning due to disrupted gas lines. There is always a risk for thermal injury due to the use of candles and other flame sources. Exposure

Table 5.9 Death Toll by disaster type (2018 vs. average twenty-first century)[a]

Event	2018	Average (2000–2017)
Drought	0	1361
Earthquake	4321	46,173
Extreme temperature	536	10,414
Flood	2859	5424
Landslide	282	929
Mass movement (dry)	17	20
Storm	1593	12,722
Volcanic activity	878	31
Wildfire	247	71
Total	**10,733**	**77,144**

[a]Used with permission from CRED, 2019 (Centre for Research on the Epidemiology of Disasters (CRED) and United Nations Office for Disaster Risk Reduction (UNISDR) 2019)

Table 5.10 Number of people affected by disaster type (2018 vs. average twenty-first century)[a]

Event	2018	Average (2000–2017)
Drought	9,368,345	58,734,128
Earthquake	1,517,138	6,783,729
Extreme temperature	396,798	6,368,470
Flood	35,385,178	86,696,923
Landslide	54,908	263,831
Mass movement (dry)	0	286
Storm	12,884,845	34,083,106
Volcanic activity	1,908,770	169,308
Wildfire	256,635	19,243
Total	**61,772,617**	**193,312,310**

[a]Used with permission from CRED, 2019 (Centre for Research on the Epidemiology of Disasters (CRED) and United Nations Office for Disaster Risk Reduction (UNISDR) 2019)

to animals (snakes) and insects (spiders) may increase the risk of envenomation. Submersion injury and drowning incidents may escalate. This will be due to lack of supervision of children around storm drains, newly formed bodies of water, or rushing waters of storm diversion systems (Sirbaugh and DiRocco 2012).

Mental health issues are often seen in children after natural disasters. Even though a child may not be injured, they may become "psychiatric casualties" due to the horrific sights they have seen during or after the disaster. Children and adolescents with behavioral or psychiatric problems may experience worsening symptoms and signs due to stress, trauma, disruption of routines, or availability of medications. This is often exacerbated if the parent, guardian, caregiver, or HCP is also

Table 5.11 Total death tolls by year (twenty-first century)[a]

Year	Death toll	Major events (500+ deaths)
2000	9609	
2001	30,844	Gujarat Earthquake
2002	12,124	
2003	109,827	Bam Earthquake, European Heatwave
2004	242,765	Indian Ocean Earthquake
2005	88,673	Kashmir Earthquake
2006	24,239	Java Earthquake
2007	16,960	
2008	235,256	Cyclone Nargis, Sichuan Earthquake
2009	10,672	
2010	297,140	Haiti Earthquake, Russian Heatwave, Somalia Drought
2011	51,434	Japan Earthquake
2012	10,319	
2013	21,859	North India Floods, Typhoon Haiyan
2014	7993	
2015	22,774	Nepal Earthquake
2016	8512	
2017	9734	
2018	10,733	
Total	**1,221,465**	

[a]Used with permission from CRED, 2019 (Centre for Research on the Epidemiology of Disasters (CRED) and United Nations Office for Disaster Risk Reduction (UNISDR) 2019)

having difficulty coping with the stress of the disaster. In general, the most common mental health problem in children is a post-traumatic stress disorder. However, separation anxiety, obsessive-compulsive symptoms, and severe stranger anxiety can also be seen in children after a traumatic event (Sirbaugh and DiRocco 2012). See Chap. 12 for more detailed information.

5.5   Man-Made Disasters

5.5.1   Terrorism

Terrorism impacts children and families all around the world (Tables 5.12 and 5.13). After the events of 9/11, much attention has been given to the possibility of another mass casualty act of terrorism, especially with weapons of mass destruction, that include chemical, biological, nuclear, radiological, and explosive devices (CBNRE), or other forms of violence such as active shooter incidents and mass shootings

Table 5.12 Terrorist and criminal attacks targeting children[a]

Date	Type	Location	Method and target	Child casualties Killed	Child casualties Injured	Total casualties Killed	Total casualties Injured
18 May 1927	Criminal	Bath, Michigan, US	Bombing of school	41	55	46	58
11 April 1956	**Terrorism**	Shafrir, Israel	Shooting attack on synagogue	3	5	4	5
15 September 1959	Criminal	Houston, Texas US	Suicide bombing of school	3	17	6	18
15 September 1963	**Terrorism**	Birmingham, Alabama US	Bombing of church	4	2+	4	23
18 March 1968	**Terrorism**	Negev desert, Israel	Landmine attack on school bus	2	28	2	28
22 May 1970	**Terrorism**	Avivim, Israel	Rocket attack on school bus	9	19	12	19
11 April 1974	**Terrorism**	Qiryat Shemona, Israel	Shooting attack on residential building	8	?	18	16
15 April 1974	**Terrorism**	Ma'alot, Israel	Hostage taking	20	66+	27	134
8 February 1975	**Terrorism**	El Arish, Sinai	Bombing	1	3	1	3
13 November 1975	**Terrorism**	Jerusalem, Israel	Bombing outside of ice cream shop	6	?	6	42
3 February 1976	**Terrorism**	Djibouti	Hostage taking of school bus	1	0	36	0
26 Jan-13 Feb 1978	**Terrorism**	Maastricht, Netherlands, and Bremen, West Germany	Poisoning of Israeli citrus products	0	5	0	13
11 March 1978	**Terrorism**	Tel Aviv, Israel	Shooting attack on beach and hostage taking on bus	13	?	51	72
20 August 1978	**Terrorism**	Abadan, Iran	Arson of movie theater	Many	0	477	10
18 November 1978	Criminal	Jonestown, Guyana	Poisoning of children during mass suicide by cult members	276	0	918	11
7 April 1980	**Terrorism**	Misgav Am Kibbutz, Israel	Hostage taking at children's dormitory	1	4	8	16
2 June 1980	**Terrorism**	Hebron, West Bank	Four bombings, including grenade attack near elementary school	0	4	0	11
2 August 1980	**Terrorism**	Bologna, Italy	Bombing at railway station	8	?	85	300
16 May 1986	**Terrorism**	Cokeville, Wyoming, US	Hostage taking and bombing of school	0	70	2	79
2 June 1988	**Terrorism**	Jerusalem, Israel	Attack in park	1	0	1	0
2 October 1988	**Terrorism**	Jerusalem, Israel	Explosion of bomb hidden in loaf of bread	0	3	0	3

(continued)

Table 5.12 (continued)

Date	Type	Location	Method and target	Child casualties		Total casualties	
				Killed	Injured	Killed	Injured
17 January 1989	Criminal	Stockton, California, US	Suicide shooting attack at school	5	29	6	30
18 April 1989	Criminal	Indianapolis, Indiana, US	Explosion of bomb hidden in toothpaste tube	0	1	0	1
17 March 1992	Terrorism	Buenos Aires, Argentina	Suicide car bombing at Israeli embassy	?	?	29	252
1 May 1992	Criminal	Olivehurst, California, US	Shooting at high school	3	9	4	10
19 April 1995	Terrorism	Oklahoma City, OK, US	Car bombing of federal office building	19	?	169	675
4 March 1996	Terrorism	Tel Aviv, Israel	Suicide bombing at Dizengoff Center	5	?	14	163
13 March 1996	Criminal	Dunblane, Scotland, UK	Suicide shooting attack at school	16	10	18	12
16 November 1996	Terrorism	Kasiysk, Dagestan, Russia	Bombing of Russian border guard housing	20	?	67	?
22 July 1997	Terrorism	Israel	Terrorist drove car into a group of teenagers, then exited and began attacking with a knife	?	?	1	12
24 March 1998	Criminal	Jonesboro, Arkansas, US	Shooting attack at school	4	9	5	11
6 May 1998	Terrorism	Jerusalem, Israel	Stabbing attack	1	0	1	0
21 May 1998	Criminal	Springfield, Oregon, US	Shooting attacks at residence and high school	2	25	4	25
29 October 1998	Terrorism	Gus Katif, Gaza	Attempted bombing of school bus	0	3	2	8
29 October 1998	Criminal	Goteborg, Sweden	Arson attack on dance hall	49	?	63	?
20 April 1999	Criminal	Littleton, Colorado, US	Suicide shooting attack at school	12	25	15	27
15 September 1999	Criminal	Fort Worth, Texas, US	Shooting attack at church service	4	4	8	8
20 November 2000	Terrorism	Gaza	Bombing of school bus	0	5	2	9
31 December 2000	Terrorism	Ramallah, West Bank	Shooting attack on civilian car	0	5	2	5
26 March 2001	Criminal	Machakos, Kenya	Arson of secondary school	67	19	67	19
5 June 2001	Terrorism	Shiloh, Israel	Stoning attack on car	1	0	1	0
8 June 2001	Criminal	Ikeda, Osaka, Japan	Knife attack on school	8	13	8	15
4 September 2001	Terrorism	Jerusalem, Israel	Attempted suicide bombing at school	0	?	1	20

Date	Type	Location	Description				
9 September 2001	Terrorism	Jerusalem, Israel	Suicide bombing at pizzeria	7	5+	15	130
1 December 2001	Terrorism	Jerusalem, Israel	Two suicide bombings in pedestrian mall	5	?	13	188
2 March 2002	Terrorism	Jerusalem, Israel	Suicide bombing outside synagogue	7	1+	11	50
26 April 2002	Criminal	Erfurt, Germany	Shooting attack in high school	2	?	17	?
9 May 2002	Terrorism	Kaspiysk, Russia	Bombing at parade	17	31	43	151
28 May 2002	Terrorism	Itamar, Israel	Shooting attack on school	3	2	4	2
3 June 2002	Terrorism	Thailand	Shooting attack on school bus	2	15	2	15
20 June 2002	Terrorism	Itamar, West Bank	Shooting attack	3	2	7	4
23 September 2002	Terrorism	Hebron, West Bank	Shooting attack	0	3	1	3
7 October 2002	Terrorism	Bowie, Maryland, US	Shooting attack by Beltway sniper	0	1	0	1
29 October 2002	Terrorism	Hermesh, West Bank	Shooting attack	2	?	4	2
11 November 2002	Criminal	Changde, P.R. China	Poisoning of food at high school	0	Many	0	193
21 November 2002	Terrorism	Jerusalem, Israel	Suicide bombing on bus	4	?	12	50
25 November 2002	Criminal	Zhanjiang City, Guangdong, P.R. China	Poisoning of food at kindergarten school	0	70	0	72
26 April 2003	Criminal	Erfurt, Germany	Shooting attack in high school	2	?	17	1
5 March 2003	Terrorism	Haifa, Israel	Suicide bombing on bus	9	?	18	53
10 August 2003	Terrorism	Near Lebanon border	Antiaircraft rocket fired from across Lebanon border	1	4	1	4
19 August 2003	Terrorism	Jerusalem, Israel	Suicide bombing on bus	8	?	24	133
7 July 2003	Terrorism	Moshav Kfar Yavetz, Israel	Suicide bombing at house	0	3	2	3
2 March 2004	Terrorism	Karbala, Iraq	Suicide bombings at shrines	15	?	121	122
21 April 2004	Terrorism	Basra, Iraq	Car bombings at police stations and police academy	13	?	74	100
2 May 2004	Terrorism	Gush Katif, Gaza	Shooting attack on vehicle	4	0	5	3
28 June 2004	Terrorism	Sderot, Gaza	Rocket attack on nursery school	1	?	2	11
4 August 2004	Criminal	Beijing, P.R. China	Knife attack at kindergarten school	1	14	1	17
1–3 Sept 2004	Terrorism	Beslan, Russia	Hostage taking and bombing at school	156	337	366	747

(continued)

Table 5.12 (continued)

Date	Type	Location	Method and target	Child casualties Killed	Child casualties Injured	Total casualties Killed	Total casualties Injured
30 September 2004	Terrorism	Baghdad, Iraq	Car bombing at public ceremony	35	72	42	69
25 November 2004	Criminal	Ruzhou, Henan, P.R. China	Knife attack at high school dormitory	8	4	8	4
28 February 2005	Terrorism	Hilla, Babil, Iraq	Car bombing outside medical clinic	8	?	135	130
21 March 2005	Criminal	Red Lake, Minnesota, US	Shooting attack at high school	6	7	10	7
4 April 2005	Criminal	Zhanjiang, Guangdong, P.R. China	Knife attack at middle school	0	8	0	8
23 April 2005	Terrorism	Pakhapani, Rolpa, Nepal	Bombing	5	3	5	3
10 June 2005	Criminal	Hikari, Yamaguchi, Japan	Bomb attack at high school	0	56	0	58
16 June 2005	Criminal	Siem Reap, Cambodia	Hostage taking at elementary school	1	0	1	0
24 June 2005	Criminal	Beit Hagai, West Bank		2	?	2	3
13 July 2005	Terrorism	Baghdad, Iraq	Car bombing of gathered children	24	20	27	50
29 September 2005	Terrorism	Balad, Salah Al-Din, Iraq	Three car bombings	25	?	95	101
12 October 2005	Criminal	Guangde, Anhui, P.R. China	Shooting at primary school	0	16	0	18
29 November 2005	Terrorism	Santa Cruz, California, US	Incendiary bombings of homes	0	2	0	4
15 June 2006	Terrorism	Kebithigollewa, Sri Lanka	Mine explosion against bus	15	?	64	80
25 June 2006	Terrorism	Beitar Illit, West Bank	Teenager kidnapped and killed	1	0	1	0
2 August 2006	Terrorism	Baghdad, Iraq	Explosion of bombs buried in soccer field	12	?	12	?
27 September 2006	Criminal	Bailey, Colorado, US	Hostage taking at school	1	?	2	?
2 October 2006	Criminal	Nickel Mines, PA, US	Hostage taking and shooting at school	5	5	6	5
6 October 2006	Terrorism	Basauti, Kailai, Nepal	Bombing of village development committee area	3	0	3	5
3 December 2006	Terrorism	Baghdad, Iraq	Mortar attack on school	0	10	0	10
28 January 2007	Terrorism	Baghdad, Iraq	Mortar attack on school	5	20	5	20
28 January 2007	Terrorism	Ramadi, Iraq	Bombing attack near school	2	10	2	10
20 February 2007	Terrorism	Taji, Iraq	Bombing of chlorine tanker truck near restaurant	0	52	9	150

Date	Type	Location	Description				
24 February 2007	**Terrorism**	Habbaniya, Al-Anbar, Iraq	Fuel truck bombing near Sunni mosque	5	?	56	48
16 March 2007	**Terrorism**	Fallujah, Iraq	Suicide bombing with dump truck carrying chlorine tanks	0	7	6	250
2 April 2007	**Terrorism**	Kirkuk, Iraq	Truck bombing of police station next to school	2	50	12	200
6 April 2007	**Terrorism**	Ramadi, Iraq	Suicide truck bombing using chlorine tanks	?	?	35	50
12 June 2007	**Terrorism**	Logar province, Afghanistan	Shooting attack on girls leaving school	2	4	2	4
15 June 2007	**Terrorism**	Tarinkot, Afghanistan	Suicide bombing near school	11	3	11	3
6 August 2007	**Terrorism**	Qubbak, Iraq	Truck bombing of residential area	19	?	28	50
14 August 2007	**Terrorism**	Al-Qataniyah and Al-Adnaniyah, Iraq	Multiple truck bombings in villages	Many	Many	520	1500
12 October 2007	**Terrorism**	Tuz Khurmato, Iraq	Bombing on playground	2	17	2	18
6 November 2007	**Terrorism**	Baghlani-jadid, Afghanistan	Suicide bombing at public ceremony	61	93	77	100
7 November 2007	Criminal	Tuusula, Finland	Shooting attack at high school	6	10	8	10
22 January 2008	**Terrorism**	Ba'qubah, Iraq	Suicide bombing at school	0	17	1	21
6 March 2008	**Terrorism**	Jerusalem, Israel	Shooting attack	7	?	9	11
12 November 2008	**Terrorism**	Kandahar City, Afghanistan	Acid attack on schoolgirls	0	14	0	15
26 December 2008	**Terrorism**	Beit Lahiya, Gaza Strip	Rocket attack	2	3	2	3
28 December 2008	**Terrorism**	Khost, Afghanistan	Suicide car bombing at checkpoint near elementary school	14	?	16	58
13 February 2009	**Terrorism**	Iskandariya, Iraq	Suicide bombing of Shiite pilgrimage	?	28	32	76
2 April 2009	**Terrorism**	Bat Ayin, West Bank	Attack by axe-wielding terrorist	1	1	1	1
26 April 2009	**Terrorism**	Charikar, Kapisa province, Afghanistan	Gas poisoning attack on girls' school	0	40	0	45
10 May 2009	**Terrorism**	Busurungi, D.R.C.	Armed attack on village	25	?	86	24
11 May 2009	**Terrorism**	Charikar, Kapisa province, Afghanistan	Gas poisoning attack on girls' school	0	61	0	62
12 May 2009	**Terrorism**	Afghanistan	Gas poisoning attack on girls' school	0	98	0	104

(continued)

Table 5.12 (continued)

Date	Type	Location	Method and target	Child casualties		Total casualties	
				Killed	Injured	Killed	Injured
9 July 2009	Terrorism	Logar province, Afghanistan	Truck bombing near highway	16	?	25	5
8 September 2009	Terrorism	Muqdadiyah, Diyala, Iraq	Kidnapping and killing of 10-year-old son of politician	1	0	1	0
25 October 2009	Terrorism	Baghdad, Iraq	Twin vehicle bombing of government buildings	20	6+	155	540
28 October 2009	Terrorism	Peshawar, Pakistan	Car bombing at marketplace	13	?	118	213
4 December 2009	Terrorism	Rawalpindi, Punjab, Pakistan	Attack on mosque with guns, grenades, and suicide bombs	17	?	40	81
7 December 2009	Terrorism	Baghdad, Iraq	Bombing of school	6	25	8	41
23 March 2010	Criminal	Fujian, P.R. China	Attack on students at elementary school	9	?	8	?
1 April 2010	Criminal	Fujian, P.R. China	Knife attack on primary school students	0	16	0	17
21 April 2010	Terrorism	Kunduz, Afghanistan	Gas poisoning attack on girls' school	0	23	0	23
24 April 2010	Terrorism	Kunduz, Afghanistan	Gas poisoning attack on girls' school	0	48	0	51
25 April 2010	Terrorism	Kunduz, Afghanistan	Gas poisoning attack on girls' school	0	13	0	13
4 May 2010	Terrorism	Kunduz, Afghanistan	Gas poisoning attack on girls' school	0	22	0	25
11 May 2010	Terrorism	Kunduz, Afghanistan	Gas poisoning attack on girls' school	0	30	0	30
11 May 2010	Terrorism	Kunduz, Afghanistan	Gas poisoning attack on girls' school	0	6	0	6
12 May 2010	Criminal	Shaanxi, P.R. China	Knife attack on kindergarten students	7	?	9	?
13 May 2010	Terrorism	Israel	Shooting attack	1	0	1	0
June 2010	Terrorism	Afghanistan	Gas poisoning attack on girls' school	0	30	0	30
12 June 2010	Terrorism	Ghazni City, Afghanistan	Gas poisoning attack on girls' school	0	60	0	60
3 August 2010	Criminal	Zibo, Shandong, P.R. China	Knife attack at kindergarten school	3	?	4	20
21 August 2010	Terrorism	Kabul, Afghanistan	Gas poisoning attack on girls' school	0	23	0	23
25 August 2010	Terrorism	Kabul, Afghanistan	Gas poisoning attack on girls' school	0	60	0	74

28 August 2010	Terrorism	Kabul, Afghanistan	Gas poisoning attack on girls' school	0	48	0	52
31 August 2010	Terrorism	Kabul, Afghanistan	Gas poisoning attack on girls' school	0	74	0	74
22 October 2010	Criminal	Zamboanga City, Philippines	Knife attack at elementary school	1	4	2	6
2010	Terrorism	Afghanistan	Gas poisoning attack on girls' school	0	?	0	?
2010	Terrorism	Afghanistan	Gas poisoning attack on girls' school	0	?	0	?
2010	Terrorism	Afghanistan	Gas poisoning attack on girls' school	0	?	0	?
2010	Terrorism	Afghanistan	Gas poisoning attack on girls' school	0	?	0	?
2010	Terrorism	Afghanistan	Gas poisoning attack on girls' school	0	?	0	?
11 March 2011	Terrorism	Itamar, West Bank	Knife attack on residence	3	0	5	0
11 March 2011	Criminal	Panjwayi district, Afghanistan	Shooting attack on villages by U.S. soldier	9	0	16	0
7 April 2011	Criminal	Rio de Janeiro, Brazil	Shooting attack at elementary school	12	12	13	12
7 April 2011	Terrorism	Sa'ad, Israel	Antitank missile attack on school bus	1	0	1	1
17 June 2011	Terrorism	Sirkanay, Kunar, Afghanistan	Strike of rocket fired across border from Pakistan	4	?	4	?
19 June 2011	Terrorism	Kapisa province, Afghanistan	Rocket strike on school during gunbattle	0	5	1	7
3 July 2011	Terrorism	Faryab province, Afghanistan	Grenade attack on high school	0	17	0	25
22 July 2011	Terrorism	Utøya and Oslo, Norway	Shooting attack and bombing	50	40?	77	151
13 September 2011	Terrorism	Peshawar, Khyber-Pakhtunkhwa, Pakistan	Attack on school bus	4	12	5	18
28 November 2011	Criminal	Kunduz, Afghanistan	Acid attack on family in home	0	3	0	4
31 March 2012	Terrorism	Esfandi area, Ghazni province, Afghanistan	Acid attack on children	2	0	2	0
17 April 2012	Terrorism	Rustaq district, Takhar province, Afghanistan	Water poisoning attack on girls' school	0	150	0	171

(continued)

Table 5.12 (continued)

Date	Type	Location	Method and target	Child casualties		Total casualties	
				Killed	Injured	Killed	Injured
22 May 2012	**Terrorism**	Taloqan, Takhar province, Afghanistan	Water poisoning attack on girls' school	0	80	0	84
26 May 2012	**Terrorism**	Taloqan, Takhar province, Afghanistan	Poisoning attack on girls' school	0	40	0	40
28 May 2012	**Terrorism**	Takhar province, Afghanistan	Poisoning attack on girls' school	0	121	0	124
2 June 2012	**Terrorism**	Taloqan, Takhar province, Afghanistan	Poisoning attack on girls' school	0	20	0	20
3 June 2012	**Terrorism**	Farkhar district, Takhar province, Afghanistan	Poisoning attack on girls' school	0	65	0	65
5 June 2012	**Terrorism**	Rustaq district, Takhar province, Afghanistan	Poisoning attack on girls' school	0	60	0	60
June 2012	**Terrorism**	Shirin Hazara, Bamyan province, Afghanistan	Gas poisoning attack on girls' school	0	2+	0	2+
19 June 2012	**Terrorism**	Bamyan province, Afghanistan	Gas poisoning attack on girls' school	0	47	0	47
22 June 2012	**Terrorism**	Sar-e-Pul province, Afghanistan	Poisoning attack on girls' high school	0	118	0	118
23 June 2012	**Terrorism**	Sar-e-Pul, Sar-e-Pul province, Afghanistan	Poisoning attack on girls' school	0	94	0	94
25 June 2012	**Terrorism**	Sar-e-Pul province, Afghanistan	Poisoning attack on girls' high school	0	90	0	90
30 June 2012	**Terrorism**	Sar-e-Pul, Sar-e-Pul province, Afghanistan	Poisoning attack on girls' school	0	53	0	53
2 July 2012	**Terrorism**	Sheberghan province, Afghanistan	Poisoning attack on girls' school	0	255	0	255

July 2012	Terrorism	Jawzjan province, Afghanistan	Poisoning attack on girls' school	0	100	0	100
7 July 2012	Terrorism	Jawzjan province, Afghanistan	Poisoning attack on girls' school	0	60	0	60
9 October 2012	Terrorism	Mingora, Pakistan	Shooting attack on school bus	0	3	0	3
26 October 2012	Terrorism	Maimana, Faryab, Afghanistan	Suicide bombing by 15-year-old	6	4	40	59
15 November 2012	Terrorism	Kiryat Malachi, Israel	Rocket attack from Gaza on apartment building	0	4	3	4
14 December 2012	Criminal	Chengping, Henan, P.R. China	Knife attack on children outside primary school	0	22	0	23
14 December 2012	Criminal	Newtown, Connecticut, US	Shooting attack on primary school	20	0	28	3
18 March 2013	Terrorism	Maiduguri, Eorno, Nigeria	Armed attack on three schools	0	3	3	3
15 April 2013	Terrorism	Boston, Massachusetts, US	Two bombings at Boston Marathon	1	14	3	264
18 April 2013	Terrorism	Taloqan, Takhar, Afghanistan	Poisoning attack on girls' school	0	18	0	18
21 April 2013	Terrorism	Taloqan, Takhar, Afghanistan	Poisoning attack on girls' school	0	74	0	74
1 May 2013	Terrorism	Kabul, Afghanistan	Poisoning attack on girls' school	0	150	0	150
1 May 2013	Terrorism	Makhachkala, Dagestan, Russia	Bombing at shopping mall	2	0	2	2
14 May 2013	Terrorism	Balkh, Afghanistan	Poisoning attack on girls' school	0	150	0	150
15 May 2013	Terrorism	Faryab, Afghanistan	Poisoning attack on girls' school	0	80	0	80
1 June 2013	Terrorism	Behsud, Afghanistan	Poisoning attack on girls' school	0	22	0	22
1 June 2013	Terrorism	Maimana, Faryab, Afghanistan	Poisoning attack on girls' school	0	77	0	77
3 June 2013	Terrorism	Paktika, Afghanistan	Suicide bombing targeting school children on lunch break	10	16	14	26
16 June 2013	Terrorism	Damaturu, Yobe, Nigeria	Attack on school	7	?	9	?

(continued)

Table 5.12 (continued)

Date	Type	Location	Method and target	Child casualties		Total casualties	
				Killed	Injured	Killed	Injured
17 June 2013	Terrorism	Maiduguri, Borno, Nigeria	Attack on school	9	?	9	?
30 June 2013	Terrorism	Baghdad, Iraq	Bombing at soccer game	10	?	12	?
6 July 2013	Terrorism	Mamudo, Yobe, Nigeria	Attack on boarding school	41	?	42	?
9 July 2013	Terrorism	Herat, Afghanistan	Roadside bombing	4	?	17	?
19 November 2013	Terrorism	Khairkot, Paktika, Afghanistan	Roadside bombing	7	3	7	3
20 January 2014	Terrorism	Rawalpindi, Pakistan	Suicide bombing at market	3	?	14	29
2 March 2014	Terrorism	Maiduguri, Borno, Nigeria	Truck bombing in market	Many	?	50	?
8 April 2014	Terrorism	Sibi, Pakistan	Bombing at market	5	?	17	46
14 April 2014	Terrorism	Chibok, Borno, Nigeria	Attack and kidnapping at girls' boarding school	?	276	1	276
28 April 2014	Terrorism	Karachi, Sindh, Pakistan	Grenade attack on seminary	3	11	3	11
12 June 2014	Terrorism	West bank	Kidnapping and killing of teenagers	3	0	3	0
2 July 2014	Terrorism	West Bank	Kidnapping and killing of teenager	1	0	1	0
6 September 2014	Criminal	Mediterranean Sea off Malta	Ramming and sinking of refugee ship	100	1	450	8
22 October 2014	Terrorism	Jerusalem, Israel	Vehicle driven into crowd at rail station	1	?	3	13
16 December 2014	Terrorism	Peshawar, Pakistan	Shooting/bomb attack on school	132	121	148	124
16 December 2014	Terrorism	Radaa, Bayda, Yemen	Two bombings, once striking a school bus	20	?	31	12
3–4 January 2015	Terrorism	Baga, Borno, Nigeria	Armed attack and arson destroying most of Baga	?	?	700	300
4 February 2015	Terrorism	Fotokol, Cameroon	Armed attack on town	?	?	90	500
24 March 2015	Criminal	Prads-Haute-Bleone, Alpes-de-Haute-Provence, France	Intentional crash of airliner by copilot	17	0	150	0
13 July 2015	Terrorism	Camp Chapman, Khost, Afghanistan	Suicide car bombing at checkpoint near Camp Chapman	12	?	33	10

Date	Type	Location	Description				
2 October 2015	**Terrorism**	Maiduguri, Borno, Nigeria	Five suicide bombings at a mosque and home of local leader; the five bombers were girls aged 9–15; three bombers attacked the mosque, one ran into a nearby bush, and one attacked the home	5	?	15	36
10 October 2015	**Terrorism**	N'Djamena, Chad	Five suicide bombings, multiple each at a marketplace where 16 were killed and at a refugee camp where 22 were killed	?	14	41	50
30 January 2016	**Terrorism**	Dalori, Borro, Nigeria	Attack on village including suicide bombings by three females, shootings, and firebombing of huts	Many	?	86	62
31 January 2016	**Terrorism**	Sayyida, Zeinab, Syria	Bombings at a bus station and a military headquarters	5	?	71	99
27 March 2016	**Terrorism**	Lahore, Pakistan	Suicide bombing attack on amusement park	29	?	72	200
14 July 2016	**Terrorism**	Nice, France	Vehicular attack on crowds celebrating Bastille Day; truck was driven down a 2 km stretch of crowded boardwalk	10	54	87	434
20 August 2016	**Terrorism**	Gaziantep, Turkey	ISIS suicide bombing of wedding	34	?	57	90
16 February 2017	**Terrorism**	Sehwan, Pakistan	Suicide bombing at Lal Shahbaz Qalandar, a Sufi shrine	9	?	88	343
11 March 2017	**Terrorism**	Damascus, Syria	Bombings targeting Shia pilgrims	8	?	74	120
15 April 2017	**Terrorism**	Rashindin, Syria	Suicide car bombing targeting buses carrying refugees	80	?	126	100
25 April 2017	**Terrorism**	Godar district, Parachinar, Pakistan	Passenger van struck by landmine explosion	4	?	14	9
2 May 2017	**Terrorism**	Al-Lataminah, Hama, Syria	?	5	?	6	?

(continued)

Table 5.12 (continued)

Date	Type	Location	Method and target	Child casualties		Total casualties	
				Killed	Injured	Killed	Injured
22 May 2017	**Terrorism**	Manchester, England, UK	Suicide bombing outside concert at Manchester Arena	7	16	23	119
5 October 2017	**Terrorism**	Jhal Magsi district, Pakistan	Suicide bombing at Shiite shrine	5	?	25	20
31 October 2017	**Terrorism**	New York City, New York, US	Vehicular attack on pedestrians, bikers, and a school bus	0	4	8	12
4 November 2017	**Terrorism**	Deir ez-Zor, Syria	Suicide car bombing at refugee center; most victims were women and children	Many	Many	100	140
5 November 2017	Criminal	Sutherland Springs, Texas, US	Shooting attack on church during worship service	9	4	27	30
17 November 2017	**Terrorism**	Deir ez-Zor, Syria	Car bombing at rally	12	?	26	30
23 November 2017	**Terrorism**	Bir al-Abed, Sinai, Egypt	Attack on mosque with bombs followed by shooting attack on fleeing survivors	27	?	305	128

[a]The table describes terrorist and criminal acts targeting children from May 1927 to December 2017. It includes the following types of incidents: terrorist attacks in which the targets were preferentially children; attempted terrorist attacks preferentially targeting children; terrorist attacks which produced very high casualties among children; and nonterrorist criminal acts which are relevant in terms of methodology and child victims. The full table, description of incidents and data resources, can be viewed at http://www.johnstonsarchive.net/terrorism/wrjp39ch.html. Used with permission from Wm. Robert Johnston PhD (2017)

Table 5.13 Summary of historical attacks using chemical or biological weapons[a]

Date	Location	Attacker	Agent	Affected population	Casualties	Description
21–27 October 2016	Near Mosul, Iraq	Islamic State militants	Sulfur	Civilians, soldiers	**2 killed**, 1500 injured	Sulfur mine set on fire, producing widespread sulfur dioxide plumes
8 March 2016	Taza, Kirkuk, Iraq	Islamic State	Blistering agent	Civilians	**1 killed**, 600 injured	Attack on town; fatality was 3-year-old child
23 January 2015	Between Mosul, Iraq, and Syrian Border	Islamic State militants	Chlorine	Kurdish soldiers	Approximately 30 injured	Truck bomb with chlorine-filled tanks against troops
September–October 2014	Duluiya and Balad, Iraq	Islamic State militants	Chlorine, possibly mustard gas	Iraqi and Shiite soldiers	40 injured	Bombs filled with chlorine-filled cylinders used against defending troops
27 March–22 April 2014	Syria–Damascus, Kafr Zita in Hama, and Talmenes in Idlit	Syrian military suspected	Chlorine, others	Civilians	**104 killed**, 200 injured	Chlorine bombs used on civilians in two towns
21 August 2013	Damascus suburbs, Syria	Syrian military	Sarin nerve gas?	Civilian in urban areas	**1429 killed (including 426 children)**, 2200 injured	Rockets with chemical agents fired at about 12 areas in suburbs south and east of Damascus, targeting rebel-held areas
19 March–13 April 2013	Syria–Damascus, Al-Otaybeh, Khan al-Assal, Adra, Aleppo, Sheikh Maqsoud, and Saraqeb	Syrian military?	Multiple chemical agents?	rebel soldiers and civilians	**At least 44 killed**, 76 injured	Multiple attacks, mostly blamed on Syrian government; Syrian government accuses rebels of the attacks

(continued)

Table 5.13 (continued)

Date	Location	Attacker	Agent	Affected population	Casualties	Description
April 2012–June 2013	Afghanistan—Takhar province (American College of Surgeons Committee on Trauma, American College of Emergency Physicians, National Association of EMS Physicians, Pediatric Equipment Guidelines Committee Emergency Medical Services for Children (EMSC) Partnership for Children Stakeholder Group, American Academy of Pediatrics 2009), Sar-e-Pul province (American Academy of Pediatrics (AAP) 2003), others	Islamist terrorists	Pesticides?	Schoolchildren	1952 injured (including 1924 children)	23 poison attacks on girls' schools, some cases of water poisoning
March 2012–April 2013	Afghanistan	Islamist terrorists	Rat poison?	Police, other civilians	**53 killed**, 40 injured	9 attacks involving poisoning of food at police stations/academies
April–August 2010	Afghanistan—Kabul (American Academy of Pediatrics and American Heart Association et al. 2016), Kunduz (American Academy of Pediatrics (AAP) 2003), others	Islamist terrorists	Pesticides?	Schoolchildren	672 injured (including 636 children)	20 gas attacks on girls' schools
11 March 2007	Iraq	Islamist terrorists	Mustard gas	U.S. soldiers	2 injured	Failed improvised explosive device using chemical weapon artillery shells

Date	Location	Perpetrator	Agent	Target	Casualties	Description
October 2006–June 2007	Iraq cities--Ramadi (American Academy of Pediatrics and American Heart Association et al. 2016), Baghdad (Advanced Hazmat Life Support (AHLS) 2003), Falluja (Advanced Hazmat Life Support (AHLS) 2003), others	Islamist terrorists	Chlorine	Civilian targets	**115 killed**, 854 injured (including 85 children)	15 car/truck bombings with chlorine tanks used; most fatalities were from the explosions, most injuries from the chemical releases
8 October 2006	Numaniyah, Iraq	Islamist terrorists	Poison	Policemen	**7 killed**, 700 injured	Poisoning of food at meal on police base (unconfirmed)
25 September 2006	Baghdad, Iraq	Islamist terrorists	Mustard gas	U.S. soldiers	2 injured	Improvised explosive device using chemical weapon artillery shells
15 May 2004	Baghdad, Iraq	Islamist terrorists	Sarin nerve gas	U.S. soldiers	2 injured	Failed improvised explosive device using chemical weapon artillery shell near Baghdad airport
24 June–July 2003	Near Mosul, Iraq	Islamist terrorists	Sulfur	Civilians, soldiers	At least 41 soldiers injured	Sulfur stockpiles at mine set on fire, producing widespread sulfur dioxide plumes
11 November 2002	Changde, PR China	Criminal	Poison	Schoolchildren	193 injured (mostly children)	Poisoning of food at high school

(continued)

Table 5.13 (continued)

Date	Location	Attacker	Agent	Affected population	Casualties	Description
26 October 2002	Moscow, Russia	Russian soldiers	Fentanyl incapacitating agent	Terrorists and civilian hostages	**124 killed**, 501 injured	Chechen terrorists took 800 hostages at Moscow theater, 23 Oct; Russian forces used fentanyl when storming the theater and killing all the terrorists on 26 Oct, but many hostages were killed or injured by the gas
18 September–9 October 2001	United States–Washington, DC, New York City, NY, others	Bruce Ivins?	Anthrax	Government and civilian media individuals; postal employees and customer	**5 killed**, 17 injured	Anthrax-laced letters mailed to federal officials in Washington DC and new media offices in multiple locations; many casualties among postal workers
20 March 1995	Tokyo, Japan	Aum Shinrikyo cult	Sarin nerve gas	Tokyo subway	**12 killed**, 5511 injured	Nerve gas releases in subway; many permanent injuries
28 June 1994	Matsumoto, Japan	Aum Shinrikyo cult	Sarin nerve gas	Civilians	**7 killed**, 270 injured	Overnight release of nerve gas in city
21 January 1994	Ormancik, Turkey	Terrorists	Chemical agent	Civilians	**16 killed**	Attack on village using chemical grenades

Date	Location	Perpetrator	Agent	Target	Casualties	Description
16 March 1988	Halabja, Iraq	Iraqi military	Cyanide, mustard gas, nerve agents	Iraqi Kurdish civilians	**5000 killed**, 8000 injured	Use of chemical agents against civilians in village; additional use of agents by Iranian military possible
6 September 1987	Zamboanga City, Philippines	Terrorists	Poison	Policemen	**19 killed**, 140 injured	Water poisoning with pesticide at constabulary
1987–August 1988	Iraq–Iran	Iranian military	Mustard gas, cyanide	Iraqi soldiers	?;?	Some use
2–3 December 1984	Bhopal, India	Accidental	Methyl isocynate gas	Civilians	**3787 killed**, 558,125 injured (including 200,000 children)	Accidental release from pesticide plant with gas plume blown across city of Bhopal
9–19 September 1984	The Dalles, Oregon, United States	Bhadwan Shree Rajneesh cult	Salmonella	Civilian restaurants	751 injured	Food poisoning in several restaurants; was experiment in preparation to interfere with upcoming election
August 1983–July 1988	Iraq–Iran	Iraqi military	Chemical agents	Iranian soldiers and civilians	**21,000 killed**, 92,000 injured	Extensive use against soldiers and civilians

(continued)

Table 5.13 (continued)

Date	Location	Attacker	Agent	Affected population	Casualties	Description
June 1979–mid 1981	Afghanistan	Soviet and Afghan militaries	Multiple chemical agents	Civilians and rebel soldiers	**3042 killed**	Used in at least 47 instances in the invasion of Afghanistan
April 1979	suburbs southeast of Sverdlovsk, USSR	Accidental	Anthrax	Civilians	**68 killed**, 300 injured	Accidental release from bioweapons production facility caused anthrax outbreak in Sverdlovsk; cause of outbreak was denied by Soviet government

[a]The table summarizes known historical instances of the use of chemical or biological weapons, in reverse chronological order, 1979–2016. A full list of all chemical or biological events since 1900 (with references and sources of data) can be found at http://www.johnstonsarchive.net/terrorism/chembioattacks.html. Although there were some earlier instances of chemical/biological warfare prior to 1900, these instances were generally of very limited effectiveness. Note that some incidents are disputed, and casualty figures in some cases are very uncertain. The following events are included: **use in warfare:** multiple attacks within a war are grouped together; **use by terrorists:** includes attacks with larger numbers of casualties; and **other:** several criminal incidents and accidental chemical releases are included because of their significance. Used with permission from Wm. Robert Johnston PhD (2017)

(Jacobson and Severin 2012). Since then, other incidents, both foreign and domestic, have involved children and complicates the concept of and the response to terrorism. Johnston (2017) said it best in his review of *Terrorist and Criminal Attacks Targeting Children*: "One of the more accepted defining characteristics of terrorism is that it targets noncombatants including men, women, and children. However, terrorist attacks specifically targeting children over other noncombatants are uncommon. This is for the same reason that most terrorists have historically avoided mass casualty terrorism: the shock value is so great that such attacks erode support for the terrorists' political objectives. The 9/11 attacks represent an increasing trend in mass casualty terrorism. At the same time, policymakers are examining this evolving threat, they must increasingly consider the threat of terrorist attacks targeting children." Based on historical events, it is clear infants, toddlers, children, and adolescents have been victims of terrorism. This global trend of terrorists targeting children seems to be escalating (Johnston 2017). Therefore, it is imperative to understand terrorism and ways it impacts the children and families served by the health care community.

Combs (2018) defines *terrorism* as "an act of violence perpetrated on innocent civilian noncombatants in order to evoke fear in an audience". However, she goes on to argue that to become an operational definition, there must also be the addition of a "political purpose" of the violent act. Therefore, "terrorism, then, is an act composed of at least four crucial elements: 1) it is an act of violence, 2) it has a political motive or goal, 3) it is perpetrated against civilian noncombatants, and 4) it is staged to be played before an audience whose reaction of fear and terror is the desired result."(Combs 2018).

There are different typologies of terrorism. At least five types of terror violence have been suggested by Feliks Gross: "*Mass terror* is terror by a state, where the regime coerces the opposition in the population, whether organized or unorganized, sometimes in an institutionalized manner. *Dynastic assassination* is an attack on a head of state or a ruling elite. *Random terror* involves the placing of explosives where people gather (such as post offices, railroads, and cafes) to destroy whoever happens to be there. *Focused random terror* restricts the placing of explosives, for example to where significant agents of oppression are likely to gather. Finally, *tactical terror* is directed solely against the ruling government as a part of a 'broad revolutionary strategic plan'" (Combs 2018). An additional typology offered is "*lone wolf terror*" which involves someone who commits violent acts in support of some group, movement, or ideology, but who does stand alone, outside of any command structure and without material assistance from any group" (Combs 2018).

Martin (2017) reviews eight different terrorism typologies in the ever shifting, multifaceted world of modern terrorism. *The New Terrorism* "is characterized by the threat of mass casualty attacks from dissident terrorist organizations, new and creative configurations, transnational religious solidarity, and redefined moral justifications for political violence" (Martin 2017). *State Terrorism* is "committed by governments against perceived enemies and can be directed externally against adversaries in the international domain or internally against domestic enemies" (Martin 2017). *Dissident Terrorism* is "committed by nonstate movements and groups against governments, ethno-national groups, religious groups, and other perceived enemies" (Martin 2017). *Religious Terrorism* is "motivated by an absolute belief that an otherworldly power has sanctioned and commanded the application of terrorist violence for the greater glory of the faith…[it] is usually conducted in defense of what believers consider to be the one true faith" (Martin 2017). *Ideological Terrorism* is "motivated by political systems of belief (ideologies), which champion the self-perceived inherent rights of a particular group or interest in opposition to another group or interest. The system of belief incorporates theoretical and philosophical justifications for violently asserting the rights of the championed group or interest" (Martin 2017). *International Terrorism* "spills over onto the world's stage. Targets are selected because of their value as symbols of international interests, either within the home country or across state boundaries" (Martin 2017). *Criminal Dissident Terrorism* "is solely profit-driven, and can be some combination of profit and politics. For instance, traditional organized criminals accrue profits to fund their criminal activity and for personal interests, while criminal-political enterprises acquire profits to sustain their movement" (Martin 2017). *Gender-Selective Terrorism* "is directed against an enemy population's men or women because of their gender. Systematic violence is directed against men because of the perceived threat posed by males as potential soldiers or sources of opposition. Systematic violence is directed against women to destroy an enemy group's cultural identity or terrorize the group into submission" (Martin 2017).

The all-hazards National Planning Scenarios are an integral component of DHS's capabilities-based approach to implementing Homeland Security Presidential Directive 8: National Preparedness (HSPD-8). The National Planning Scenarios are planning tools and are representative of the range of potential terrorist and natural disasters and the related impacts that face the nation. The federal interagency community has developed 15 all-hazards planning scenarios for use in national, federal, state, and local homeland security preparedness activities. The objective was to develop a minimum number of credible scenarios to establish the range of response requirements to facilitate disaster planning (DHS 2006) (Table 5.14).

Twelve of the scenarios represent terrorist attacks while three represent natural disasters or naturally occurring epidemics. This ratio reflects the fact that the nation has recurring experience with natural disasters but faces newfound dangers, including the increasing potential for use of weapons of mass destruction by terrorists. The scenarios form the basis for coordinated federal planning, training, exercises, and grant investments needed to prepare for all hazards. DHS employed the scenarios as the basis for a rigorous task analysis of prevention, protection, response, and recovery missions and identification of key tasks that supported the development of essential all-hazards capabilities (United States Department of Homeland Security, Federal Emergency Management Agency 2019) (Table 5.15).

Each of the 15 scenarios follows the same outline to include a detailed scenario description, planning considerations, and implications. For each of the 12 terrorism-related scenarios, FEMA National Preparedness Directorate (NPD) partnered with DHS Office of Intelligence and Analysis (I&A) and other intelligence community and law enforcement experts to develop and validate prevention prequels. The

Table 5.14 DHS national planning scenarios[a]

	Category	Scenario description
Scenario 1	Nuclear Detonation	10-kiloton Improvised Nuclear Device
Scenario 2	Biological Attack	Aerosol Anthrax
Scenario 3	Biological Disease Outbreak	Pandemic Influenza
Scenario 4	Biological Attack	Plague
Scenario 5	Chemical Attack	Blister Agent
Scenario 6	Chemical Attack	Toxic Industrial Chemicals
Scenario 7	Chemical Attack	Nerve Agent
Scenario 8	Chemical Attack	Chlorine Tank Explosion
Scenario 9	Natural Disaster	Major Earthquake
Scenario 10	Natural Disaster	Major Hurricane
Scenario 11	Radiological Attack	Radiological Dispersal Devices
Scenario 12	Explosives Attack	Bombing Using Improvised Explosive Devices
Scenario 13	Biological Attack	Food Contamination
Scenario 14	Biological Attack	Foreign Animal Disease (Foot-and-Mouth Disease)
Scenario 15	Cyber Attack	Cyber Attack Against Critical Internet Related Infrastructures

[a]Reference: (United States Department of Homeland Security 2006)

Table 5.15 DHS FEMA key scenarios and corresponding national planning scenarios[a]

Key scenarios	National planning scenarios
1. Explosives Attack-Bombing Using Improvised Explosive Device	Scenario 12: Explosives Attack-Bombing Using Improvised Explosive Device
2. Nuclear Attack	Scenario 1: Nuclear Detonation-Improvised Nuclear Device
3. Radiological Attack-Radiological Dispersal Device	Scenario 11: Radiological Attack-Radiological Dispersal Device
4. Biological Attack-With annexes for different pathogens	Scenario 2: Biological Attack-Aerosol Anthrax Scenario 4: Biological Attack-Plague Scenario 13: Biological Attack-Food Contamination Scenario 14: Biological Attack-Foreign Animal Disease
5. Chemical Attack-With annexes for different agents	Scenario 5: Chemical Attack-Blister Agent Scenario 6: Chemical Attack-Toxic Industrial Chemicals Scenario 7: Chemical Attack-Nerve Agent Scenario 8: Chemical Attack: Chlorine Tank Explosion
6. Natural Disaster-With annexes for different disasters	Scenario 9: Natural Disaster-Major Earthquake Scenario 10: Natural Disaster-Major Hurricane
7. Cyber Attack	Scenario 15: Cyber Attack
8. Pandemic Influenza	Scenario 3: Biological Disease Outbreak-Pandemic Influenza

[a]References: United States Department of Homeland Security, Federal Emergency Management Agency 2019; United States Department of Homeland Security 2006)

prequels provide an understanding of terrorists' motivation, capability, intent, tactics, techniques and procedures, and technical weapons data. The prequels also provide a credible adversary based on known threats to test the homeland security community's ability to understand and respond to indications and warnings of possible terrorist attacks (United States Department of Homeland Security, Federal Emergency Management Agency 2019).

5.6 Chemical Agents

A chemical agent of terrorism is defined as any chemical substance intended for use in military operations to kill, seriously injure, or incapacitate humans (or animals) through its toxicological effects. Chemicals excluded from this list are riot-control agents, chemical herbicides, and smoke/flame materials. Chemical agents are classified as toxic agents (producing injury or death) or incapacitating agents (producing temporary effects). Toxic agents are further described as nerve agents (anticholinesterases), blood agents (cyanogens), blister agents (vesicants), and lung-damaging agents (choking agents). Incapacitating agents include stimulants, depressants, psychedelics, and deliriants (Banks 2014; Departments of the Army, the Navy, and the Air Force, and Commandant, Marine Corps 1995).

5.6.1 Nerve Agents

Nerve agents are organophosphate anticholinesterase compounds. They are used in various insecticide, industrial, and military applications. Military-grade agents include tabun (GA), sarin (GB), soman (GD), cyclosarin (GF), Venom X (VX), and the Novichok series. These are all major military threats. The only known battlefield use of nerve agents was the Iraq–Iran war. However, other nerve agent incidents, such as the 1995 Tokyo subway attack (sarin), the chemical attacks in Syria (chlorine, sarin, mustard), and the attempted assassination of Sergei Skripal in Salisbury, UK (Novichok), support that civilian threats also exist.

Nerve agents are volatile chemicals and can be released in liquid or vapor form. However, the liquid form can become vapor depending upon its level of volatility (e.g, G-agents are more volatile than VX). The level of toxicity depends on the agent, concentration of the agent, physical form, route and length of exposure, and environmental factors (temperature and wind) (Tables 5.16 and 5.17).

Nerve agents exert their effects by the inhibition of esterase enzymes. Acetylcholinesterase inhibition prevents the hydrolysis of acetylcholine. The clinical result is a cholinergic crisis and subsequent overstimulation of muscarinic and nicotinic receptors throughout the body including the central nervous system. Clinical muscarinic responses include SLUDGE (salivation, lacrimation, urination, defecation, gastrointestinal distress, and emesis) and DUMBELS (diarrhea, urinary incontinence, miosis/muscle fasciculation, bronchorrhea/bronchospasm/bradycardia, emesis, lacrimation, and salivation). Nicotinic responses vary by site. Preganglionic sympathetic nerve stimulation produces mydriasis, tachycardia,

Table 5.16 Comparative nerve agent vapor toxicity[a]

Agent	LCt_{50}	ICt_{50}	MCt_{50}
GA	400	300	2–3
GB	100	75	3
GD	70	Unknown	<1
GF	Unknown	Unknown	<1
VX	50	35	0.04

[a]For this table, one concentration of VX = 50, and one concentration of GB = 100, meaning it would take 2 times more GB to have the same median lethal dose as one concentration of VX (LCt_{50}:median lethal concentration/time; ICt_{50}:median incapacitation concentration/time; MCt_{50}: median first noticeable effect (of miosis) concentration/time) (Banks 2014)

Table 5.17 Comparative median lethal dose values on skin (liquid)[a]

Agent	Amount
GA	100
GB	170
GD	5
GF	3
VX	1

[a]For this table, one dose of VX = 1, and 170 doses of GB = 170, meaning it would take 170 times more GB to have the same median lethal dose as one dose of VX (Banks 2014)

hypertension, and pallor. However, stimulation at the neuromuscular junction leads to muscular fasciculation and cramping, weakness, paralysis, and diaphragmatic weakness. Central nervous system presentations range from anxiety and restlessness to seizures, coma, and death (Banks 2014; Rotenberg and Newmark 2003; Rotenberg 2003b).

Pediatric manifestations (Table 5.19) may vary from the classic clinical responses due to their unique vulnerabilities (Hilmas et al. 2008):

- Children may manifest symptoms earliest and possibly more severe presentations.
- Could be hospitalized for similarly related illnesses and diseases.
- Smaller mass.
- Lower baseline cholinesterase activity.
- Tendency to bronchospasm.
- Pediatric airway and respiratory differences.
- Altered pulmonary compensation.
- Lower reserves of cardiovascular system and fluids.
- Isolated central nervous system signs (stupor, coma).
- Less miosis.
- Vulnerability to seizures and neurotransmitter imbalances (excitability).
- Immature metabolic systems.

Differential diagnoses include upper or lower airway obstruction, bronchiolitis, status asthmaticus, cardiogenic shock, acute gastroenteritis, seizures, and poisonings (carbon monoxide, organophosphates, and cyanide). Diagnostic tests include acetylcholinesterase levels, red blood cell cholinesterase levels, and an arterial blood gas.

Treatment (Tables 5.20 and 5.21) includes decontamination (Reactive Skin Decontamination Lotion® [potassium 2,3-butanedione monoximate], soap and water, and 0.5% hypochlorite solution), supportive care, and administration of nerve agent antidotes (atropine, pralidoxime chloride, and diazepam). Atropine is a competitive antagonist of acetylcholine muscarinic receptors and reverses peripheral muscarinic symptoms. It does not restore function at the neuromuscular junction nicotinic receptors. It does, however, treat early phases of convulsions. Pralidoxime chloride separates the nerve agent from acetylcholinesterase and restores enzymatic function. It also binds free nerve agent. The major goal is to prevent "aging" of the enzyme (e.g., GD). Diazepam provides treatment of nerve agent-induced seizures and prevents secondary neurologic injury. Typically, associated seizures are refractory to other antiepileptic drugs. The antiseizure effect of diazepam is enhanced by atropine (Banks 2014; Cieslak and Henretig 2016; Messele et al. 2018). Potential medical countermeasures include trimedoxime (TMB4), HI-6 (an H-series oxime), obidoxime, "bioscavengers" (butyrylcholinesterase, carboxylesterase, organophosphorus acid anhydride hydrolase, and human serum paraoxonase), novel anticonvulsant drugs, N-methyl-D-aspartate (NMDA) receptor antagonists (ketamine, dexanabinol), and common immunosuppressants such as cyclosporine A (Jokanovic 2015; Merrill et al. 2015; National Institutes of Health 2007; United States Department of Health and Human Services 2017). All patients should be observed closely for electroencephalographic changes and neuropsychiatric pathologies. Polyneuropathy, reported after organophosphate insecticide poisoning, has not been reported in humans exposed to nerve agents and has been produced in animals only at unsurvivable doses. The intermediate syndrome has not been reported in humans after nerve agent exposure, nor has it been produced in animals. Muscular necrosis has occurred in animals after high-dose nerve agent exposure but reversed within weeks; it has not been reported in humans (Banks 2014).

5.6.2 Novichok Series

On March 4, 2018, Sergei Skripal, a former Russian double agent, and his daughter, Yulia Skripal, were found unresponsive on a park bench in Salisbury, UK. They were brought to a nearby hospital and treated for signs consistent with a cholinergic crisis due to a nerve agent exposure. Analysis of the Skripals found the presence of a secret nerve agent called Novichok. Further testing found high concentrations of the agent on the front-door handle of his home. One of the investigating police officers, Detective Sergeant Nick Bailey, unknowingly touched the door-handle and also became ill. All three survived due to rapid recognition of the nerve agent exposure by hospital personnel. Four months later, two other people, Dawn Sturgess and

Charlie Rowley, became ill with identical symptoms in the town of Amesbury, 7 miles from Salisbury. They were later confirmed to have high concentrations of Novichok on their hands from a perfume bottle found in a recycling bin. Both were immediately treated, but Dawn Sturgess later died. Charlie Rowley survived. It was believed the discarded perfume bottle contained Novichok and was discarded by the assailants after the attempt on Sergei Skripal. On September 5, 2018, the UK government revealed that their investigation uncovered two suspects from closed circuit television (CCTV) footage near the Skripal's home. The suspects entered the UK on Russian passports using the names Alexander Petrov and Ruslan Boshirov, stayed in a London hotel for 2 days, visited Salisbury briefly, and then returned to Moscow. Minute traces of Novichok were also found in the London hotel where they had stayed. The UK Prime Minister, Teresa May, said that the suspects are thought to be officers from Russia's military intelligence service the Glavnoye Razvedyvatel'noye Upravleniye (GRU), and that this showed that the poisoning was "not a rogue operation" and was "almost certainly" approved at a senior level of the Russian state. The two suspects later appeared on Russian TV denying the accusations and saying they were just "tourists" who had traveled all the way from Moscow to Salisbury just to see the "famous cathedral". However, CCTV of the cathedral area found no evidence of the two men visiting the cathedral, although they were captured on CCTV near the Skripal's home. In a development in September 2018, one of the men was revealed as actually being a Russian intelligence officer named Colonel Anatoliy Chepiga and was a decorated veteran of Russian campaigns in Chechnya and Ukraine. And later in October, the second man was named as Dr. Alexander Mishkin, a naval medical doctor allegedly recruited by the GRU (Chai et al. 2018; May 2018).

Novichok (Новичóк: Russian for "newcomer") is a highly potent nerve agent developed from the Russian classified nerve agent program known as FOLIANT. Almost everything known about these agents is due to a Russian defector, Vil Mirzayanov (2009) who was an analytical chemist at the Russian State Research Institute of Organic Chemistry and Technology (GosNIIOKhT). He has described the details of the Novichok program in his book "*State Secrets: An Insider's Chronicle of the Russian Chemical Weapons Program*". The first three nerve agents of the Novichok series developed in the program were Substance-33, A-230, and A-232 (Table 5.18). They were synthesized as unitary agents, like VX, tabun, soman, and sarin. Unitary means that the chemical structure was produced at its maximum potency. However, the Novichok agents were developed as binary agents: maximum potency when two inert substances are combined together prior to deployment to create the active nerve agent (Cieslak and Henretig 2003). Very little is known about the chemistry of these weaponized organophosphate agents. However, they appear to be more potent than current nerve agents. For example, the LD_{50} of Novichok agents is reported 0.22 µg/kg similar to 2-(dimethylamino)ethyl *N,N*-dimethylphosphoramidofluoridate (VG), a novel fourth generation nerve agent. Furthermore, Novichok-5 is 8× more effective than VX and Novichock-7 is 10× more effective than soman (Cieslak and Henretig 2003; Hoenig 2007).

Clinically, they behave like other organophosphates by binding to acetylcholinesterase preventing the breakdown of acetylcholine thereby leading to a cholinergic

Table 5.18 A list of known Novichok agents attributed to the GosNIIOKhT research program and their status[a]

Agent	Type	Current status
Substance-33	Unitary	Estimated 15,000 tons produced Designated as chemical weapon
A-230	Unitary	Experimental quantities produced Designated as chemical weapon (1990)
A-232	Unitary	Experimental agent Not designated, or officially approved
A-234	Unitary analog of A-232	Unknown
Novichok-5	Binary analog of A-232 8× more effective than VX	Experimental agent Designated as chemical weapon (1989)
Novichok-7	Binary analog of A-234 10× more effective than soman	Experimental agent Not designated
Novichok-#	Binary analog of Substance-33	Adopted as chemical weapon (1990)

[a]VX = Venom X (Cieslak and Henretig 2003)

crisis. There appears to be a similar "aging" process as seen with other nerve agents. In addition, the Novichok agents binding to peripheral sensory nerves distinguishes this class of organophosphates. Prolonged or high-dose exposure results in debilitating peripheral neuropathy. Exposure to these agents is fatal unless aggressively managed (Cieslak and Henretig 2003). Decontamination is essential to prevent ongoing exposure to the patient and medical personnel. Clothing should be removed and quickly placed in a sealed bag (prevents ongoing exposure to the emission of vapors) followed by thorough washing with soap and water. Application of dry bleach powder should be avoided as it may hydrolyze nerve agents into toxic metabolites that can produce ongoing cholinergic effects. Supportive care is essential. Antidote therapy should be given as usual for nerve agents, including atropine, diazepam, and pralidoxime chloride (United States Department of Health and Human Services, Office of the Assistant Secretary for Preparedness and Response, National Library of Medicine 2019; United States Department of Health and Human Services, Chemical Hazards Emergency Medical Management (CHEMM) 2019). Of note, the toxicity of the Novichok agents may not rely on anticholinesterase inhibition. Some have suggested that reactive oximes like potassium 2,3-butanedione monoximate are preferred oximes for antidotal therapy (Cieslak and Henretig 2003).

5.6.3 Blood Agents

Cyanide is a naturally occurring chemical. It can be found in plants and seeds. It is also used in many industrial applications and is a common product of combustion of synthetic materials. Typical cyanogens include hydrogen cyanide (AC) and cyanogen chloride (CK). Low levels of cyanide are detoxified by a natural reaction in the human body using the rhodanese system. There is reversible metabolism with Vitamin B12a to Vitamin B12 (cyanocobalamin). An irreversible reaction occurs with sulfanes to produce thiocyanates and sulfates. The former is excreted via the urinary tract. When cyanide overwhelms this natural process, cyanide binds to cytochrome oxidase within the mitochondria and disrupts cellular respiration. Cyanide has an affinity for Fe+3 in the cytochrome a3 complex and oxidative phosphorylation is interrupted. Cells can no longer use oxygen to produce ATP and lactic acidosis ensues from resultant anaerobic metabolism.

When inhaled, cyanide produces rapid onset of clinical signs. Findings include transient tachypnea and Kussmaul breathing (from hypoxia of carotid and aortic bodies), hypertension and tachycardia (from hypoxia of aortic body), and neurologic findings such as seizures, muscle rigidity (trismus), opisthotonus, and decerebrate posturing. Other findings include cherry red flush, acute respiratory failure/ arrest, bradycardia, dissociative shock, and cardiac arrest. Venous blood samples exhibit a bright red color. Arterial blood gas may demonstrate a metabolic acidosis with an increased anion gap due to lactic acid (Banks 2014; Cieslak and Henretig 2016; Rotenberg 2003a).

Pediatric manifestations (Table 5.19) may vary from the classic clinical responses due to their unique vulnerabilities (Hilmas et al. 2008):

- Thinner integument leading to shorter time from exposure to symptom development.
- Higher vapor density (CK) and concentration accumulation in living zone of children,
- Higher minute ventilation and metabolism.
- Abdominal pain, nausea, restlessness, and giddiness are common early findings.
- Cyanosis mostly noted other than classic cherry red flushing of the skin.
- Resilient with recovery even when just using supportive measures alone.

Differential diagnoses include meningitis, encephalitis, gastroenteritis, ischemic stroke, methemoglobinemia, and poisonings (nerve agents, organophosphates, methanol, hydrogen sulfide, and carbon monoxide). Diagnostic tests include arterial blood gas, lactic acid, and thiocyanate levels.

Treatment (Tables 5.20 and 5.21) includes decontamination, supportive care, and administration of cyanide antidote kit (nitrites and thiosulfate). The nitrites facilitate the production of methemoglobinemia (Fe+3) which attracts cyanide molecules forming cyanmethemoglobin. Amyl nitrite pearls are crushed into gauze and placed over the mouth/nose or in a mask used for bag/mask ventilation. Sodium nitrite is given parenterally and dosed according to the patient's estimated hemoglobin so as to prevent severe methemoglobinemia. Since the formation of cyanmethemoglobin is a reversible reaction, and sodium thiosulfate is given to extract the cyanide. Dosing is also dependent upon estimated hemoglobin. Along with the naturally occurring rhodanese enzymatic system, the irreversible reaction forms thiocyanate. Thiocyanate is water soluble and is excreted harmlessly via the kidneys (Banks 2014; Cieslak and Henretig 2016). Potential medical countermeasures (National Institutes of Health 2007; United States Army Medical Research Institute of Infectious Diseases (USAMRIID) 2014) include hydroxocobalamin, cobinamide (a cobalamin precursor), dicobalt edetate, cyanohydrin-forming compounds (alpha-ketoglutarate and pyruvate), S-substituted crystallized rhodanese, sulfur-containing drugs (N-acetylcysteine), and methemoglobin inducers (4-dimethylaminophenol and others).

Table 5.19 Pediatric vulnerabilities and implications for clinical management

	Unique vulnerability in children	Implications and impact from chemical toxicity
Body composition	Larger BSA compared to body mass Lower total body lipid/fat content	Greater dermal absorption Less partitioning of lipid-soluble components
Volume status	More prone to dehydration Chemical agents lead to diarrhea and vomiting	Can be more symptomatic and show signs of severe dehydration
Respiratory	Increased basal metabolic rate compared to greater minute volume	Enhance toxicity via inhalational route
Blood	Limited serum protein binding capacity Greater cutaneous blood flow	Potential for greater amount of free toxicant and greater distribution Greater percutaneous absorption
Skin	Thinner epidermis in preterm infants Greater cutaneous blood flow	Increased toxicity from percutaneous absorption of chemical agents
Organ size and enzymatic function	Larger brain mass Immature renal function Immature hepatic enzymes	Greater CNS exposure Slower elimination of renally cleared toxins, chemicals, and metabolites Decreased metabolic clearance by hepatic phase I and II reactions
Anatomical considerations	Shorter stature means breathing occurs closer to the ground where aerosolized chemical agents settle Smaller airway Greater deposition of fine particles in the upper airway Higher proportion of rapidly growing tissues	Exposure to chemicals can have significant impact on bone marrow and developing CNS Increased airway narrowing from chemical agent-induced secretions Mustard significantly affects rapidly growing tissue
Central nervous system	Higher BBB permeability Rapidly growing CNS	Increased risk of CNS damage
Miscellaneous	Immature cognitive function Unable to flee emergency Immature coping mechanisms	Inability to discern threat, follow directions, and protect self High risk for developing PTSD

BBB blood-brain barrier, *BSA* body surface area, *CNS* central nervous system, *PTSD* post-traumatic stress disorder (Hilmas et al. 2008)

5.6.4 Blister Agents

Blistering agents, or vesicants, promote the production of blisters. Typical examples include sulfur mustard (HD), nitrogen mustard (HN), and Lewisite (L). These agents, especially sulfur mustard, are considered capable chemical weapons since illness may not occur until hours or days later. Vesicants are alkylating agents that affect rapidly reproducing and poorly differentiated cells in the body. However, they can also produce cellular oxidative stress, deplete glutathione stores, and promote intense inflammatory responses. Clinical findings are initially cutaneous (erythema, pruritus, yellow blisters, ulcers, and sloughing), respiratory (hoarseness, cough, voice changes, pneumonia, respiratory failure, acute lung injury, and acute respiratory distress syndrome), and ophthalmologic (pain, irritation, blepharospasm, photophobia, conjunctivitis, corneal ulceration, and globe perforation) in nature. After exposure through these primary portals of entry, other sites are affected, including the gastrointestinal tract (nausea, vomiting, and mucosal injury), the hematopoietic system (bone marrow suppression), the cardiovascular system (L), reproductive system (HD, HN), and the central nervous system (lethargy, headache, malaise, and depression) (Banks 2014; Yu et al. 2003).

Pediatric manifestations (Table 5.19) may vary from the classic clinical responses due to their unique vulnerabilities (Hilmas et al. 2008):

- Thinner integument leading to shorter time from exposure to symptom development.
- Higher vapor density and concentration accumulation in the living zone.
- Higher minute ventilation and metabolism.
- Greater pulmonary injury.
- Ocular findings more frequent (less self-protection and more hand/eye contact).
- Gastrointestinal manifestations more prominent.
- Unable to escape and decontaminate.
- Unable to verbalize complaints (i.e., pain).

Treatment (Tables 5.20 and 5.21) includes decontamination and supportive care. Currently, there are no antidotes for mustard toxicity (Cieslak and Henretig 2016). Agents under investigation include antioxidants (Vitamin E), anti-inflammatory drugs (corticosteroids), mustard scavengers (glutathione, *N*-acetylcysteine), and nitric oxide synthase inhibitors (L-nitroarginine methyl ester). Other therapeutics under investigation include the use of British Anti-Lewisite (BAL), reactive skin protectants, and ocular therapies (National Institutes of Health 2007; USAMRIID 2014).

5.6.5 Lung-Damaging Agents

Lung-damaging agents are toxic inhalants and potentially can affect the entire respiratory tract. Typical examples include chlorine (Cl_2), phosgene (carbonyl chloride), oxides of nitrogen, organofluoride polymers, hydrogen fluoride, and zinc oxide. Since many of these chemicals are readily available and have multiple industrial applications, they are considered terrorist weapons of opportunity. Toxicity is dependent upon agent particle size, solubility, and method of release. Large particles produce injury in the nasopharynx (sneezing, pain, and erythema). Midsize particles affect the central airways (painful swelling, cough, stridor, wheezing, and rhonchi). Small particles cause injury at the level of the alveoli (dyspnea, chest tightness, and rales). Highly soluble agents, such as chlorine, dissolve with mucosal moisture and immediately produce strong upper airway reactions. Less soluble

Table 5.20 Recommended treatment and management of chemical agents used in terrorism

Agent	Toxicity	Clinical findings	Onset	Decontamination[a]	Management
Nerve agents					
Tabun, Sarin, Soman, VX	Anticholinesterase: muscarinic, nicotinic, and CNS effects	Vapor: miosis, rhinorrhea, dyspnea	Vapor: seconds	Vapor: fresh air, remove clothes, wash hair	ABCs
		Liquid: Diaphoresis, emesis	Liquid: minutes to hours	Liquid: remove clothes, copious washing of skin and hair with soap and water, ocular irrigation	Atropine[b,c,d]: 0.05 mg/k IV, IM (min 0.1 mg, max 5 mg), repeat q2–5 min prn for marked secretions, bronchospasm
		Both: coma, paralysis, seizures, apnea			Pralidoxime[e]: 25 mg/kg IV, IM (max 1 g IV; 2 g IM), may repeat within 30–60 min prn, then again q1 h for 1 or 2 doses prn for persistent weakness, high atropine requirement
					Diazepam: 0.3 mg/kg (max 10 mg) IV; Lorazepam 0.1 mg/kg IV, IM (max 4 mg); Midazolam: 0.2 mg/kg (max 10 mg) IM prn seizures, or severe exposure
Blistering (Vesicant) agents					
Mustard	Alkylation	Skin: erythema, vesicles	Hours	Skin: soap and water	Symptomatic care
Lewisite	Arsenical	Eye: inflammation	Immediate pain	Eyes: irrigation with water (major impact only if done within minutes of exposure)	Possibly British Anti-Lewisite (BAL) 3 mg/kg IM q4–6 h for systemic effects of lewisite in severe cases
		Respiratory tract: inflammation, respiratory distress, acute respiratory distress syndrome			
Pulmonary agents					

					Symptomatic care
Chlorine, phosgene	Liberate HCl, alkylation	Eyes, nose, throat, irritation (especially chlorine)	Minutes	Fresh air Skin: water	Symptomatic care
		Bronchospasm, pulmonary edema (especially phosgene)	Bronchospasm: minutes Pulmonary edema: hours		
Blood agents					
Cyanide	Cytochrome oxidase inhibition: cellular anoxia, lactic acidosis	Tachypnea, coma, seizures, apnea	Seconds	Fresh air Skin: soap and water	Airway, breathing, circulatory support, 100% oxygen Sodium bicarbonate prn for metabolic acidosis Sodium nitrite (3%): Dose (mL/kg)—Est. Hb (g/dL) 0.27—10 0.33—12 0.39—14 Max 10 mL Sodium thiosulfate (25%) 1.65 mL/kg (max 50 mL) Need to consider hydroxocobalamin, which may be very useful especially during a terrorist incident (Cyanokit)

Used with permission from Society of Critical Care Medicine

References: (Markenson et al. 2006; Berger and Burns 2012; Cieslak and Henretig 2016; Jacobson and Severin 2012; Markenson and Redlener 2007)

[a]Decontamination, especially for patients with significant nerve agent or vesicant exposure, should be performed by nurses or HCPs garbed in adequate personal protective equipment. For Emergency Department staff, this consists of nonencapsulated, chemically resistant body suit, boots, and gloves with a full-face air purifier mask/hood

[b]Intraosseous route is likely equivalent to intravenous

[c]Atropine might have some benefit via endotracheal tube or inhalation, as might aerosolized ipratropium

[d]As of September 2004, the FDA has approved pediatric autoinjectors of atropine in 0.25, 0.5, and 1 mg sizes. Recommendations are:

Approximate age	Approximate weight (kg)	Approximate weight (lb)	Autoinjector size
Less than 6 months	Less than 7.5 kg	Less than 15 lb	0.25 mg
6 months–4 years	7.5–18 kg	15–40 lb	0.5 mg
5–10 years	18–30 kg	41–90 lb	1 mg
Greater than 10 years	Greater than 30 kg	Greater than 90 lb	2 mg (adult size)

ᵉPralidoxime is reconstituted to 50 mg/mL (1 g in 20 mL water) for IV administration, and the total dose infused over 30 min, or may be given by continuous infusion (loading dose 25 mg/kg over 30 min, then 10 mg/kg/h). For IM use, it might be diluted to a concentration of 300 mg/mL (1 g added to 3 mL water—by analogy to the US Army's Mark-1 autoinjector concentration) to effect a reasonable volume for injection. Pediatric autoinjectors of pralidoxime are not FDA approved or available; however, for mass casualty situations, consider the following:

Approximate age (yr)	Approximate weight (kg)	Number of autoinjectors	Pralidoxime dose (mg/kg)
3–7	13–25	1	24–46 mg/kg
8–14	26–50	2	24–46 mg/kg
Older than 14	Over 50 kg	3	Less than 35 kg

agents, such as phosgene, travel to the lower airway before dissolving and subsequently causing toxicity. It is important, however, to realize that very few lung-damaging agents affect only the upper or lower airway (e.g., Cl_2). If the agent is aerosolized, solid or liquid droplets suspend in the air and distribute by size. If it is a gas or vapor release, there is uniform distribution throughout the lungs and toxicity will be based on solubility and reactivity of the agent (Banks 2014; Burklow et al. 2003; Cieslak and Henretig 2016).

Pediatric manifestations (Table 5.19) may vary from the classic clinical responses due to their unique vulnerabilities (Hilmas et al. 2008):

- Pediatric airway and respiratory tract issues (obligate nose breathers, relatively small mouth/large tongue, copious secretions, anterior/cephalad vocal cords, Omega or horseshoe-shaped epiglottis, tendency of laryngospasm and bronchospasm, and anatomically small, "floppy" airways).
- High vapor density and concentration accumulation in the living zone.
- Unable to verbalize or localize physical complaints.
- Rapid dehydration and shock secondary to pulmonary edema.
- Increased minute ventilation and metabolism.

Differential diagnoses include smoke inhalation injury, cardiogenic shock, heart failure, traumatic injury, asthma, bronchiolitis, and poisoning (cyanide). Treatment (Tables 5.20 and 5.21) includes decontamination and supportive care. Currently, there are no antidotes for lung-damaging agent toxicity (Cieslak and Henretig 2016). Potential countermeasures include novel positive-pressure devices, drugs to prevent lung inflammation, and treatments for chemically induced pulmonary edema (beta agonists, dopamine, insulin, allopurinol, and ibuprofen). In addition, drugs are being investigated that act at complex molecular pathways of the lung

Table 5.21 Decontamination for patients exposed to chemical agents of terrorism

Agent	Decontamination[a]
Nerve agents (tabun, sarin, soman, VX)	Vapor: fresh air, remove clothes, wash hair Liquid: remove clothes, wash skin, hair with copious soap and water, ocular irrigation
Vesicants (mustard, Lewisite)	Skin: soap and water Eyes: water (effective only if done within minutes of exposure)
Pulmonary agents (chlorine, phosgene)	Fresh air Skin: water
Cyanide	Fresh air Skin: soap and water

[a]Decontamination, especially for patients with significant nerve agent or vesicant exposure, should be performed by nurses or HCPs garbed in adequate personal protective equipment. For Emergency Department staff, this equipment consists of a nonencapsulated, chemically resistant body suit, boots, and gloves with a full-face air-purifier mask/hood (Cieslak and Henretig 2016)

(i.e., modulate the activity of ion channels that control fluid transport across lung membranes or supports surfactant) (National Institutes of Health 2007; USAMRIID 2014).

5.7 Biological Agents

The Centers for Disease Control and Prevention (CDC) has delineated bioterrorism agents and diseases into three categories based on priority. Category A agents include organisms with the highest risk because the ease of dissemination or transmission from person-to-person, result in high mortality rates, have the potential for major public health impact, promote public panic and social disruption, and require special action of public health preparedness. These agents/diseases include smallpox (*Variola major*), anthrax (*Bacillus anthracis*), plague (*Yersinia pestis*), viral hemorrhagic fevers (filoviruses [Ebola, Marburg] and arenaviruses [Lassa, Macupo]), botulinum toxin (from *Clostridium botulinum*), and tularemia (*Francisella tularensis*). Category B agents, the second highest priority, include those that are moderately easy to disseminate, result in moderate morbidity and low mortality rates, and require specific enhancements of diagnostic capacity and enhanced disease surveillance. These agents/diseases include ricin toxin (*Ricinus communis*), brucellosis (*Brucella* species), epsilon toxin of *Clostridium perfringens*, food safety threats (*Salmonella* species, *Escherichia coli* O157:H7, *Shigella*), glanders (*Burkholderia mallei*), meliodosis (*Burkholderia pseudomallei*), psitticosis (*Chlamydia psittaci*), typhus fever (*Rickettsia prowazekii*), Q fever (*Coxiella burnetii*), Staphylococcal enterotoxin B, trichothecenes mycotoxin, viral encephalitis (alphaviruses, such as eastern equine encephalitis, Venezuelan equine encephalitis, and western equine encephalitis), and water safety threats (*Vibrio cholera*, *Cryptosporidium parvum*). Category C agents have the next priority and include emerging pathogens that could be engineered for mass dissemination because of availability, ease of production and dissemination, and have the potential for high morbidity and mortality rates and major health impact.

These agents include Nipah virus, hantavirus, yellow fever virus, drug resistant tuberculosis, and tick-borne encephalitis (Markenson et al. 2006; Centers for Disease Control and Prevention 2019a; Cieslak 2018). Based on biological threats to national security, the National Institute of Allergy and Infectious Disease has developed a strategic plan that outlines priority areas of biodefense research including infrastructure, basic research, and medical countermeasure development for these agents/diseases (National Institutes of Health 2005). The strategic efforts have since been expanded by a collaborative effort among the CDC, Food and Drug Administration (FDA), Biomedical Advanced Research and Development Authority (BARDA), Public Health Emergency Medical Countermeasure Enterprise (PHEMCE), National Institutes of Health (NIH), and other key stakeholders (Fagbuyi et al. 2016; U.S. Department of Health and Human Services, Assistant Secretary for Preparedness and Response Biomedical Advanced Research and Development Authority 2016; U.S. Department of Health and Human Services, Assistant Secretary for Preparedness and Response 2017; USAMRIID 2014).

Recognition of a biologic attack is essential. There are various epidemiologic clues to consider when determining whether the outbreak is natural or man-made (Markenson et al. 2006; Cieslak 2018; USAMRIID 2014):

- The appearance of a large outbreak of cases of a similar disease or syndrome, or especially in a discrete population.
- Many cases of unexplained diseases or deaths.
- More severe disease than is usually expected for a specific pathogen or failure to respond to standard therapy.
- Unusual routes of exposure for a pathogen, such as the inhalational route for disease that normally occur through other exposures.
- A disease case or cases that are unusual for a given geographic area or transmission season.
- Disease normally transmitted by a vector that is not present in the local area.
- Multiple simultaneous or serial epidemics of different diseases in the same population.
- A single case of disease by an uncommon agent (smallpox, some viral hemorrhagic fevers, inhalational anthrax, pneumonic plague).
- A disease that is unusual for an age group.
- Unusual strains or variants of organisms or antimicrobial resistance patterns different from those known to be circulating.
- A similar or identical genetic type among agents isolated from distinct sources at different times and/or locations.
- Higher attack rates among those exposed in certain areas, such as inside a building if released indoors, or lower rates in those inside a sealed building if released outside.
- Outbreaks of the same disease occurring in noncontiguous areas.
- Zoonotic disease outbreaks.
- Intelligence of a potential attack, claims by a terrorist or aggressor of a release, and discovery of munitions, tampering, or other potential vehicle of spread (spray device, contaminated letter).

One should know the cellular, physiological, and clinical manifestations of each biologic agent. Furthermore, knowledge of distinct presentation patterns of children will be helpful to diagnosis. In any event, the ten steps in the management of biologic attack victims, pediatric, or otherwise, should be applied (Cieslak and Henretig 2003; Cieslak 2018; USAMRIID 2014):

1. Maintain an index of suspicion.
2. Protect yourself.
3. Assess the patient.
4. Decontaminate as appropriate.
5. Establish a diagnosis.
6. Render prompt treatment.
7. Practice good infection control.
8. Alert the proper authorities.
9. Assist in the epidemiologic investigation and manage the psychological consequences.
10. Maintain proficiency and spread the word.

5.7.1   Smallpox (Variola major)

Smallpox is caused by the Orthopoxvirus variola and was declared globally eradicated in 1980. The disease is highly communicable from person-to-person and remains a threat due to its potential for weaponization. The only stockpiles are at the CDC and at the Russian State Centre for Research on Virology and Biotechnology. However, clandestine stockpiles in other parts of the world are unknown. Since the cessation of smallpox vaccination, the general population has little or no immunity.

The three clinical forms of smallpox include ordinary, flat, and hemorrhagic. Another form, modified type, occurred in those previously vaccinated who were no longer protected. The asymptomatic incubation period is from 7 to 17 days (average 12 days) after exposure. A prodrome follows that lasts for 2–4 days and is marked by fever, malaise, and myalgia. Lesions start on the buccal and pharyngeal mucosa. The rash then spreads in a centrifugal fashion, and the lesions are synchronous. Initially, there are macules followed by papules, pustules, and scabs in 1–2 weeks. Other clinical features include extensive fluid loss and hypovolemic shock, nausea, vomiting, diarrhea, bacterial superinfections, viral bronchitis and pneumonitis, corneal ulceration with or without keratitis, and encephalitis. Death, if it occurs, is typically during the second week of clinical disease. *Variola minor* caused a mortality of 1% in unvaccinated individuals. However, the *Variola major* type caused death in 3% and 30% in those vaccinated and unvaccinated, respectively. Flat (mostly children) and hemorrhagic (pregnant women and immunocompromised) types caused severe mortality in those populations infected.

The differential diagnoses for smallpox include chickenpox (varicella), herpes, erythema multiforme with bullae, or allergic contact dermatitis. Varicella typically has a longer incubation period (14–21 days) and minimal or no prodrome. Furthermore, the rash distributes in a centripetal fashion and the progression is asynchronous (Images 5.1 and 5.2). Diagnosis of smallpox is mostly clinical

EVALUATING PATIENTS FOR SMALLPOX
ACUTE, GENERALIZED VESICULAR OR PUSTULAR RASH ILLNESS PROTOCOL

Patients with Acute, Generalized Vesicular or Pustular Rash Illness

Institute Airborne & Contact Precautions Alert Infection Control on Admission

Low Risk of Smallpox (see "Risk of Smallpox" below)
- History and Exam Highly Suggestive of Varicella
  - Varicella Testing Optional
- Diagnosis Uncertain
  - Test for Varicella and Other Conditions as Indicated

Moderate Risk of Smallpox (see "Risk of Smallpox" below)
- ID and/or Derm Consultation Varicella +/- Other Lab Testing as Indicated
  - Non-Smallpox Diagnosis Confirmed Report Result to Infection Control
  - No Diagnosis Made Ensure Adequacy of Specimen ID/Derm Consultant Re-Evaluates Patient
    - Cannot R/O Smallpox Classify as High Risk

High Risk of Smallpox (see "Risk of Smallpox" below)
- ID and/or Derm Consultation Alert Local and States Health Departments Immediately (contact information below)
  - Response Team Advises on Management & Specimen Collection
    - Testing at CDC
      - NOT Smallpox Further Testing
      - SMALLPOX

RISK OF SMALLPOX

High Risk of Smallpox → Report Immediately

1. Febrile prodrome (defined below) AND
2. Classic smallpox lesion (defined below & photo at top right) AND
3. Lesions in same stage of development (defined below)

Moderate Risk of Smallpox → Urgent Evaluation

1. Febrile prodrome (defined below) AND
2. One other MAJOR smallpox criterion (defined below)

OR

1. Febrile prodrome (defined below) AND
2. ≥4 MINOR smallpox criteria (defined below)

Low Risk of Smallpox → Manage as Clinically Indicated

1. No febrile prodrome

OR

1. Febrile prodrome AND
2. <4 MINOR smallpox criteria (defined below)

There have been no naturally occuring cases of smallpox anywhere in the world since 1977. A high risk case of smallpox is a public health and medical emergency.

Report all HIGH RISK CASES immediately (without waiting for lab result) to:

1. Hospital Infection Control _____ ( ) _____ - _____

2. _____ health department ( ) _____ - _____
   ( ) _____ - _____

3. _____ health department ( ) _____ - _____
   ( ) _____ - _____

MAJOR SMALLPOX CRITERIA

- **FEBRILE PRODROME:** occurring 1-4 days before rash onset: fever ≥101°F and at least one of the following: prostration, headache, backache, chills, vomiting or severe abdominal pain
- **CLASSIC SMALLPOX LESIONS:** deep-seated, firm/hard, round well-circumscribed vesicles or pustules; as they evolve, lesions may become umbilicated or confluent
- **LESIONS IN SAME STAGE OF DEVELOPMENT:** on any one part of the body (e.g., the face, or arm) all the lesions are in same stage of development (i.e., all are vesicles, or all are pustules)

MINOR SMALLPOX CRITERIA

- Centrifugal distribution: greatest concentration of lesions on face and distal extremities
- First lesions on the oral mucosa/palate, face, or forearms
- Patient appears toxic or moribund
- Slow evolution: lesions evolve from macules to papules→ pustules over days (each stage lasts 1-2 days)
- Lesions on the palms and soles

For more information, please go to the CDC website www.cdc.gov/smallpox

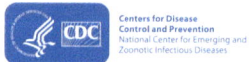

Centers for Disease Control and Prevention
National Center for Emerging and Zoonotic Infectious Diseases

CS205116-A

Image 5.1 CDC Evaluating Patients for Smallpox Algorithm. (Used with permission from Centers for Disease Control and Prevention; Source: https://www.cdc.gov/smallpox/pdfs/small-pox-diagnostic-algorithm-poster-2-pages.pdf)

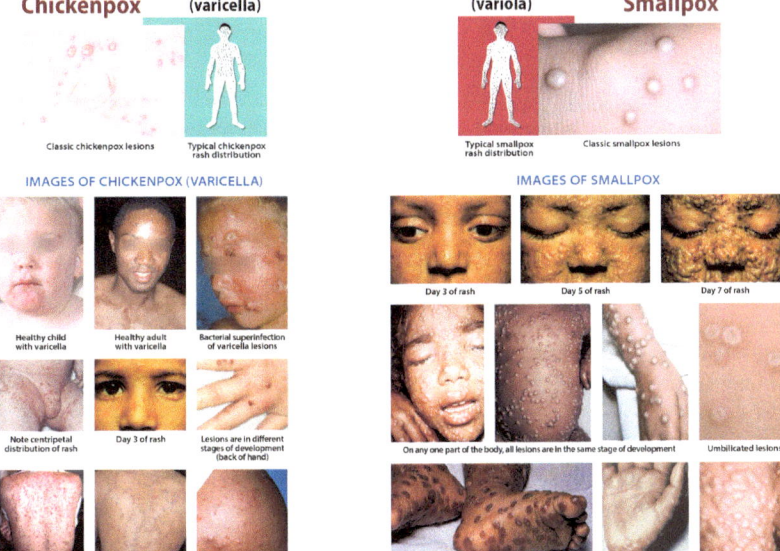

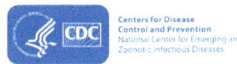

Image 5.2 CDC Evaluating Patients for Smallpox Algorithm. (Used with permission from Centers for Disease Control and Prevention; Photo Credits: Dr. Thomas Mack, Dr. Barbara Watson, Dr. Scott A. Norton, Dr. Patrick Alguire, World Health Organization, Philadelphia Department of Public Health, American Academy of Pediatrics, American Academy of Dermatology, American College of Physicians; Source: https://www.cdc.gov/smallpox/pdfs/smallpox-diagnostic-algorithm-poster-2-pages.pdf)

(Centers for Disease Control and Prevention 2019a). If considered, contact public health immediately. Laboratory confirmation (CDC or WHO) can be done by DNA sequencing, polymerase chain reaction (PCR), restriction fragment-length polymorphism (RFLP), real-time PCR, and microarrays. These are more sensitive and specific than the conventional virological and immunological approaches (Goff et al. 2018).

Generally, treatment is largely supportive (Table 5.23). Fluid losses and hypovolemic shock must be addressed. Also, due to electrolyte and protein loss, replacement therapy will be required. Bacterial superinfections must be aggressively treated with appropriate antibiotics. Biologic countermeasures and antivirals against smallpox are under investigation, including cidofovir, brincidovir (CMX-001), and tecovirimat (ST-246). These agents have shown efficacy in orthopoxvirus animal models and have been used to treat disseminated vaccinia infection under emergency use. Cidofovir has activity against poxviruses in animal studies (in vitro and in vivo) and some humans (eczema vaccinatum and molluscum contagiosum). Brincidovir is an oral formulation of cidofovir with less nephrotoxicity and has recently been announced as an addition to the Strategic National Stockpile (SNS) for patients with smallpox. Tecovirimat is a potent and specific inhibitor of orthopoxvirus replication. A recent study found that treatment with tecovirimat resulted in 100% survival of cynomolgus macaques challenged with intravenous variola virus. The disease was milder in tecovirimat-treated survivors and viral shedding was reduced compared to placebo-treated survivors. Prophylaxis comes in the form of the smallpox vaccine (vaccinia virus), ACAM2000®, which replaced Wyeth Dryvax™ in 2007. Safety profile of the two vaccines appears to be similar. Side effects of vaccination range from low-grade fever and axillary lymphadenopathy to inadvertent inoculation of the virus to other body sites to generalized vaccinia and cardiac events (myopericarditis). Rare, but typically fatal complications include progressive vaccinia, eczema vaccinatum, postvaccination encephalomyelitis, and fetal vaccinia. Modified Vaccinia Ankara (MVA) Smallpox Vaccine (Bavarian Nordic's IMVAMUNE®) is a live, highly attenuated, viral vaccine that is under development as a future nonreplicating smallpox vaccine (Greenberg et al. 2016; Kennedy and Greenberg 2009). Passive immunoprophylaxis exists in the form of vaccinia immune globulin (VIG) and is used for primarily treating complications from smallpox vaccine. Limited information suggests that VIG may be of use in postexposure prophylaxis of smallpox if given the first week after exposure and with vaccination. Monoclonal antibodies may represent another form of immunoprophylaxis. Postexposure administration of human monoclonal antibodies has protected rabbits from a lethal dose of an orthopoxvirus. As mentioned, smallpox is highly communicable person-to-person (Table 5.25). Contact precautions with full personal protective equipment (PPE) are required. Airborne isolation with the use of an N-95 mask is needed for baseline protection. An N-95 mask or powered air-purifying respirator (PAPR) is recommended for protection during high risk procedures (Beigel and Sandrock 2009; Goff et al. 2018; Rotz et al. 2005; Pittman et al. 2018; USAMRIID 2014).

5.7.2   Anthrax (*Bacillus anthracis*)

Anthrax is caused by the aerobic, spore-forming, nonmotile, encapsulated gram-positive rod *Bacillus anthracis*. It is a naturally occurring disease in herbivores. Humans contract the illness by handling contaminated portions of infected animals, especially hides and wool. Infection is introduced by scratches or abrasions on the skin. There is concern for potential aerosol dispersal leading to intentional infection through inhalation: it is fairly easy to obtain, capable of large quantity production, stable in aerosol form, and highly lethal.

Anthrax spores enter the body via skin, ingestion, or inhalation. The spores germinate inside macrophages and become vegetative bacteria. The vegetative form is released, replicates in the lymphatic system, and produces intense bacteremia. The production of virulence factors leads to overwhelming sepsis. The main virulence factors are encoded on two plasmids. One produces an antiphagocytic polypeptide capsule. The other contains genes for the synthesis of three proteins it secretes: protective antigen, edema factor, and lethal factor. The combination of protective antigen with lethal factor or edema factor forms binary cytotoxins, lethal toxin, and edema toxin. The anthrax capsule, lethal toxin, and edema toxin act in concert to drive the disease. Three clinical syndromes occur with anthrax: cutaneous, gastrointestinal, and inhalational.

Cutaneous anthrax is the most common naturally occurring form. After an individual is exposed to infected material or the agent itself, there is a 1–12 day (average 7 days) incubation period. A painless or pruritic papule forms at the site of exposure. The papule enlarges and forms a central vesicle, which is followed by erosion into a coal-black but painless eschar. Edema surrounds the area and regional lymphadenopathy may occur.

Gastrointestinal anthrax is rare. Typically, it develops after ingestion of viable vegetative organisms found in undercooked meats of infected animals. The two forms of gastrointestinal anthrax, oropharyngeal and intestinal, have incubation periods of 1–6 days. The oropharyngeal form is marked by fever and severe pharyngitis followed by ulcers and pseudomembrane formation. Other findings include dysphagia, regional lymphadenopathy, unilateral neck swelling, airway compromise, and sepsis. The intestinal form begins with fever, nausea, vomiting, and abdominal pain. Bowel edema develops which leads to mesenteric lymphadenitis with necrosis, shock, and death.

Endemic inhalational anthrax (Woolsorters' disease) is also extremely rare and is due to inhaling spores. Therefore, any case of inhalational anthrax should be assumed to be due to intentional exposure until proven otherwise. The incubation period is 1–5 days but can be up to 43 days. There is a prodrome of 1–2 days consisting of fever, malaise, and cough. Within 24 h, the disease rapidly progresses to respiratory failure, hemorrhagic mediastinitis (wide mediastinum), septic shock, multiorgan failure, and death. Patients with inhalational anthrax may also have hemorrhagic meningitis. Mortality is greater than 80% in 24–36 h despite aggressive treatment of inhalational anthrax.

The differential diagnoses of ulceroglandular lesions include antiphospholipid antibody syndrome, brown recluse spider bite, coumadin/heparin necrosis, cutaneous leishmaniasis, cutaneous tuberculosis, ecthyma gangrenosum, glanders, leprosy, mucormycosis, orf, plague, rat bite fever, rickettsial pox, staphylococcal/ streptococcal ecthyma, tropical ulcer, tularemia, and typhus. The differential diagnoses of ulceroglandular syndromes include cat scratch fever, chancroid, glanders, herpes, lymphogranuloma venereum, melioidosis, plague, staphylococcal and streptococcal adenitis, tuberculosis, and tularemia. The differential diagnoses for inhalational anthrax include influenza and influenza-like illnesses from other causes. The differential diagnoses of mediastinal widening include normal variant, aneurysm, histoplasmosis, sarcoidosis, tuberculosis, and lymphoma.

The diagnosis of anthrax is by culture and Gram stain of the blood, sputum, pleural fluid, cerebrospinal fluid, or skin. Specimens must be handled carefully, especially by lab personnel and those performing autopsies. ELISA and PCR are available at some reference laboratories. The chest radiograph of inhalational anthrax shows the classic widening of the mediastinum. Additional findings include hemorrhagic pleural effusions, air bronchograms, and/or consolidation (Purcell et al. 2018).

Supportive treatment is indicated, including mechanical ventilation, pleural effusion drainage, fluid and electrolyte support, and vasopressor administration. For inhalational anthrax, antibiotic treatment is unlikely to be effective unless started before respiratory symptoms develop. Treatment (Table 5.22) includes ciprofloxacin (or levofloxacin or doxycycline), clindamycin, and penicillin G. Raxibacumab, a monoclonal antibody, was approved by the FDA in 2012 for the treatment of inhalational anthrax in combination with recommended antibiotic regimens and prophylaxis for inhalational anthrax when other therapies are unavailable or inappropriate. It works by inhibiting anthrax antigen binding to cells and, therefore, prevents toxins from entering cells (Kummerfeldt 2014). The adult dose is 40 mg/kg given IV over 2 h and 15 min. The dose for children is weight based; ≤15 kg: 80 mg/kg; >15–50 kg: 60 mg/kg; >50 kg: 40 mg/kg. Premedication with diphenhydramine IV or PO is recommended 1 h before the infusion. It can also be used as postexposure prophylaxis in high risk spore exposure cases (Cieslak and Henretig 2016; Migone et al. 2009; The Medical Letter 2013). Obiltoxaximab (Anthim) is a recently approved monoclonal antibody treatment for inhalational anthrax in combination with recommended antibiotic regimens and prophylaxis for inhalational anthrax when other therapies are unavailable or inappropriate. Adults and children >40 kg should receive a single obiltoxaximab dose of 16 mg/kg. The recommended dose is 24 mg/kg for children >15–40 kg and 32 mg/kg for those weighing ≤15 kg. Premedication with diphenhydramine is recommended to reduce risk of hypersensitivity reactions (The Medical Letter 2018). In patients with inhalational anthrax, intravenous anthrax immune globulin (Anthrasil) should be considered in addition to appropriate antibiotic therapy (Mytle et al. 2013; The Medical Letter 2016; USAMRIID 2014). Postexposure prophylaxis includes ciprofloxacin (or levofloxacin or doxycycline) for 60 days plus administration of vaccine; since spores can persist in human

Table 5.22 Recommended therapy and prophylaxis of anthrax in children

Form of anthrax	Category of treatment (therapy or prophylaxis)	Agent and dosage
Inhalation	Therapy[a,b]	Ciprofloxacin[c] 10–15 mg/kg IV q12 h (max 400 mg/dose) **or** Doxycycline 2.2 mg/kg IV (max 100 mg) q12 h *and* Clindamycin[d] 10–15 mg/kg IV q8 h *and* Penicillin G[e] 400–600 k μ/kg/day IV divided q4 h *plus* raxibacumab Patients who are clinically stable after 14 days can be switched to a single oral agent (ciprofloxacin or doxycycline) to complete a 60-day course[f] of therapy
Inhalation	Postexposure prophylaxis (60-day course[f])	Ciprofloxacin[g] 10–15 mg/kg PO (max 500 mg/dose) q12 h **or** Doxcycline 2.2 mg/kg (max 100 mg) PO q12 h
Cutaneous, endemic	Therapy[h]	Penicillin V 40–80 mg/kg/day PO divided q6 h **or** Amoxicillin 40–80 mg/kg/d PO divided q8h **or** Ciprofloxacin 10–15 mg/kg PO (max 1 g/day) q12 h **or** Levofloxacin 10–15 mg/kg IV q24 h **or** Doxycycline 2.2 mg/kg PO (max 100 mg) q12 h
Cutaneous (in setting of terrorism)	Therapy[a]	Ciprofloxacin 10–15 mg/kg PO (max 1 g/day) q12 h **or** Levofloxacin 10–15 mg/kg IV q24 h Doxycycline 2.2 mg/kg PO (max 100 mg) q12 h
Gastrointestinal	Therapy[a]	Same as inhalational

Used with permission from Society of Critical Care Medicine
References: (Berger and Burns 2012; Cieslak and Henretig 2016; Markenson and Redlener 2007; Pittman et al. 2018; USAMRIID 2014)
[a]In a mass casualty setting, in which resources are severely limited, oral therapy may need to be substituted for the preferred parenteral option
[b]In addition to appropriate antibiotic regimen, monoclonal antibody therapy (see text for dosing) and intravenous anthrax immune globulin should be administered for inhalational anthrax
[c]Levofloxacin or ofloxacin may be an acceptable alternative to ciprofloxacin
[d]Rifampin or clarithromycin may be acceptable alternatives to clindamycin as a drug that targets bacterial protein synthesis. If ciprofloxacin or another quinolone is employed, doxycycline may be used as a second agent because it also targets protein synthesis
[e]Ampicillin, imipenem, meropenem, or chloramphenicol may be acceptable alternatives to penicillin as drugs with good CNS penetration
[f]Assuming the organism is sensitive, children may be switched to oral amoxicillin (40–80 mg/kg/d divided q8 h) to complete a 60-day course. The first 14 days of therapy of postexposure prophylaxis, however, should include ciprofloxacin or levofloxacin and/or doxycycline regardless of age. Vaccination should also be provided; if not, antibiotic course will need to be longer
[g]According to most experts, ciprofloxacin is the preferred agent for oral prophylaxis
[h]Ten days of therapy may be adequate for endemic cutaneous disease. A full 60-day course is recommended in the setting of terrorism, however, because of the possibility of concomitant inhalational exposure

tissues for a long time, antibiotics must be given for a longer period if vaccine is not also given. The Anthrax Vaccine Adsorbed (AVA BioThrax™) is derived from sterile culture fluid supernatant taken from an attenuated strain of *Bacillus anthracis* and does not contain any live or dead organisms. The vaccine is given 0.5 mL intramuscularly at 0 and 4 weeks then at 6, 12, and 18 months followed by yearly boosters (Pittman et al. 2018; USAMRIID 2014). Consult with CDC for current pediatric recommendations.

Anthrax is not contagious in the vegetative form during clinical illness (Table 5.25). Contact with infected animals increases likelihood of spread. Therefore, contact should be limited and the use of appropriate PPE in endemic areas is indicated (Beigel and Sandrock 2009; Carbone 2005; Purcell et al. 2018; USAMRIID 2014).

5.7.3 Plague (*Yersinia pestis*)

Plague is caused by *Yersinia pestis*, a nonmotile, nonsporulating gram-negative bacterium. It is a zoonotic disease of rodents. It is typically found worldwide and is endemic in western and southwestern states. Humans develop the disease after contact with infected rodents, or being bitten by their fleas. After a rodent population dies off, the fleas search for other sources of blood, namely humans. This is when large outbreaks of human plague occur. Pneumonic plague is a very rare disease and when it is present in a patient, it may be highly suspicious for intentional dispersal of this deadly agent. Three clinical syndromes occur with plague: bubonic plague (85%), septicemic plague (13%), and primary pneumonic plague (1–2%).

Bubonic plague occurs after an infected flea bites a human. After an incubation period of 2–8 days, there is onset of high fever, severe malaise, headache, myalgias, and nausea with vomiting. Almost 50% have abdominal pain. Around the same time, a characteristic bubo forms which is tender, erythematous, and edematous without fluctuation. Buboes typically form in the femoral or inguinal lymph nodes, but other areas can be involved as well (axillary, intraabdominal). The spleen and liver can be tender and palpable. The disease disseminates without therapy. Severe complications can ensue, including pneumonia, meningitis, sepsis, and multiorgan failure. Pneumonia is particularly concerning since these patients are extremely contagious. Mortality of untreated bubonic plague is 60%, but 5% with efficient and effective treatment.

Septicemic plague is characterized by acute fever followed by sepsis without bubo formation. The clinical syndrome is very similar to other forms of gram-negative sepsis: chills, malaise, tachycardia, tachypnea, hypotension, nausea, vomiting, and diarrhea. In addition to sepsis, disseminated intravascular coagulation can ensue leading to thrombosis, necrosis, gangrene, and the formation of black appendages. Multiorgan failure can quickly follow. Untreated septicemic plague is almost 100% fatal versus 30–50% in those treated.

Pneumonic plague is very rare and should be considered due to an intentional aerosol release until proven otherwise. The incubation period is relatively short at

1–3 days. Sudden fever, cough, and respiratory failure quickly follow. This form produces a fulminant pneumonia with watery sputum that usually progresses to bloody. Within a short period of time, septic shock and disseminated intravascular coagulation develop. ARDS and death may occur. Mortality rate of pneumonic plague is very high but may respond to early treatment.

Plague meningitis is a rare complication of plague. It can occur in 6% of patients with septicemia and pneumonic forms and is more common in children. Usually occurring a few weeks into the illness, it affects those receiving subtherapeutic doses of antibiotics or bacteriostatic antibiotics that do not cross the blood-brain barrier (tetracyclines). Fever, meningismus, and other meningeal signs occur. Plague meningitis is virtually indistinguishable from meningococcemia.

The differential diagnoses of bubonic plague include tularemia, cat scratch fever, lymphogranuloma venereum, chancroid, scrub typhus, and other staphylococcal and streptococcal infections. The differential diagnoses of septicemic plague should include meningococcemia, other forms of gram-negative sepsis, and rickettsial diseases. The differential diagnosis of pneumonic plague is very broad. However, sudden appearance of previously healthy individuals with rapidly progressive gram-negative pneumonia with hemoptysis should strongly suggest pneumonic plague due to intentional release.

Diagnosis can be made clinically as previously described. Demonstration of *Yersinia pestis* in blood or sputum is paramount. Methylene blue or Wright's stain of exudates may reveal the classic safety-pin appearance of *Yersinia pestis*. Culture on sheep blood or MacConkey agar demonstrates beaten-copper colonies (48 h) followed by fried-egg colonies (72 h). Detection of *Yersinia pestis* F1-antigen by specific immunoassay is available, but the result is available retrospectively. Chest radiograph of patients will demonstrate patchy infiltrates (Centers for Disease Control and Prevention 2018a; Worsham et al. 2018).

Treatment includes mechanical ventilation strategies for ARDS, hemodynamic support (fluid and vasopressor administration), and antimicrobial agents (Table 5.23). Gentamicin or streptomycin is the preferred antimicrobial treatment. Alternatives include doxycycline or ciprofloxacin or levofloxacin or chloramphenicol. In cases of meningitis, chloramphenicol is recommended due to its ability to effectively cross the blood-brain barrier. Streptomycin is in limited supply and is available for compassionate use. It should be avoided in pregnant women. Postexposure prophylaxis includes doxycycline or ciprofloxacin. No licensed plague vaccine is currently in production. A previous licensed vaccine was used in the past. It only offered protection against bubonic plague but not aerosolized *Yersinia pestis*. The plague bacterium secretes several virulence factors (Fraction 1 (F1) and V (virulence) proteins) that as subunit proteins are immunogenic and possess protective properties. Recently, an F1-V antigen (fusion protein) vaccine developed by USAMRIID provided 100% protection in monkeys against high-dose aerosol challenge. There is no passive immunoprophylaxis (i.e., immune globulin) available for pre- or postexposure of plague (USAMRIID 2014).

Use of standard precautions for patients with bubonic and septicemic plague is indicated. Suspected pneumonic plague will require strict isolation with respiratory

Table 5.23 Recommended therapy and prophylaxis in children for diseases associated with bioterrorism

Disease	Therapy or prophylaxis	Treatment[a], agent and dosage
Smallpox	Therapy	Supportive care
	Prophylaxis	Vaccination may be effective if given with the first several days after exposure
Plague	Therapy	Gentamicin 2.5 mg/kg IV q8 h *or* Streptomycin 15 mg/kg IM q12 h (max 2 g/day, although only available for compassionate usage and in limited supply) *or* Doxycycline 2.2 mg/kg IV q12 h (max 200 mg/day) *or* Ciprofloxacin[b] 15 mg/kg IV q12 h *or* Levofloxacin 10–15 mg/kg IV q24 h *or* Chloramphenicol[c] 25 mg/kg q6 h (max 4 g/day)
	Prophylaxis	Doxycycline 2.2 mg/kg PO q12 h *or* Ciprofloxacin[b] 20 mg/kg PO q12 h
Tularemia	Therapy	Same as for plague
	Prophylaxis	Same as for plague
Botulism	Therapy	Supportive care, antitoxin and/or botulism immune globulin may halt progression of symptoms but are unlikely to reverse them
	Prophylaxis	None
Viral hemorrhagic fevers	Therapy	Supportive care, ribavirin may be beneficial in select cases[d]
	Prophylaxis	None

Used with permission from Society of Critical Care Medicine
References: (Berger and Burns 2012; Cieslak and Henretig 2016; Markenson and Redlener 2007; Pittman et al. 2018; USAMRIID 2014)
[a]In a mass casualty setting, parenteral therapy might not be possible. In such cases, oral therapy (with analogous agents) may need to be used
[b]Ofloxacin (and possibly other quinolones) may be acceptable alternatives to ciprofloxacin or levofloxacin; however, they are not approved for use in children
[c]Concentration should be maintained between 5 and 20 μg/mL. Some experts have recommended that chloramphenicol be used to treat patients with plague meningitis, because chloramphenicol penetrates the blood-brain barrier. Use in children younger than 2 may be associated with adverse reactions but might be warranted for serious infections
[d]Ribavirin is recommended for arenavirus or bunyavirus infections and may be indicated for a viral hemorrhagic fever of an unknown etiology although not FDA approved for these indications. For intravenous therapy use a loading dose: 30 kg IV once (max dose, 2 g), then 16 mg/kg IV q6 h for 4 days (max dose, 1 g), and then 8 mg/kg IV q8 h for 6 days (max dose, 500 mg). In a mass casualty setting, it may be necessary to use oral therapy. For oral therapy, use a loading dose of 30 mg/kg PO once, then 15 mg/kg/day PO in 2 divided doses for 10 days

droplet precautions for at least 48 h after initiation of effective antimicrobial therapy, or until sputum cultures are negative in confirmed cases. An N-95 respirator should be used for baseline protection (Table 5.25). It is also recommended to use an N-95 respirator or PAPR for high risk procedures (Beigel and Sandrock 2009; Carbone 2005; Centers for Disease Control and Prevention 2017; Centers for Disease Control and Prevention 2018b; Pittman et al. 2018; USAMRIID 2014).

5.7.4 Viral Hemorrhagic Fevers

Viral hemorrhagic fever has a variety of causative agents. However, the syndromes they produce are characterized by fever and bleeding diathesis. The etiologies include RNA viruses from four distinct families: Arenaviridae, Bunyaviridae, Filoviridae, and Flaviviridae. The Filoviridae (includes Ebola and Marburg) and Arenaviridae (includes Lassa fever and New World viruses) are Category A agents. Based on multiple identified characteristics, there is strong concern for the weaponization potential of the viral hemorrhagic fevers. Specifically, there has been demonstration of high contagiousness in aerosolized primate models.

There are five identified Ebola species, but only four are known to cause disease in humans. The natural reservoir host of Ebola virus remains unknown. However, on the basis of evidence and the nature of similar viruses, researchers believe that the virus is animal-borne and that bats are the most likely reservoir. Four of the five virus strains occur in an animal host native to Africa. Marburg virus has a single species. Geographic distribution of Ebola and Marburg is Africa (Fitzgerald et al. 2016). Both diseases are very similar clinically. Incubation period is typically 5–10 days with a range of 2–16 days. Symptoms may include fever, chills, headache, myalgia, nausea, and vomiting. There is rapid progression to prostration, stupor, and hypotension. The onset of a maculopapular rash on the arms and trunk is classic. Disseminated intravascular coagulation and thrombocytopenia develops with conjunctival injection, petechiae, hemorrhage, and soft tissue bleeding. There is a possible central nervous system and hepatic involvement. Bleeding, uncompensated shock, and multiorgan failure are seen. High viral load early in course is associated with poor prognosis. Death usually occurs during the second week of illness. Mortality rate of Marburg is 25–85% and for Ebola 50–90%.

In a retrospective cohort study of children during the 2014/2105 Ebola outbreak in Liberia and Sierra Leone (all less than 18 years with a median age of 7 years with one-third less than 5 years of age), the most common features upon presentation were fever, weakness, anorexia, and diarrhea. About 20% were initially afebrile. Bleeding was rare upon initial presentation. The overall case fatality rate was 57%. Factors associated with death included children less than 5 years of age, bleeding at any time during hospitalization, and high viral load (Smit et al. 2017). In another retrospective cohort study of children at two Ebola centers in Sierra Leone in 2014 (all less than 5 years of age), presenting symptoms included weakness, fever, anorexia, diarrhea, and cough. About 25% were afebrile on presentation. The case fatality rate was higher in children less than 2 years (76%) versus 2–5 years of age (46%) and 9 times more likely to die if child had a higher viral load. Signs associated with death included fever, emesis, and diarrhea. Interestingly, hiccups, bleeding, and confusion were only observed in children who died (Shah et al. 2016).

Lassa virus and New World viruses (Junin, Machupo, Sabia, and Guanarito) are transmitted from person-to-person. The vector in nature is the rodent. The incubation period is from 5 to 16 days. The geographical distribution is West Africa and South America, respectively. The South American hemorrhagic fevers are quite similar but differ from Lassa fever. The onset of the South American viruses is insidious and results in high fever and constitutional symptoms. Petechiae or vesicular enanthem with conjunctival injection is common. These fevers are associated with neurologic disease (hyporeflexia, gait abnormalities, and cerebellar dysfunction). Seizures portend a poor prognosis. Mortality ranges from 15% to over 30%. On the contrary, Lassa viruses are mild. Less than 10% of infections result in severe disease. Signs include chest pain, sore throat, and proteinuria. Hemorrhagic disease is uncommon. Other features include neurologic disease such as encephalitis, meningitis, cerebellar disease, and cranial nerve VIII deafness (common feature). Mortality can be as high as 25%.

Differential diagnoses include malaria, meningococcemia, hemolytic uremic syndrome, thrombotic thrombocytopenic purpura, and typhoid fever. Diagnosis is through detection of the viral antigen testing by ELISA or viral isolation by culture at the CDC. No specific therapy is present and generally involves supportive care, especially mechanical ventilation strategies for ARDS, hemodynamic support, and renal replacement therapy. For the Arenaviridae and Bunyaviridae groups, ribavirin may be indicated (Table 5.24). For Ebola, there has been anecdotal success with immune serum transfusion. Additional potential therapies under investigation include favipiravir (Ebola), BCX4430 (Ebola, Marburg, and other viral hemorrhagic fevers), interferons (IFN α-2b or IFN-β for viral hemorrhagic fevers), and small molecule therapeutics (antisense phosphorodiamidate morpholino oligomers [AVI-6002, AVI-6003] and lipid nanoparticle/small interfering RNA [TKM-Ebola]) (Pittman et al. 2018).

There is no current vaccine for Ebola that is licensed by the FDA. An experimental vaccine called rVSV-ZEBOV was found to be highly protective against Ebola virus in a trial conducted by the World Health Organization (WHO) and other international partners in Guinea in 2015. FDA licensure for the vaccine is expected in 2019. Until then, 300,000 doses have been committed for an emergency use stockpile under the appropriate regulatory mechanism in the event and an outbreak occurs before FDA approval is received (Centers for Disease Control and Prevention 2019b; Henao-Restrepo et al. 2015). Another Ebola vaccine candidate, the recombinant adenovirus type-5 Ebola vaccine, was evaluated in a phase 2 trial in Sierra Leone in 2015. An immune response was stimulated by this vaccine within 28 days of vaccination and

Table 5.24 Recommended ribavirin dosing for treatment of viral hemorrhagic fevers[a]

		Intravenous	Oral
Adults	Loading dose	30 mg/kg IV (max 2 g once)	2000 mg PO once
	Maintenance dose	Day 1–4: 16 mg/kg IV (max 1 g) q6 h for 4 days Day 5–7: 8 mg/kg IV (max 500 mg) q8 for 6 days	Weight > 75 kg: 600 mg PO BID for 10 days Weight < 75 kg: 400 mg PO qAM, 600 mg PO in PM for 10 days
Children	Loading dose	Same as adult	30 mg/kg PO once
	Maintenance dose	Same as adult	7.5 mg/kg PO BID for 10 days

[a]For confirmed or suspected arenavirus or bunyvirus or viral hemorrhagic fever of unknown etiology (USAMRIID 2014)

Table 5.25 Isolation precautions for critical biologic agents of terrorism

Disease	Isolation precautions
Anthrax (inhalational)	Standard
Plague (pneumonic)	Droplet (for first 3 days of therapy)
Tularemia	Standard
Smallpox	Airborne plus contact
Botulism	Standard
Viral hemorrhagic fevers	Contact (consider airborne in cases of massive hemorrhage)

References: (Centers for Disease Control and Prevention 2019a; Cieslak and Henretig 2016)

the response decreased over 6 months after injection. Research on this vaccine is ongoing (Centers for Disease Control and Prevention 2019b; Zhu et al. 2017).

Strict contact precautions (hand hygiene, double gloves, gowns, shoe and leg coverings, and face shield or goggles) and droplet precautions (private room or cohorting, surgical mask within 3 ft) are mandatory for viral hemorrhagic fevers. Airborne precautions (negative-pressure isolation room with 6–12 air exchanges per h) should also be instituted to the maximum extent possible and especially for procedures that induce aerosols (e.g., bronchoscopy). At a minimum, a fit-tested, HEPA filter-equipped respirator (e.g., an N-95 mask) should be used, but a battery-powered PAPR or a positive pressure-supplied air respirator should be considered for personnel sharing an enclosed space with, or coming within 6 ft of, the patient. Multiple patients should be cohorted in a separate ward or building with a dedicated air-handling system when feasible (Table 5.25). Environmental decontamination is accomplished with hypochlorite or phenolic disinfectants (Beigel and Sandrock 2009; Radoshitzky et al. 2018; USAMRIID 2014; Won and Carbone 2005).

5.7.5 Tularemia (*Francisella tularensis*)

Francisella tularensis, a small aerobic, nonmotile gram-negative coccobacillus, causes tularemia (rabbit fever). Clinical disease is caused by two isolates, Biovars Jellison Type A and B. This organism can be stabilized for weaponization and delivered in a wet or dry form. The incubation period is usually 3–6 days (range 1–21 days). Initial symptoms are nonspecific and mimic the flu-like symptoms or other upper respiratory tract infections. There is acute onset of fever with chills, myalgias, cough, fatigue, and sore throat. The two clinical forms of tularemia are typhoidal and ulceroglandular diseases.

Typhoidal tularemia (5–15%) occurs after inhalational exposure and sometimes intradermal or gastrointestinal exposures. There is abrupt onset of fever, headache, malaise, myalgias, and prostration. It presents without lymphadenopathy. Nausea, vomiting, and abdominal pain are sometimes present. Untreated, there is a 35% mortality rate in naturally acquired cases (vs. 1–3% in those treated). It is higher if pneumonia is present. This form would be most likely seen during an aerosol release of the agent.

Ulceroglandular tularemia (75–85%) occurs through skin or mucus membrane inoculation. There is abrupt onset of fever, chills, headache, cough, and myalgias along with a painful papule at the site of exposure. The papule becomes a painful ulcer with tender regional lymph nodes. Skin ulcers have heaped up edges. In 5–10%, there is focal lymphadenopathy without an apparent ulcer. Lymph nodes may become fluctuant and drain when receiving antibiotics. Without treatment, they may persist for months or even years.

In some cases (1–2%), the primary entry port is the eye leading to oculoglandular tularemia. Patients have unilateral, painful, and purulent conjunctivitis with local lymphadenopathy. Chemosis, periorbital edema, and small nodular granulomatous lesions or ulceration may be found. Oropharyngeal tularemia with pharyngitis may occur in 25% of patients. Findings include exudative pharyngitis/tonsillitis, ulceration, and painful cervical lymphadenopathy. The differential diagnosis is antibiotic unresponsive pharyngitis, infectious mononucleosis, and viral pharyngitis. Pulmonary involvement (47–94%) is seen in naturally occurring disease. It ranges from mild to fulminant. Various processes include pneumonia, bronchiolitis, cavitary lesions, bronchopleural fistulas, and chronic granulomatous diseases. Left untreated, 60% will die.

Differential diagnoses include those for typhoidal (typhoid fever, rickettsia, and malaria) or pneumonic (plague, mycoplasma, influenza, Q-fever, and staphylococcal enterotoxin B) tularemia. Diagnosis should be considered when there is a cluster of nonspecific, febrile, systemically ill patients who rapidly progress to fulminant pneumonitis. Tularemia can be diagnosed by recovering the organism from sputum (PCR or DFA) or serology at a state health laboratory. Chest radiograph is nonspecific with possible hilar adenopathy. Treatment is streptomycin or gentamicin (Table 5.23). Alternatives include doxycycline, ciprofloxacin, or chloramphenicol. A live-attenuated vaccine (NDBR 101) exists and typically used for laboratory personnel working with *Francisella tularensis*. There is no passive immunoprophylaxis. Ciprofloxacin or doxycycline can be given as pre- and postexposure prophylaxis (Beigel and Sandrock 2009; Hepburn et al. 2018; Pittman et al. 2018; USAMRIID 2014).

5.7.6 Botulinum Toxin (*Clostridium botulinum*)

Botulinum neurotoxins (BoNT) are produced from the spore-forming, Gram-positive, obligate anaerobe *Clostridium botulinum*. It is the most potent toxin known to man. A lethal dose is 1 ng per kilogram. It is 100,000 times more toxic than sarin (GB). There are seven serotypes of botulinum toxin (A through G). A new serotype (H) has been tentatively identified in a case of infant botulism but has not been fully investigated. Most common are serotypes A, B, and E. The toxin acts on the presynaptic nerve terminal of the neuromuscular junction and cholinergic autonomic synapses. This disrupts neurotransmission and leads to clinical findings. There are three forms of botulism: foodborne, wound, and intestinal (infant or adult intestinal). Botulinum toxin can also be released as an act of bioterrorism via ingestion or aerosol forms.

Incubation can be from 12 h after exposure to several days later. Clinical findings of botulism include cranial nerve palsies such as ptosis, diplopia, and dysphagia. This is followed by symmetric descending flaccid paralysis. However, the victim remains afebrile, alert, and oriented. Death is typically due to respiratory failure. Prolonged respiratory support is often required (1–3 months).

Differential diagnoses include Guillain-Barre syndrome, myasthenia gravis, tick paralysis, stroke, other intoxications (nerve gas, organophosphates), inflammatory myopathy, congenital and hereditary myopathies, and hypothyroidism. Diagnosis is mostly clinical. Laboratory confirmation can be obtained by bioassay of patient's serum. Other assays include immunoassays for bacterial antigen, PCR for bacterial DNA, and reverse transcriptase-PCR for mRNA to detect active synthesis of toxin. Cerebrospinal fluid demonstrates normal protein (unlike Guillain-Barre syndrome). EMG reveals augmentation of muscle action potential with repetitive nerve stimulation at 20–30 Hz.

Treatment (Table 5.23) is mainly supportive including intubation and ventilator support. Tracheostomy may be required due to prolonged respiratory weakness and failure. Antibiotics do not play a role in treatment. Botulism Antitoxin Heptavalent [A, B, C, D, E, F, G]-Equine (BAT) was approved by the FDA in 2013. BAT was developed at USAMRIID as one of two equine-derived heptavalent BoNT antitoxins. BAT is approved to treat individuals with symptoms of botulism following a known or suspected exposure. It has the potential to cause hypersensitivity reactions in those sensitive to equine proteins. The safety of BAT in pregnant and lactating women is unknown. Evidence regarding safety and efficacy in the pediatric population is limited. In 2003, the FDA approved Botulinum Immune Globulin Intravenous (BabyBIG), a human botulism immune globulin derived from pooled plasma of adults immunized with pentavalent botulinum toxoid. It is indicated for the treatment of infants with botulism from toxin serotypes A and B. Immediately after clinical diagnosis of botulism, adults (including pregnant women) and children should receive a single intravenous infusion of antitoxin (BAT or, for infants with botulism from serotypes A or B, BabyBIG) to prevent further disease progression. The administration of antitoxin should not be delayed for laboratory testing to confirm the diagnosis. The pentavalent toxoid vaccine (previously for protection against A, B, C, D, and E; but not F or G) is no longer available as of 2011. No replacement vaccine is currently available. Standard isolation precautions (Table 5.25) should be followed (Beigel and Sandrock 2009; Dembek et al. 2018; Pittman et al. 2018; Timmons and Carbone 2005; USAMRIID 2014).

5.7.7 Ricin (from *Ricinus communis*)

Ricin is a potent cytotoxin derived from the castor bean plant *Ricinus communis*. It is related in structure and function to Shiga toxins and Shiga-like toxin of *Shigella dysenteriae* and *Escherichia coli*, respectively. It consists of two glycoprotein subunits, A and B, connected by a disulfide bond. The B-chain allows the toxin to bind to cell receptors and gain entrance into the cell. Once ricin enters the cell, the disulfide chemical linkage is broken. The free A chain then acts as an enzyme and inactivates ribosomes thereby disrupting normal cell function. Cells are incapable of survival and soon die. Ricin has a high terrorist potential due to it characteristics: readily available, ease of extraction, and notoriety (Maman and Yehezkelli 2005).

Three modes of exposure exist: oral, inhalation, and injection. Four to eight hours after inhalation exposure, the victim develops fever, chest tightness, cough, dyspnea, nausea, and arthralgias. Airway necrosis and pulmonary capillary leak ensues within 18–24 h. This is followed quickly by severe respiratory distress, ARDS, and death due to hypoxemia within 36–72 h. Injection may cause minimal pulmonary vascular leak. Pain at the site and local lymphadenopathy may occur. However, it may be followed by nausea, vomiting, and gastrointestinal hemorrhage. Ingestion leads to necrosis of the gastrointestinal mucosa, hemorrhage, and organ necrosis (spleen, liver, and kidney).

Diagnosis is suspected when multiple cases of acute lung injury occur in a geographic cluster. Serum and respiratory secretions can be checked for antigen using ELISA. Pulmonary intoxication is managed by mechanical ventilation. Gastrointestinal toxicity is managed by gastric lavage and use of cathartics. Activated charcoal has little value due to the size of ricin molecules. Supportive care is indicated for injection exposure. In general, treatment is largely supportive, especially for pulmonary edema that can result from the capillary leak. There is no vaccine available or prophylactic antitoxin for human use. However, there are two ricin vaccines in the development that focus on the ricin toxin A (RTA) chain subunit. A mutant recombinant RTA chain vaccine, RiVax, has been shown to be safe and immunogenic in humans. The other vaccine is another recombinant RTA chain vaccine, RVEc (RTA 1–33/44–198). It has shown effectiveness in animal models by producing protective immunity against aerosol challenge with ricin in animal models. Standard precautions are advised for health care workers (Pittman et al. 2018; Roxas-Duncan et al. 2018; Traub 2005; USAMRIID 2014).

5.8   Radiological/Nuclear

Recent events which include the nuclear reactor meltdown at Fukushima and international tension between nuclear powers, spark concern over potential devastation from nuclear catastrophes. There are numerous examples of radiation disasters in history. Sixty-six thousand people were killed in Hiroshima and thirty-nine thousand people were killed in Nagasaki from nuclear bombs detonated over these cities in 1945 (Avalon Project—Documents in Law, History and Diplomacy n.d.). Many other people suffered from long-term consequences of radiation poisoning. In 1986, 21,000 square kilometers of land in Russia, Ukraine, and Belarus were contaminated with radiation from a meltdown at a nuclear power plant in Chernobyl, Ukraine. One hundred and thirty-five thousand people were permanently evacuated from their homes (Likhtarev et al. 2002). Long-term health consequences included many children who developed thyroid cancer several years later. Many of these children died.

A tsunami pummeled the east coast of Japan in March of 2011. The power outage that ensued at the Fukushima power plant led to a failure of the cooling system of the fuel rods, leading to a meltdown of four of the reactors at the plant. A massive quantity of radiation was released into the atmosphere, forcing people to evacuate their homes indefinitely. Creative thinking and heroic actions by the Tokyo fire department prevented entire populations of cities from being poisoned with radiation.

Terrorism experts are concerned that terrorist organizations will produce and detonate a radiological dispersion device (RDD), sometimes referred to as a dirty bomb. This is a conventional explosive, loaded with radioactive material which would be dispersed upon detonation. This would likely involve only one radioisotope. Fewer people would be exposed and a smaller area would be contaminated than what would transpire with the detonation of a nuclear weapon. Spreading fear and panic would be the primary purpose of such a device (Mettler Jr and Voelz 2002).

5.8.1 Principles of Ionizing radiation

Radiation is the emission and propagation of energy through space or through a medium in the form of waves. Radiation can be ionizing or nonionizing depending on the amount of energy released. Most radiation that people encounter is low energy and, therefore, nonionizing with no biological effects. Ionizing radiation emits enough energy to strip electrons from an atom, which provokes cellular changes and thereby, results in biological effects. Radiation emitted from nuclear decay is always ionizing (Radiation Emergency Assistance Center/Training Site (REACT/S-CDC) 2006).

Atomic nuclei are held together by a very powerful binding energy despite positively charged protons repelling each other. This energy is released from unstable nuclei in the form of electromagnetic waves or particles. When ionizing radiation reaches biological tissue, chemical bonds are disrupted, free radicals are produced, and DNA is broken.

Electromagnetic waves are of two types, X-rays and gamma rays. X-rays are relatively low energy and less penetrating. Gamma rays have a shorter wavelength and contain relatively higher energy, making them more penetrating of biological tissue. Ionizing radiation in the form of particles consists of alpha particles, beta particles, and neutrons. Alpha particles are the largest of the forms of particulate radiation. They are composed of two neutrons and two protons. They do not easily penetrate solid surfaces, including clothes and skin. However, they can cause severe damage to an organism if internalized. In 2006, in the United Kingdom, Alexander Litvienko, an ex KGB agent was poisoned with a radioactive element called polonium (McPhee and Leikin 2009). A small amount of polonium was sprinkled into his food. Polonium releases alpha particles when it decays. It was relatively safe for the assassin to carry this element with him because of the relatively poor ability of alpha particles to penetrate clothing and skin. Once it is ingested, however, alpha particles have profound biological effects. Mr. Litvienko became very ill, and ultimately died.

Beta particles are high energy electrons discharged from the nucleus and are highly penetrating. Neutrons emitted from a nucleus are also highly penetrating. In general, neutrons are only released by the detonation of a nuclear weapon.

Ionizing radiation of any form cannot be detected by our senses. It is not smelled, felt by touch, tasted, or seen. It is possible to be exposed to a lethal dose of radiation without realizing it. In Goiania, Brazil, in 1987, children found a canister of radio-active Cesium (^{137}Cs) that had been looted from a medical center and left in the street. The children liked the appearance of the substance but were not able to sense any abnormalities or danger with it. They began to rub it on their bodies because they liked the way it made them glow in the dark. The children all became ill. Ultimately, 250 people were exposed to this radioisotope. It took 10 days before physicians recognized that the people had radiation poisoning. Four people died of acute radiation syndrome.

Four factors determine the severity of exposure to ionizing radiation: time, distance, dose, and shielding. Time is the time of exposure to the radiation source. Distance is the distance from the radiation source. Based on the inverse square law, exposure is reduced exponentially with increasing distance from the radiation source. Dose is measured by the amount of energy released by the source and is numerically described by how many disintegrations per second occur, in Curies (Ci) or Becquerels (Bq). Shielding is the efficacy of the barrier to the radioactive source. Lead is well-known to be a very effective shield to X-rays. In a radiation exposure, injury to skin from trauma or burns may cause a greater degree of contamination because of loss of the shielding of the skin.

There are four important principles for the nurse or HCP to understand with regard to exposure to ionizing radiation: external exposure, external contamination, internal contamination, and incorporation. External contamination occurs when radioactive material is carried on a person after exposure. This person can then con-taminate others. Removing contaminated clothing eliminates 90% of the toxin. Others are then less vulnerable to exposure. Internal contamination is when a radio-active substance enters the body through inhalation, ingestion, or translocation through open skin. Incorporation is internalization of the toxin into body organs. Incorporation is dependent on the chemical and not the radiological properties of the radioactive toxin. Radioactive iodine, ^{131}I, is taken up by the thyroid gland because iodine enters the gland as part of normal physiology (Advanced Hazmat Life Support (AHLS) 2003).

5.8.2   Biological and Clinical Effects

Ionizing radiation can damage chromosomes directly and indirectly, causing ravaging biological effects. Indirect damage comes from the production of H^+ and OH^-. Free radical formation upsets biochemical processes and causes inflammation. These effects can take anywhere from seconds to hours to be expressed. Clinical changes can take from hours to years to be realized (Zajtchuk et al. 1989).

Immediately after a major radiation exposure, the clinical matters of most concern are those related to trauma from blast and thermal injuries. These injuries may be life-threatening and must be addressed first.

After thermal and traumatic injuries are addressed, attention should be paid to the severity of radiation exposure. Severe exposure can cause acute radiation syndrome. "The acute radiation syndrome is a broad term used to describe a range of signs and symptoms that reflect severe damage to specific organ systems and that can lead to death within hours or up to several months after exposure" (National Council on Radiation Protection (NCRP) and Measurements 2001; National Council on Radiation Protection (NCRP) and Measurements 2009). The mechanism of cell death from toxic radiation exposure is related to the inhibition of mitosis. Organs with the most rapidly dividing cells are the most susceptible. The gastrointestinal and the hematopoietic are the organ systems most notably affected. The organs of pediatric patient have a higher mitotic index, in general, to those of adults and are more vulnerable to injury from radiation poisoning. The time of onset and the severity of acute radiation syndrome are controlled by the total radiation dose, the dose rate, percent of total body exposed, and associated thermal and traumatic injuries. There is a 50% death rate (LD_{50}) within 60 days for people exposed to a dose of radiation of 2.5–4.0 Gy. The LD_{50} is lower for the pediatric population.

The acute radiation syndrome is composed of four phases: prodromal, latent, manifest illness, and death or recovery. Inflammatory mediator release during the prodromal phase causes damage to cell membranes. This phase occurs during the first 48 h after exposure to radiation. Nausea and vomiting and fever can occur during this time. If these symptoms occur during the first 2 h after exposure, there is a poor prognosis.

The onset of the latent phase is usually in the first 4 days post exposure but can ensue anytime during the first 21 days thereafter. All cell lines of the hematopoietic system are affected. Lymphocytes and platelets, the most rapidly dividing cells of the bone marrow, are most severely affected.

The illness phase manifests after 30 days since radiation exposure. Infection, impaired wound healing, anemia, and bleeding occur during this time of illness. The hematopoietic, gastrointestinal, central nervous, and integumentary are the organ systems affected. There is a marked reduction of cells from all cell lines of the bone marrow. There is a direct correlation with the drop in absolute lymphocyte count with the dose of radiation received. The absolute lymphocyte count is commonly used to estimate the dose of radiation received.

The gastrointestinal (GI) epithelial lining, one of the most rapidly dividing cell lines of the body is the second most vulnerable to radiation poisoning. The radiation dose required to affect the GI system is 8 Gy. Vomiting, diarrhea, and a capillary leak syndrome for GI tract are common manifestations. Hypovolemia and electrolyte instability ensue. Translocation of bacteria into the bloodstream, combined with the diminished immunity caused by the decimation of the hematopoietic system, place victims at high risk for septic shock.

Another organ system affected by the acute radiation syndrome is the central nervous system. This requires a large dose of at least 30 Gy. Manifestations include cerebral edema, disorientation, hyperthermia, seizures, and coma. Acute radiation syndrome that involves the central nervous system is always fatal.

The integumentary system is frequently affected by the acute radiation syndrome, especially if the skin is in direct contact with a radioisotope. Epilation, erythema, dry desquamation, wet desquamation, and necrosis occur respectively with increasing severity associated with increasing doses of radiation. Radiation burns can be distinguished from thermal or chemical burns by their delayed onset. It can take days to weeks for radiation burns to affect victims. Thermal and chemical burns cause signs and symptoms more acutely.

5.8.3 Immediate Clinical Management

Hospitals that anticipate victims of radiation should prepare areas of triage with decontamination supplies and techniques ready to be deployed. An Emergency Department (ED) should be divided into "clean" and "dirty" areas. The dirty area is created for the purpose of decontamination to prevent the spread of radioisotopes.

All health care personnel should wear PPE including surgical scrubs and gowns, face shields, shoe covers, caps, and two pairs of gloves. The inner pair of gloves is taped to the sleeves of the gown. Each health care worker should be monitored for the exposure of the radiation and its dose with a dosimeter worn underneath the gown. The radiation safety officer of the hospital should take a leadership role in health care worker protection and decontamination procedures. Consultation from the Radiation Emergency, Assistance Center (REACT/TS) is imperative. REACT/TS is a subsidiary of the U.S. Department of Energy. Its contact information is as follows:

Phone number during business hours is 865-576-3131. The phone number is 865-576-1005 after business hours. The REACT/TS website is http://orise.orau.gov/reac/ts/.

As victims arrive, triage protocols of mass casualty scenarios should be implemented. It should be noted that radiation exposure is not "immediately" life-threatening. Initial clinical management should focus on the ABCDE (Airway, Breathing, Circulation, Disability, and Exposure) of basic trauma protocol. The "D" in the above acronym can also be a symbol for decontamination. After airway, breathing, and circulation are addressed, initial phase of decontamination entails careful removal of potentially contaminated clothing. Caution should be exercised to remove the clothing gently, while rolling garments outward to prevent the release of dust of radioactive material that could contaminate people in the treatment area. Further decontamination procedures take place after initial stabilization.

Skin decontamination procedures are identical to those of toxic chemical exposure with the following exceptions:

- PPE are slightly different as described above.
- Gentle skin rubbing is done to prevent provocation of an inflammatory response and further absorption of the radioactive toxin.

- Only soap and water are used. Rubbing alcohol and bleach should be avoided. It is advisable to shampoo the hair first, because it is usually the site of the highest level of contamination of the body, and runoff onto the body can then be cleansed during skin decontamination (Radiation Event Medical Management (REMM) of the U.S. Dept. of Health and Human Services n.d.).

It should be noted that health care workers are not at risk for contamination if they wear proper PPE during the resuscitation and decontamination process. The lack of knowledge of this point may lead to reluctance to treat patients and increase morbidity and mortality for victims. "No HCP has ever received a significant dose of radiation from handling, treating, and managing patients with radiation injuries and/or contamination."(REACT/S-CDC 2006).

5.8.4 Ongoing Clinical Management

When initial resuscitation and decontamination have been completed, attention should be paid to ongoing support of ventilation, oxygenation, the management of fluid and electrolytes, and treatment of traumatic and burn injuries. Infection control procedures are important due to the impending immunocompromised state of the victims.

It is important to ascertain the details of the catastrophic event. Data on the nature and size of the exposure and the types of radioactive agents involved are vital for ongoing management and decontamination.

After the details of the nature of the exposure are uncovered, diagnostic tests should be done, including serial CBC and cytogenetic analysis of lymphocytes, otherwise known as cytogenic dosimetry (REACT/S-CDC 2006). Measurements of change in lymphocyte counts and cytogenetic dosimetry are sensitive markers for the dose of radiation received by a victim. Measurements of internal decontamination are done by the sampling and analysis of nasal and throat swabs, stool, and 24 h urine. Wound samples and irrigation fluid should also be sampled.

5.8.5 Treatment of Internal Contamination

After initial stabilization, external decontamination, and diagnostic testing, internal decontamination is performed. External decontamination involves removal of clothes and cleaning the skin and hair. Internal decontamination removes radioisotopes that are internalized via inhalation, ingestion, and entry into open wounds. Because ionizing radiation is being released inside the body, internal decontamination must be performed promptly after initial resuscitation. Since radioisotopes behave identically to their nonradioactive counterparts, antidotes are chosen based on the chemical, and not the radiological properties of the element. Basic strategies of internal decontamination include chelation, competitive inhibition, enhanced gastrointestinal elimination, and enhanced renal elimination.

Specific agents are used for chelation of different radioisotopes. DTPA (diethyen-etriaminepentaacetic acid) is administered for the elimination of heavy metals such as americium, californium, curium, and plutonium. DTPA comes in two forms, Calcium DTPA (Ca-DTPA) and Zinc-DTPA (Zn-DTPA). Ca-DTPA is ten times more effective than Zn-DTPA. For adults and adolescents, administration is as follows:

- 1 g of Ca-DTPA IV initially in the first 24 h, followed by 1 g Zn-DTPA IV daily for maintenance.
- For children less than 12 years of age administer:
- Fourteen mg/kg Ca-DTPA IV initially, followed by fourteen mg/kg of Zn-DTPA IV daily thereafter (National Council on Radiation Protection (NCRP) and Measurements 2009).
- The initial dose of DTPA may be administered via inhalation to adolescents and adults if the contamination occurred via inhalation. This method of administration is not approved for pediatric use.

Chelation with dimercaprol (BAL) is used to eliminate polonium. BAL is a highly toxic drug and should be administered with caution.

The dose is 2.5 mg per kg IM four times a day for 2 days, then twice a day on the third day and once a day for 5–10 days, thereafter (National Council on Radiation Protection (NCRP) and Measurements 2009). Alkalinization of the urine is renal protective during administration. A less toxic alternative to BAL, Dimercaptosuccinic acid (DMSA), otherwise known as Chemet® is also available. The dose of DMSA is ten mg per kg po every 8 h for 5 days. The same dose is given every 12 h for 14 days, thereafter (National Council on Radiation Protection (NCRP) and Measurements 2009).

Another mechanism for internal decontamination is competitive inhibition. The radioisotope, ^{131}I, is released during a meltdown of a reactor at a nuclear power plant. Potassium iodide (KI) is widely recognized as a competitive inhibitor to its radioactive counterpart, ^{131}I, from being incorporated into the thyroid gland. KI blocks 90% of ^{131}I uptake into the thyroid gland if KI is given within the first hour of exposure. It will block 50% of incorporation if given within 5 h of exposure. Its protective effect lasts for 24 h. With administration of this drug, thyroid function should be monitored closely. Dosing guidelines (Table 5.26) are included in the table below (U.S. Food and Drug Administration n.d.).

Gastrointestinal elimination is another mechanism of internal decontamination (Table 5.27). An ion exchanger, Prussian Blue, (ferric ferrocyanide), binds elements that circulate through the enterohepatic cycle. Since it is not absorbed through the gastrointestinal tract, Prussian Blue carries the toxins into the stool. It is highly effective in the elimination of ^{137}Cs or thallium and was used during the ^{137}Cs incident in Goiania, Brazil. The dosing of Prussian Blue is as follows:

- Infants: 0.2–0.3 mg per kg po three times a day (not FDA approved).
- Children 2–12 years of age: 1 g po three times a day.
- Children $\geq$12 years of age: 3 g po three times a day.

Table 5.26 Potassium Iodide (KI) dosing for [131]Iodine contamination

	Predicted thyroid exposure, Gy	KI dose, mg	No. of 130-mg tablets	No. of 65-mg tablets
Adults >40 years	≥5	130	1	2
Adults >18 to 40 years	≥0.1	130	1	2
Pregnant/lactating women	≥0.05	130	1	2
Adolescents >12 to 18 years	≥0.05	65	½	1
Children >3 to 12 years	≥0.05	65	½	1
Children >1 month to 3 years	≥0.05	32	¼	½
Children birth to 1 month	≥0.05	16	1/8	¼

Reproduced with permission from the US Department of Health and Human Services, Food and Drug Administration, Center for Drug Evaluation and Research (U.S. Food and Drug Administration n.d.)

Table 5.27 Table of most common radionuclides and decontamination strategies

Radionuclides	Organ of incorporation	Decontamination strategy	Antidote
Heavy metals: Americium Californium Curium Plutonium	Bone	Chelation	IV Ca-DTPA Or IV Zn-DTPA
Polonium	Total body	Chelation	BAL with IV alkalinization Or IM DMSA
[131]Iodine	Thyroid	Competitive inhibition	PO Potassium Iodide
[137]Cesium	Total body	Enhanced GI elimination	PO Prussian Blue
Tritium	Total body	Enhanced urinary elimination	IV fluids
Uranium	Kidneys, bone	Alkalinization of urine	Sodium Bicarbonate

Doses are included in the text (Jacobson and Severin 2012)

- Prussian Blue is administered for at least 30 days, and can be adjusted based on the degree of poisoning (National Council on Radiation Protection (NCRP) and Measurements 2009).

Urinary elimination is another useful method of internal decontamination. Tritium can be eliminated with excess fluid administration. Uranium is eliminated by alkalinizing the urine to a pH of 8–9. Sodium bicarbonate is given at a dose of 1 mEq/kg IV every 4–6 h and is titrated to effect. If renal injury occurs, dialysis may be required.

5.8.6 Treating Acute Radiation Syndrome

The basic approach to treating acute radiation syndrome is supportive therapy. GI losses from gastrointestinal difficulties are treated with IV fluids and electrolyte replacement. 5-HT3 antagonists can be used to suppress vomiting and benzodiazepines for anxiety. A patient suffering from acute radiation syndrome may be severely immunocompromised and requires a room with positive pressure isolation. Colony stimulating agents for granulocytes and erythrocytes can be used for bone anemia and leukopenia. Bone marrow transplant may be required for severe cases.

5.8.7 Treatment of Local Skin Contamination

A patient with skin contamination with radiation should be decontaminated with soap and water. A Geiger counter can be helpful to identify areas of contamination. Scrubbing is performed in a concentric matter, beginning at the outer layers of contamination and moving into the center since the area of greatest contamination is in the center. In this way, the area of contamination remains contained. Attention should be paid to good nutrition and pain control. Burn and plastic surgery service should also be consulted. More details on decontamination can be found in Chap. 9.

5.8.8 Psychosocial Implications

The psychological impact of a radiation catastrophe on the pediatric victims is likely to be devastating (American Academy of Pediatrics (AAP) 2003). Sleep disturbances, social withdrawal, altered play, chronic fear and anxiety, and developmental regression can occur. A correlation between the parent's psychological response and that of the child would occur as with other types of disaster. Mental health professionals should be consulted in the event of this type of situation. Please refer to Chap. 12 for more information.

5.9 Explosives

A lot of concern has been expressed over the possibility of terrorist attacks involving explosive devices in recent years (DePalma et al. 2005). Explosive devices are relatively simple to manufacture and easy to detonate. They can injure and kill many people and spread fear over large populations. Victims of bomb blasts sustain more body regions injured, have more body injury severity scores, and require more surgeries than victims of nonexplosive trauma incidents. Victims of explosives also have a higher mortality (Kluger et al. 2004). These observations are also true of pediatric victims (Daniel-Aharonson et al. 2003).

Many factors influence the number of people injured and the severity of the injuries in an explosion. The magnitude of the explosion and its proximity to people and the number of people in the area affect the severity and number of injuries. Other factors include the collapse of building or structure from the blast, promptness of the rescue operation, and the caliber and proximity of medical resources in the vicinity. Victims who experience explosions in closed spaces are especially vulnerable to more severe injuries. Twenty-nine case reports of injuries from terrorist bombings were reviewed (Arnold et al. 2004a). The investigators compared the injury severity of victims of explosions who sustained injuries from structural collapse, closed space explosions without structural collapse, and open space explosions. The mortality rate for these victims was 25%, 8%, and 4%, respectively. Hospitalization rates were 25%, 36%, and 15%, respectively. ED visits were 48%, 36%, and 15%, respectively. Victims of closed space explosions without structural collapse experienced greater hospitalizations rates than those involved in a structural collapse, because many of the victims involved in the structural collapse experienced immediate death.

5.9.1 Basics of Explosions

An explosion is defined as a rapid chemical conversion of a liquid or solid into a gas with energy release. Substances that are chemically predisposed to explosion, called explosives, are characterized as low or high order, depending on the speed and magnitude of energy release. Low-order explosives release energy at a relatively slow pace and explosions from these substances tend not to produce large air pressure changes or a "blast." The energy release is caused by combustion, producing heat. The involved material "goes up in flames." Gunpowder, liquid fuel, and Molotov cocktails are examples of low-order explosives (Centers for Disease Control and Prevention 2010). Explosions from high-order materials cause a blast with a pressure wave in addition to causing the release of heat and light. The blast pressure wave causes compression of the surrounding medium which is physically transformed in all directions from the exact point of explosion. When an explosion occurs on land, air is the surrounding medium compressed. In bodies of water, the surrounding medium is water. The degree of medium compression and the distance that the energy wave travels is determined by the magnitude of the explosion. The power of the blast is measured in pounds per square inch (psi). The pressure blast wave has distinctive characteristics. The amplitude of the wave reaches its highest point immediately after the blast. The blast wave then rapidly decays as it travels through space. As the blast wave propagates, and compresses the surrounding medium, it leaves a vacuum because of displaced molecules in the surrounding medium and a negative phase of the wave ensues. In a land explosion, air molecules are displaced by the initial positive pressure, after which a negative pressure occurs in the vacated space. A wave that propagates through a confined space rebounds off of the wall and reverberates. It may interact with victims in the confined space many times, causing more severe injuries (Stuhmiller et al. 1991) (Fig. 5.10).

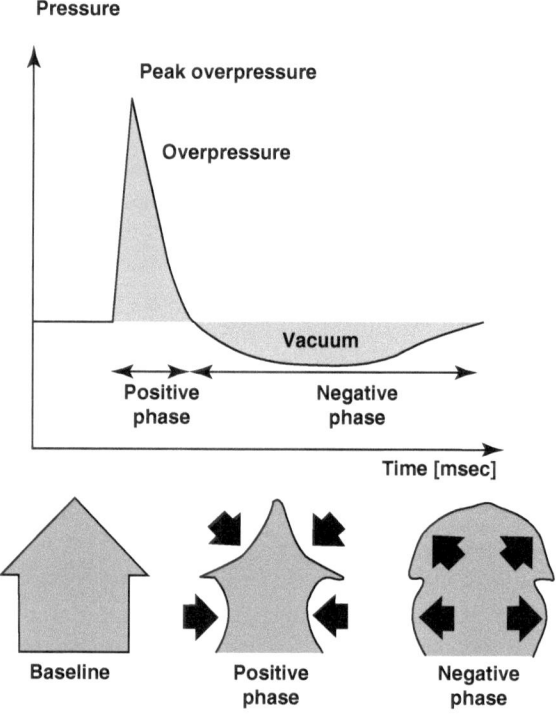

Originally described by Friedlander, a blast wave consists of a short, high-amplitude overpressure peak followed by a longer depression phase. Injury potential depends on the wave's amplitude as well as the slopes of its increase and decrease in pressure. X-axis refers to time and Y-axis refers to pressure.

Fig. 5.10 Blast Wave Physics: Friedlander Blast Wave*. *Used with permission Society of Critical Care Medicine (Jacobson and Severin 2012)

5.9.2 Mechanisms of Injury

Four kinds of injury occur in high energy explosions. Primary blast injuries occur directly from the pressure wave of the blast. Secondary injuries occur from being struck by flying objects from the blast. These injuries can be blunt or penetrating. Tertiary injuries occur when victims are displaced from a location and strike other objects or surfaces. All other injuries related to the blast are called quarternary. They include burns, inhalational injuries, toxic exposures, and traumatic injuries from structural collapse.

5.9.3 Clinical Manifestations of Primary Blast Injuries

Primary injuries from blast waves affect bodily tissues with a tissue gas interface. When a pressure wave enters the body, tissue of gas filled organs compress slower than the air inside the tissue, causing stress in the tissue, possibly damaging it. This also known as the "spalling effect." As the negative pressure phase of the blast wave propagates through, it causes more stress on the tissue and further damage.

In addition to damaging tissues with an air tissue interface, pressure blasts can cause injury to the brain and can lead to limb detachments. Despite the fact that primary blast injuries can be ravaging, they are less common than other types of injury from blasts. The tympanic membranes, lungs, and gastrointestinal tract are the most common organs sustaining injury from pressure waves. The tympanic membrane is the most vulnerable of these three organ systems (DePalma et al. 2005; Garth 1997). Five psi, which is considered a weak blast, will rupture 50% of tympanic membranes. To put this in perspective, C4, a commonly used explosive generates a pressure of four million psi. Otoscopy can reveal ruptured tympanic membranes. Neuropraxia, deafness, tinnitus, and vertigo are symptoms that can be experienced. Severe blast injuries of the ear can result in damage to the organ of Corti, resulting in permanent hearing loss.

The second most common organ injured from a blast wave is the lung. Fifteen psi are required to cause injury to this organ. Lung injuries are more likely to occur from a blast within a closed space, or when victims sustain burns (burns commonly cause acute lung injury from release of inflammatory mediators). Direct alveolar damage, blood vessel with bleeding, and inflammation are the three different manifestations of lung injury from blasts. Alveolar damage can cause pneumothorax and pulmonary interstitial emphysema. When air dissects along the bronchovascular sheath, pneumomediastinum, pneumopericardium, and subcutaneous emphysema can occur. Air that enters the pulmonary venous system can result in a systemic arterial air embolism, and possibly, a stroke. Inflammation of the lungs from direct pressure damage to the tissue, cause acute lung injury and possibly, disseminated intravascular coagulation. Clinical signs of lung injury include tachypnea, chest pain, hypoxia, rales, and dyspnea. If there is vascular disruption, hemoptysis can occur. Air leaks from alveolar injury can result in diminished breath sounds, subcutaneous crepitance, increased resonance, and tracheal deviation. Hemodynamic compromise will occur with tracheal deviation.

Alveolar damage, leading to air in the pulmonary venous system, can lead to a systemic arterial air embolism. Air in the coronary arteries can lead to coronary ischemia with ST and/or T waves changes on ECG. Air embolism to cerebral arteries leads to cerebral vascular accidents (strokes) with focal neurological deficits. Other manifestations of systemic air embolism include mottling of the skin, demarcated tongue blanching, and/or air in the retinal vessels (the most common sign of arterial air embolus). Rapid death after initial survival is most often caused by arterial air embolus. Initiation of positive pressure ventilation may trigger this event (Ho and Ling 1999). A lung injury from a blast can also precipitate a vagal reflex resulting in bradycardia and hypotension. It is postulated that this occurs from the stimulation of C fibers in the lungs (Guy et al. 1998).

The gastrointestinal system is the third most common organ system affected by primary blast injury. Physical stress and/or mesenteric infarct leads to weakening of the bowel wall with possible rupture. Hemorrhage can also occur (Paran et al. 1996; Sharpnack et al. 1991). The most common site of injury is the colon. Injury to the bowel can be delayed and occur up to several days after the inciting incident. Solid organs are spared because of their homogeneity and lack of air tissue interface.

Brain injury is becoming increasingly recognized as a result of primary blast. Shearing injuries of the brain occur as a result of wave reverberation in the skull. Hippocampal injury causing cognitive impairment has been shown in animal studies (Cernak 2017; Cernak et al. 2001; Singer et al. 2005). Observations in humans have revealed electroencephalographic abnormalities and attention deficit disorder (Born 2005). Human autopsies have revealed punctate hemorrhages and disintegration of Nissl substance in victims who sustained blast injury without direct head trauma (Guy et al. 1998).

Research involving Yucatan minipigs revealed that the brain sustains neuronal loss in the hippocampus after being subjected to primary blast injury. Brain injury also occurred from the inflammation that ensued post blast (Goodrich et al. 2016).

Novel therapeutic approaches may be on the horizon for treatment of traumatic brain injury, including that caused by primary blast. Intranasal insulin administered to rats subjected to traumatic brain injury resulted in enhanced neuronal glucose uptake and utilization, and subsequently improved motor function and memory. Decreased neuroinflammation and preservation of the hippocampus were also noted (Brabazon et al. 2017). In a different investigation, a neuroprotective nucleotide, guanosine, was administered to rats subjected to traumatic brain injury. The treatment group of rats had better locomotor and cognitive outcomes than did the placebo group. Programmed cell death and inflammation were also attenuated in the treatment group (Gerbatin et al. 2017).

The leading cause of death from blast is from flying objects striking victims (secondary blast injury). Eyes are particularly vulnerable. Injuries resulting from displacement of the victims who strike objects are known as tertiary injuries. Lighter weight children are particularly susceptible to this type of injury.

Burns, toxic exposures, and crush injuries constitute quaternary injuries. Crush injuries commonly occur in explosions with structural collapse. The "crush syndrome" can occur when a trapped limb sustains prolonged compromise to the circulation, leading to rhabdomyolysis. Tissue destruction and inflammatory response then occur. Life-threatening electrolyte abnormalities including hyperkalemia, renal failure, hyperuricemia, metabolic acidosis, acute respiratory distress syndrome, disseminated intravascular coagulation, and shock can result from crush syndrome (Gonzalez 2005).

The crush syndrome is commonly seen in natural disasters that result in a lot of structural collapse. Structural collapse and fires can cause the release of toxic materials such as carbon monoxide and cyanide.

5.9.4   Clinical Management of Blast Injuries

Knowledge of the details of a blast can greatly enhance the ability of nurses and HCPs to care for victims of a blast in a hospital setting. Knowledge of whether a blast occurred in a closed or open space, whether structural collapse occurred, or if a victim was rescued from a collapsed area are details that can alert nurses and HCPs as to what kind of injuries that they may anticipate. If toxic substances are released with a blast, nurses and HCPs can prepare for decontamination techniques and antidote therapies. It would be advantageous for a hospital to be aware of the number of victims that are arriving for care. A mass casualty incident will stress the resources of the institution. Hospital personnel should take stock of the resources that are available. The number of available ventilators and O-blood are examples of finite resources that should be considered.

Advanced Trauma Life Support (ATLS) principles should be applied to all blast injury victims. ABCD of initial resuscitation is applied. The "D" stands for disability as well as decontamination. Decontamination techniques should be deployed if there is uncertainty about toxic exposure as described elsewhere in this chapter. On completion of ABCD of initial resuscitation a secondary survey is performed, as described by ATLS protocol. Attention should be paid to potential injuries that occur with blast injuries. Ruptured tympanic membranes should alert the nurse or HCP of problems from primary blast injury. Impaled objects should remain in place and removed in the operating room by surgical staff so that bleeding may be controlled. A thoracoscopy tube should be placed with an open three point seal over a wound on the side of the chest with an open pneumothorax. A hemothorax is also treated with a thoracoscopy tube. An autotransfusion setup can be applied to recirculate the blood from the pleural cavity of a hemothorax (Wightman and Gladish 2001) that would help preserve donor blood for other victims.

For severe respiratory distress and/or impending respiratory failure, endotracheal intubation should be performed and positive pressure ventilation should be instituted. Because lung tissue could be weakened from primary blast injury, caution should be exercised because of a high risk of pneumothorax, hemorrhage, or arterial air embolus. Gentle application of positive pressure ventilation should be applied to avoid these complications. If only one lung is injured unilateral lung ventilation can be considered for larger children and adults. This technique is not suitable for babies and small children.

Supplemental oxygen with an FiO_2 of 100% should be administered to patients suspected of having an arterial air embolus. Hyperbaric oxygen therapy could even be considered to help accelerate the removal of air from the arteries. Placement of the patient in the left lateral recumbent position may reduce the likelihood of the air lodging in the coronary arteries.

5.9.5 Postresuscitation Management

Victims of blast injuries should be treated identically to those of other types of trauma after initial resuscitation is completed. If primary blast injury occurred, frequent chest and abdominal X-rays should be performed in consideration of the possibility of lung or gastrointestinal injuries. Limbs with open fractures should be immobilized and covered with sterile dressings. Systemic, broad spectrum antibiotics should be administered to patients with open limb injuries. Eyes that sustained chemical injury should be irrigated with water for an hour. All injured eyes should be covered. Most ruptured tympanic membranes will heal spontaneously. Victims with tympanic membrane injury should be advised to avoid swimming for some time. Topical antibiotics are prescribed if dirt or debris is seen in the ear canal. Oral prednisone is prescribed for hearing loss. Victims with crush injuries should be treated with large volumes of IV fluids to treat inflammatory shock and possibly rhabdomyolysis. Electrolytes should be monitored carefully as these patients are at risk for hyperkalemia, hyperphosphatemia, hyperuricemia, hypocalcemia, and acidosis. Smoke inhalation, burns, and toxic exposures should be treated according to guidelines of burn, trauma, and toxicology protocols.

5.10   Active Shooter

Mass casualty incidents (i.e. mass shootings, active shooter events, bombings, and other multifatality crimes) often attract extensive media coverage as well as the attention of policy makers. Many agencies and organizations record and publish data on these incidents. The measurement and reporting does vary based on the absence of a common definition. However, it is clearly evident that mass casualty incidents (MCIs) continue to increase in both number and scope (Federal Bureau of Investigation 2017; Office for Victims of Crime, Office of Justice Programs, U.S. Department of Justice 2019).

In the U.S., mass shootings are the most common and most closely tracked. The Congressional Research Service (CRS) defines *mass shootings* as events where more than four people are killed with a firearm "within one event, and in one or more locations in close proximity." Congress uses the term *mass killings* and describes these events as "three or more killings in a single incident." The Federal Bureau of Investigation (FBI) uses the term *active shooter*, which it defines as "an individual actively engaged in killing or attempting to kill people in a populated area." It is important to realize that nongovernmental (NGO) organizations (Mother Jones, USA Today, and the Stanford Mass Shootings in America [MSA] data project) use various combinations of these definitions. The exclusion of *gang-* or *drug-related incidents*, the *accidental discharge* of a firearm, or *family-* and *intimate partner-related shootings* further complicates the definition of mass shooting. Mother Jones, the FBI, CRS, the MSA, and Congress do not include these incidents in their definitions, but USA Today does (Office for Victims of Crime, Office of Justice Programs, U.S. Department of Justice 2019).

The FBI has released investigative reports of active shooter events occurring from 2000 to 2013 (Blair and Schweit 2014) as well as 2014 and 2015 (Schweit 2016). In April 2018, the FBI, in collaboration with the Advanced Law Enforcement Rapid Response Training (ALERRT) Center, published a supplemental report reviewing the active shooter incidents in the U.S. for 2016 and 2017. The report revealed striking differences about active shooter incidents from 2016 and 2017 as compared to 2014 and 2015 (Advanced Law Enforcement Rapid Response Training (ALERRT) Center, Texas State University and Federal Bureau of Investigation, U.S. Department of Justice 2018). The report also compared the characteristics of the active shooters from both time periods (Tables 5.28 and 5.29) (Advanced Law Enforcement Rapid Response Training (ALERRT) Center, Texas State University and Federal Bureau of Investigation, U.S. Department of Justice 2018).

Table 5.28 Active shooter incidents in the United States for 2014 and 2015 versus 2016 and 2017[a]

	2014 and 2015	2016 and 2017
Total number of incidents	40 in 26 states	50 in 21 states
Casualties	231 (excluding shooters): 92 killed and 139 wounded	943 (excluding shooters): 221 killed and 722 wounded
Law enforcement officers killed	4 killed, 10 wounded	13 killed, 20 wounded
Met "mass killing" definition	20	20

[a](Advanced Law Enforcement Rapid Response Training (ALERRT) Center, Texas State University and Federal Bureau of Investigation, U.S. Department of Justice 2018)

Table 5.29 Characteristics of the active shooters 2014 and 2015 versus 2016 and 2017[a]

	2014 and 2015	2016 and 2017
Shooters	42: 39 male; 3 female	50 (all male with 17 being teens)
Body armor	2	3
Shooter committed suicide	16	13
Shooter killed by police	14	11
Shooter stopped by citizen	6	8
Shooter apprehended by police	12	18

[a]Reference: (Advanced Law Enforcement Rapid Response Training (ALERRT) Center, Texas State University and Federal Bureau of Investigation, U.S. Department of Justice 2018)

Geographically, the 50 active shooter incidents in 2016 and 2017 occurred in 21 states: six in Texas, five in California and Florida, four in Ohio, three in Maryland and Washington, two in Colorado, Kansas, Nevada, New Mexico, New York, Pennsylvania, Tennessee, Virginia, and Wisconsin, and one in Arizona, Illinois, Louisiana, Michigan, Missouri, and South Carolina. The 50 incidents resulted in 943 casualties (221 people killed and 722 people wounding, excluding shooters). The highest number of casualties (58 killed and 489 wounded) occurred during the Route 91 Harvest Festival in Las Vegas, Nevada, in 2017. The second highest number of casualties (49 killed and 53 wounded) occurred at Pulse, a nightclub in Orlando, Florida, in 2016. The third highest number of casualties (26 killed and 20 wounded) occurred at the First Baptist Church in Sutherland Springs, Texas, in 2017 (Advanced Law Enforcement Rapid Response Training (ALERRT) Center, Texas State University and Federal Bureau of Investigation, U.S. Department of Justice 2018).

Of note, in the 2000–2013 report,(Blair and Schweit 2014) the FBI identified 11 locations where the public was most at risk during an active shooter incident. These location categories include commercial areas (divided into businesses open to pedestrian traffic, businesses closed to pedestrian traffic, and malls), education environments (divided into schools [prekindergarten through 12th grade] and institutions of higher learning), open spaces, government properties (divided into military and other government properties), residences, houses of worship, and health care facilities. For the April 2018 report of 2016 and 2017 active shooter incidents, the

Table 5.30 Summary of active shooter incident locations identified for 2016 and 2017[a]

Location category	Number of incidents	Killed	Wounded
Commercial area	17	85	98
Open space	14	79 (58 in one incident)	540 (489 in one incident)
Educational	7	5	19
Government property	3	8	12
Residencies	2	4	8
Houses of worship	2	27	27
Health care facility	4	7	8
Other location	1	1	1

[a]Reference: (Advanced Law Enforcement Rapid Response Training (ALERRT) Center, Texas State University and Federal Bureau of Investigation, U.S. Department of Justice 2018)

FBI added a new location category, Other Location, to capture events that occurred in venues not included in the 11 previously identified locations (Advanced Law Enforcement Rapid Response Training (ALERRT) Center, Texas State University and Federal Bureau of Investigation, U.S. Department of Justice 2018). The following is a summary of active shooter incident locations identified for 2016 and 2017 (Table 5.30) (Advanced Law Enforcement Rapid Response Training (ALERRT) Center, Texas State University and Federal Bureau of Investigation, U.S. Department of Justice 2018).

Ranking third of all locations for 2016 and 2017, seven of the 50 incidents occurred in educational environments resulting in five killed and 19 wounded. Two incidents occurred in elementary schools, resulting in two killed (including a first-grade student) and eight wounded (one teacher shot, three students shot, and four wounded from shrapnel). One incident occurred in a junior/senior high school, resulting in none killed and four wounded (two from shrapnel, all students). Four incidents occurred at high schools (one outside a school during prom), resulting in three killed (all students) and seven wounded (all students). Fortunately, no incident occurred at institutions of higher learning during 2016 or 2017 (Advanced Law Enforcement Rapid Response Training (ALERRT) Center, Texas State University and Federal Bureau of Investigation, U.S. Department of Justice 2018). Notably, two of the 50 incidents occurred in houses of worship, resulting in 27 killed and 27 wounded. One of these incidents occurred at the First Baptist Church in Sutherland Springs, Texas, and had the third highest number of casualties (26 killed and 20 wounded) in 2017. The dead included 10 women, 7 men, 8 children (7 girls and 1 boy), and an unborn child (Goldman et al. 2017).

A summary report has also been developed for all 250 active shooter incidents from 2000 to 2017, including incidents per year (Fig. 5.11), casualties per year (Fig. 5.12), and location (Fig. 5.13) categories (Federal Bureau of Investigation 2017; Federal Bureau of Investigation 2018). Overall, there was an increase in number of active shooter incidents and casualties per year. Location categories with number of incidents and statistics of their contribution were provided: areas of

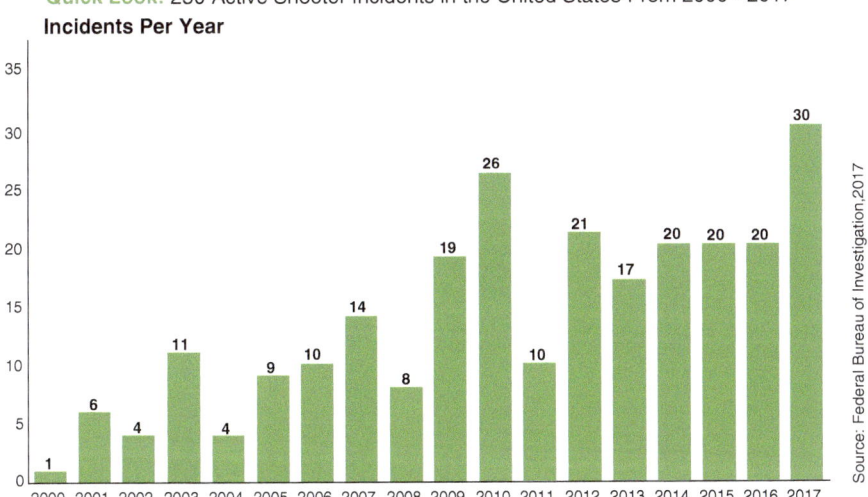

Fig. 5.11 Active shooter incident in United States: Incidents per year

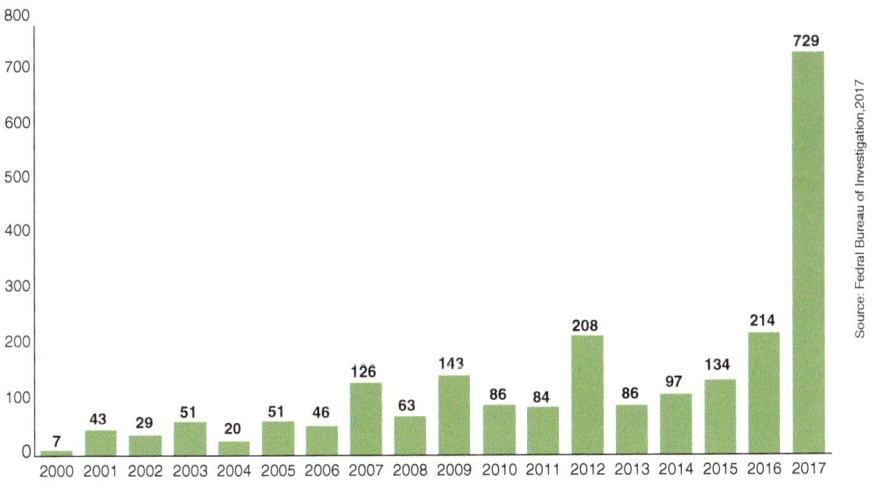

Fig. 5.12 Active shooter incident in United States: Casualties per year

commerce, 105 incidents (42%); educational environments, 52 incidents (21%); government property, 25 incidents (10%); open spaces, 35 incidents (14%); residences, 12 incidents (5%); houses of worship, ten incidents (4%); and health care facilities, ten incidents (4%) (Federal Bureau of Investigation 2017). As noted,

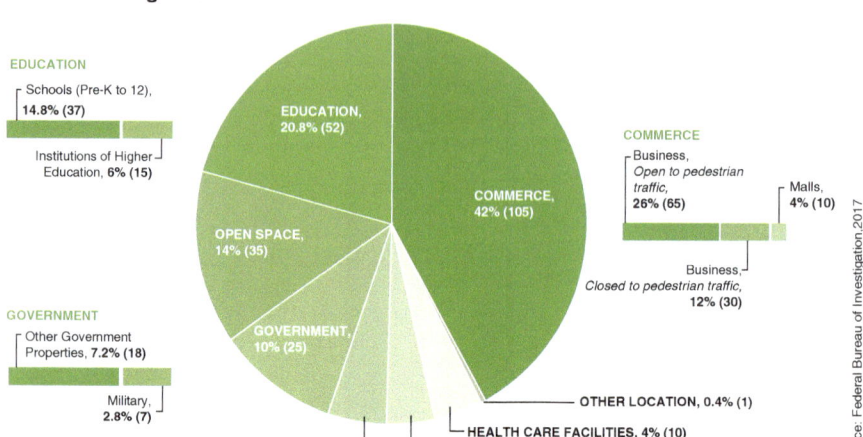

Quick Look: 250 Active Shooter Incidents in the United States From 2000 to 2017
Location Categories

Source: Federal Bureau of Investigation, 2017

Fig. 5.13 Active shooter incident in United States: Location categories

educational environments account for a large portion of locations for active shooter incidents, ranking only second to commercial areas. Of the 37 incidents (14.8%) occurring at schools, one took place at a nursery (pre-K) school and one incident occurred during a school board meeting that was being hosted on school property but no students were involved (neither perpetrator or victim). The remainder (35 incidents) were perpetrated by or against students, faculty, and/or staff at K-12 schools (Federal Bureau of Investigation 2018). Finally, 15 active shooter incidents (6%) did occur at institutions of higher learning. As a reminder, no incident occurred at institutions of higher learning during 2016 or 2017. Table 5.31 provides a detailed summary of educational environment incidents from 2000 to 2017.

Since the beginning of 2018, other tragic active shooter attacks have occurred in the U.S. and greatly impacted children and adolescents. Two of these such events have occurred in educational environments (United States Secret Service National Threat Assessment Center 2018). On February 14, 2018, a gunman opened fire at Marjory Stoneman Douglas High School. Fourteen students and three staff members were killed while fourteen others were injured (Follman et al. 2019). Twelve victims died inside the building, three died just outside the building on school premises, and two died in the hospital. The shooter was a former student of the school. Another active shooter event occurred on May 18, 2018 at Santa Fe High School in Santa Fe, Texas. The shooter killed ten individuals including eight students and two teachers while injuring 13 others. The shooter was an enrolled student at the school (Follman et al. 2019).

Based on the statistics of active shooter incidents, casualties, and locations, it is vital to prepare schools and plan for such events. National preparedness efforts, including planning, are now informed by the Presidential Policy Directive (PPD) 8 that was signed by the president in March 2011 and describes the nation's approach to preparedness. This directive represents an evolution in our collective understanding of national preparedness based on the lessons learned from terrorist attacks, hurricanes, school incidents, and other experiences. PPD-8 defines preparedness around five mission areas and can be applied to school active shooter incidents.

Table 5.31 Active shooter incidents involving education environments in the United States from 2000 to 2017[a]

Education site	Details
Santana High School (Education)	On March 5, 2001, at 9:20 a.m., Charles Andrew Williams Jr., 15, armed with a handgun, began shooting in Santana High School in Santee, California. Two people were killed; 13 were wounded. The shooter was apprehended by an off-duty officer who heard gunshots
Granite Hills High School (Education)	On March 22, 2001, at 12:55 p.m., Jason Anthony Hoffman, 18, armed with a shotgun and a handgun, began shooting in Granite Hills High School in El Cajon, California. No one was killed; five were wounded. The shooter was shot by police. He committed suicide in jail 1 week before sentencing
Appalachian School of Law (Education)	On January 16, 2002, at 1:15 p.m., Peter Odighizuma, 43, armed with a handgun, began shooting in the Appalachian School of Law located in Grundy, Virginia. Three people were killed; three were wounded. Three students—two of whom were off-duty police officers—tackled and restrained the shooter until police arrived and took him into custody
Red Lion Junior High School (Education)	On April 24, 2003, at 7:34 a.m., James Sheets, 14, armed with three handguns, shot and killed the school principal in the cafeteria at Red Lion Junior High School in Red Lion, Pennsylvania. Though others were present at the scene, the shooter committed suicide after killing the principal, before police arrived
Case Western Reserve University, Weatherhead School of Management (Education)	On May 9, 2003, at 3:55 p.m., Biswanath A. Halder, 62, armed with a rifle and a handgun, began shooting in the Weatherhead School of Management building at Case Western Reserve University in Cleveland, Ohio. One person was killed; two were wounded. The shooter was wounded during an exchange of gunfire with police
Kanawha County Board of Education (Education)	On July 17, 2003, at 7:00 p.m., Richard Dean Bright, 58, armed with two rifles and two handguns, began shooting during a Kanawha County Board of Education meeting in Charleston, West Virginia. He attempted to light a board member on fire and fired one round at board members before three administrators wrestled the gun away from him. No one was killed; one was wounded
Rocori High School (Education)	On September 24, 2003, at 11:35 a.m., John Jason McLaughlin, 15, armed with a handgun, began shooting in Rocori High School in Cold Spring, Minnesota. A teacher at the school confronted the shooter and ordered him to place his gun on the ground. The shooter complied. Two people were killed; no one was wounded. Police took the shooter into custody
Columbia High School (Education)	On February 9, 2004, at 10:30 a.m., Jon William Romano, 16, armed with a shotgun, began shooting while entering Columbia High School in East Greenbush, New York. No one was killed; one person was wounded. The shooter was restrained by administrators before police arrived and took him into custody

(continued)

Table 5.31 (continued)

Education site	Details
Red Lake High School and Residence (Education)	On March 21, 2005, at 2:49 p.m., Jeffery James Weise, 16, armed with a shotgun and two handguns, began shooting at Red Lake High School in Red Lake, Minnesota. Before the incident at the school, the shooter fatally shot his grandfather, who was a police officer, and another individual at their home. He then took his grandfather's police equipment, including guns and body armor, to the school. A total of nine people were killed, including an unarmed security guard, a teacher, and five students; six students were wounded. The shooter committed suicide during an exchange of gunfire with police
Campbell County Comprehensive High School (Education)	On November 8, 2005, at 2:14 p.m., Kenneth S. Bartley, 14, armed with a handgun, began shooting in Campbell County Comprehensive High School in Jacksboro, Tennessee. Before the shooting, he had been called to the office when administrators received a report that he had a gun. When confronted, he shot and killed an assistant principal and wounded the principal and another assistant principal. The shooter was restrained by students and administrators until police arrived and took him into custody
Pine Middle School (Education)	On March 14, 2006, at 9:00 a.m., James Scott Newman, 14, armed with a handgun, began shooting outside the cafeteria at Pine Middle School in Reno, Nevada. No one was killed; two were wounded. The shooter was restrained by a teacher until police arrived and took him into custody
Essex Elementary School and Two Residences (Education)	On August 24, 2006, at 1:55 p.m., Christopher Williams, 26, armed with a handgun, shot at various locations in Essex, Vermont. He began by fatally shooting his ex-girlfriend's mother at her home and then drove to Essex Elementary School, where his ex-girlfriend was a teacher. He did not find her, but as he searched, he killed one teacher and wounded another. He then fled to a friend's home, where he wounded one person. A total of two people were killed; two were wounded. The shooter also shot himself twice but survived and was apprehended when police arrived at the scene
Orange High School and Residence (Education)	On August 30, 2006, at 1:00 p.m., Alvaro Castillo, 19, armed with two pipe bombs, two rifles, a shotgun, and a smoke grenade, began shooting a rifle from his vehicle at his former high school, Orange High School in Hillsborough, North Carolina. He had fatally shot his father in his home that morning. One person was killed; two were wounded. The shooter was apprehended by police
Weston High School (Education)	On September 29, 2006, at 8:00 a.m., Eric Jordan Hainstock, 15, armed with a handgun and a rifle, began shooting in Weston High School in Cazenovia, Wisconsin. One person was killed; no one was wounded. The shooter was restrained by school employees until police arrived and took him into custody
West Nickel Mines School (Education)	On October 2, 2006, at 10:30 a.m., Charles Carl Roberts, IV, 32, armed with a rifle, a shotgun, and a handgun, began shooting at the West Nickel Mines School in Bart Township, Pennsylvania. After the shooter entered the building, he ordered all males and adults out of the room. After a 20-min standoff, he began firing. The shooter committed suicide as the police began to breach the school through a window. Five people were killed; five were wounded

Table 5.31 (continued)

Education site	Details
Memorial Middle School (Education)	On October 9, 2006, at 7:40 a.m., Thomas White, 13, armed with a rifle and a handgun, began shooting in Memorial Middle School in Joplin, Missouri. His rifle jammed after firing one shot. Hearing the shot, the school principal located the shooter, escorted him from the building, and turned him over to police. No one was killed or wounded
Virginia Polytechnic Institute and State University (Education)	On April 16, 2007, at 7:15 a.m., Seung Hui Cho, 23, armed with two handguns, began shooting in a dormitory at Virginia Polytechnic Institute and State University in Blacksburg, Virginia. Two-and-a-half hours later, he chained the doors shut in a classroom building and began shooting at the students and faculty inside. Thirty-two people were killed; 17 were wounded. In addition, six students were injured jumping from a second-floor classroom and were not included in other reported injury totals. The shooter committed suicide as police entered the building
SuccessTech Academy (Education)	On October 10, 2007, at 1:02 p.m., Asa Halley Coon, 14, armed with two handguns, began shooting in SuccessTech Academy in Cleveland, Ohio. No one was killed; four were wounded. The shooter committed suicide before police arrived
Louisiana Technical College (Education)	On February 8, 2008, at 8:35 a.m., Latina Williams (female), 23, armed with a handgun, began shooting in a second-floor classroom at Louisiana Technical College in Baton Rouge, Louisiana. She fired six rounds, then reloaded and committed suicide before police arrived. Two people were killed; no one was wounded
Cole Hall Auditorium, Northern Illinois University (Education)	On February 14, 2008, at 3:00 p.m., Steven Phillip Kazmierczak, 27, armed with a shotgun and three handguns, began shooting in the Cole Hall Auditorium at Northern Illinois University in DeKalb, Illinois. He had attended graduate school at the university. Five people were killed; 16 were wounded, including three who were injured as they fled. The shooter committed suicide before police arrived
Harkness Hall at Hampton University (Education)	On April 26, 2009, at 12:57 a.m., Odane Greg Maye, 18, armed with three handguns, began shooting in Harkness Hall, a residence hall at Hampton University in Hampton, Virginia, and then shot himself before police arrived. The shooter had briefly attended the university. A dormitory manager pulled the fire alarm when the shooting began, emptying the building. No one was killed; two were wounded. He was apprehended by police
Larose-Cut Off Middle School (Education)	On May 18, 2009, at 9:00 a.m., Justin Doucet, 15, armed with a handgun, fired once at a teacher at Larose-Cut Off Middle School in Cut Off, Louisiana, then went to the bathroom and shot himself. He died a week later. No one was killed or wounded
Inskip Elementary School (Education)	On February 10, 2010, at 12:49 p.m., Mark Stephen Foster, 48, armed with a handgun, began shooting inside Inskip Elementary School in Knoxville, Tennessee. He had just been informed that his teaching contract would not be renewed. The shooting occurred after he left the office and returned with a gun. No one was killed; two members of the administration were wounded. The shooter was apprehended by responding police

(continued)

Table 5.31 (continued)

Education site	Details
Shelby Center, University of Alabama (Education)	On February 12, 2010, at 4:00 p.m., Amy Bishop Anderson (female), 44, armed with a handgun, began shooting during a biology department meeting in the Shelby Center at the University of Alabama in Huntsville, Alabama. She sat in the meeting for 30 min, then stood up, and began firing. Three people were killed; three were wounded. The shooter surrendered to responding police
Deer Creek Middle School (Education)	On February 23, 2010, at 3:10 p.m., Bruco Strongeagle Eastwood, 32, armed with a rifle, began shooting in Deer Creek Middle School in Littleton, Colorado. No one was killed; two people were wounded. The shooter was restrained by teachers until police arrived and took him into custody
The Ohio State University, Maintenance Building (Education)	On March 9, 2010, at 3:30 a.m., Nathaniel Alvin Brown, 50, armed with two handguns, began shooting in the maintenance building at The Ohio State University in Columbus, Ohio. He had just been fired for allegedly lying on his job application. One person was killed; one was wounded. The shooter committed suicide before police arrived
Kelly Elementary School (Education)	On October 8, 2010, at 12:10 p.m., Brendan O'Rourke, aka Brandon O'Rourke, 41, armed with a handgun, began shooting at Kelly Elementary School in Carlsbad, California, after having jumped the school fence. No one was killed; two students were wounded. The shooter was tackled and restrained by nearby construction workers until police arrived and took him into custody
Panama City School Board Meeting (Education)	On December 14, 2010, at 2:14 p.m., Clay Allen Duke, 56, armed with a handgun, began shooting during a school board meeting in the Nelson Administrative Building in Panama City, Florida. The shooter's wife had previously been employed by the school district. After allowing several people to leave the room, the shooter fired in the direction of board members. No one was killed or wounded. The shooter committed suicide during an exchange of gunfire with the school district's armed security
Millard South High School (Education)	On January 5, 2011, at 12:44 p.m., Richard L. Butler Jr., 17, armed with a handgun, began shooting in Millard South High School in Omaha, Nebraska. Earlier that day, the assistant principal had suspended the shooter for allegedly driving his car onto the football field. The assistant principal was killed; the principal was wounded. The shooter committed suicide after fleeing the site of the shooting.
Chardon High School (Education)	On February 27, 2012, at 7:30 a.m., Thomas Michael Lane, III, 17, armed with a handgun, began shooting in the cafeteria at Chardon High School in Chardon, Ohio. The shooter was chased out of the building by a school coach. Three people were killed; three were wounded. The shooter was apprehended by police near the school
University of Pittsburgh Medical Center, Western Psychiatric Institute and Clinic (Education)	On March 8, 2012, at 1:40 p.m., John Schick, 30, armed with two handguns, began shooting inside the lobby of the Western Psychiatric Institute and Clinic at the University of Pittsburgh Medical Center in Pittsburgh, Pennsylvania. One person was killed; seven were wounded, including one police officer. The shooter was killed by University of Pittsburgh police
Oikos University (Education)	On April 2, 2012, at 10:30 a.m., Su Nam Ko, aka One L. Goh, 43, armed with a handgun, began shooting inside Oikos University in Oakland, California. He then killed a woman to steal her car. Seven people were killed; three were wounded. The shooter was arrested by police later that day

Table 5.31 (continued)

Education site	Details
Perry Hall High School (Education)	On August 27, 2012, at 10:45 a.m., Robert Wayne Gladden Jr., 15, armed with a shotgun, shot a classmate in the cafeteria of Perry Hall High School in Baltimore, Maryland. The shooter had an altercation with another student before the shooting began. He left the cafeteria and returned with a gun. No one was killed; one person was wounded. The shooter was restrained by a guidance counselor before being taken into custody by the school's resource officer
Sandy Hook Elementary School and Residence (Education)	On December 14, 2012, at 9:30 a.m., Adam Lanza, 20, armed with two handguns and a rifle, shot through the secured front door to enter Sandy Hook Elementary School in Newtown, Connecticut. He killed 20 students and six adults, and wounded two adults inside the school. Prior to the shooting, the shooter killed his mother at their home. In total, 27 people were killed; two were wounded. The shooter committed suicide after police arrived
Taft Union High School (Education)	On January 10, 2013, at 8:59 a.m., Bryan Oliver, 16, armed with a shotgun, allegedly began shooting in a science class at Taft Union High School in Taft, California. No one was killed; two people were wounded. An administrator persuaded the shooter to put the gun down before police arrived and took him into custody
New River Community College, Satellite Campus (Education)	On April 12, 2013, at 1:55 p.m., Neil Allen MacInnis, 22, armed with a shotgun, began shooting in the New River Community College satellite campus in the New River Valley Mall in Christiansburg, Virginia. No one was killed; two were wounded. The shooter was apprehended by police after being detained by an off-duty mall security officer as he attempted to flee
Santa Monica College and Residence (Education)	On June 7, 2013, at 11:52 a.m., John Zawahri, 23, armed with a handgun, fatally shot his father and brother in their home in Santa Monica, California. He then carjacked a vehicle and forced the driver to take him to the Santa Monica College campus. He allowed the driver to leave her vehicle unharmed but continued shooting until he was killed in an exchange of gunfire with police. Five people were killed; four were wounded
Sparks Middle School (Education)	On October 21, 2013, at 7:16 a.m., Jose Reyes, 12, armed with a handgun, began shooting outside Sparks Middle School in Sparks, Nevada. A teacher was killed when he confronted the shooter; two people were wounded. The shooter committed suicide before police arrived
Arapahoe High School (Education)	On December 13, 2013, at 12:30 p.m., Karl Halverson Pierson, 18, armed with a shotgun, machete, and three Molotov cocktails, began shooting in the hallways of Arapahoe High School in Centennial, Colorado. As he moved through the school and into the library, he fired one additional round and lit a Molotov cocktail, throwing it into a bookcase and causing minor damage. One person was killed; no one was wounded. The shooter committed suicide as a school resource officer approached him
Berrendo Middle School (Education)	On January 14, 2014, at 7:30 a.m., Mason Andrew Campbell, 12, armed with a shotgun, began shooting in Berrendo Middle School in Roswell, New Mexico. A teacher at the school confronted and ordered him to place his gun on the ground. The shooter complied. No one was killed; 3 were wounded: 2 students and an unarmed security guard. The shooter was taken into custody

(continued)

Table 5.31 (continued)

Education site	Details
Seattle Pacific University (Education)	On June 5, 2014, at 3:25 p.m., Aaron Rey Ybarra, 26, armed with a shotgun, allegedly began shooting in Otto Miller Hall at Seattle Pacific University in Seattle, Washington. He was confronted and pepper sprayed by a student as he was reloading. One person was killed; 3 were wounded. Students restrained the shooter until law enforcement arrived
Reynolds High School (Education)	On June 10, 2014, at 8:05 a.m., Jared Michael Padgett, 15, armed with a handgun and a rifle, began shooting inside the boy's locker room at Reynolds High School in Portland, Oregon. One student was killed; 1 teacher was wounded. The shooter committed suicide in a bathroom stall after law enforcement arrived
Marysville-Pilchuck High School (Education)	On October 24, 2014, at 10:39 a.m., Jaylen Ray Fryberg, 15, armed with a handgun, began shooting in the cafeteria of Marysville-Pilchuck High School in Marysville, Washington. Four students were killed, including the shooter's cousin; 3 students were wounded, including one who injured himself while fleeing the scene. The shooter, when confronted by a teacher, committed suicide before law enforcement arrived
Florida State University (Education)	On November 20, 2014, at 12:00 a.m., Myron May, 31, armed with a handgun, began shooting in Strozier Library at Florida State University in Tallahassee, Florida. He was an alumnus of the university. No one was killed; 3 were wounded. The shooter was killed during an exchange of gunfire with campus law enforcement.
Umpqua Community College (Education)	On October 1, 2015, at 10:38 a.m., Christopher Sean Harper-Mercer, 26, armed with several handguns and a rifle, began shooting classmates in a classroom on the campus of Umpqua Community College in Roseburg, Oregon. Nine people were killed; 7 were wounded. The shooter committed suicide after being wounded during an exchange of gunfire with law enforcement.
Madison Junior/ Senior High School (Education)	On February 29, 2016, at 11:30 a.m., James Austin Hancock, 14, armed with a handgun, allegedly began shooting in the cafeteria of Madison Junior/Senior High School in Middletown, Ohio. He shot two students before fleeing the building. No one was killed; four students were wounded (two from shrapnel). The shooter was apprehended near the school by law enforcement officers
Antigo High School (Education)	On April 23, 2016, at 11:02 p.m., Jakob Edward Wagner, 18, armed with a rifle, began shooting outside a prom being held at his former school, Antigo High School in Antigo, Wisconsin. Two law enforcement officers, who were on the premises, heard the shots and responded immediately. No one was killed; two students were wounded. The shooter was wounded in an exchange of gunfire with law enforcement officers and later died at the hospital
Townville Elementary School (Education)	On September 28, 2016, at 1:45 p.m., Jesse Dewitt Osborne, 14, armed with a handgun, allegedly began shooting at the Townville Elementary School playground in Townville, South Carolina. Prior to the shooting, the shooter, a former student, killed his father at their home. Two people were killed, including one student; three were wounded, one teacher and two students. A volunteer firefighter, who possessed a valid firearms permit, restrained the shooter until law enforcement officers arrived and apprehended him

Table 5.31 (continued)

Education site	Details
West Liberty-Salem High School (Education)	On January 20, 2017, at 7:36 a.m., Ely Ray Serna, 17, armed with a shotgun, allegedly began shooting inside West Liberty Salem High School, in West Liberty, Ohio, where he was a student. After assembling the weapon in a bathroom, the shooter shot a student who entered, then shot at a teacher who heard the commotion. The shooter shot classroom door windows before returning to the bathroom and surrendering to school administrators. No one was killed; two students were wounded. School staff members subdued the shooter until law enforcement arrived and took the shooter into custody
Freeman High School (Education)	On September 13, 2017, at 10:00 a.m., Caleb Sharpe, 15, armed with a rifle and a pistol, allegedly began shooting at Freeman High School in Rockford, Washington, where he was a student. One student was killed; three students were wounded. A school employee confronted the shooter, ordered him to the ground, and held him there until law enforcement arrived and took him into custody
Rancho Tehama Elementary School and Multiple Locations in Tehama County, California (Education)	On November 14, 2017, at 7:53 a.m., Kevin Janson Neal, 44, armed with a rifle and two handguns, began shooting at his neighbors, the first in a series of shootings occurring in Rancho Tehama Reserve, Tehama County, California. After killing three neighbors, he stole a car and began firing randomly at vehicles and pedestrians as he drove around the community. After deliberately bumping into another car, the shooter fired into the car and wounded the driver and three passengers. The shooter then drove into the gate of a nearby elementary school. He was prevented from entering the school due to a lockdown, so he fired at the windows and doors of the building, wounding five children. Upon fleeing the school, the shooter continued to shoot at people as he drove around Rancho Tehama Reserve. Law enforcement pursued the shooter; they rammed his vehicle, forced him off the road, and exchanged gunfire. The shooter's wife's body was later discovered at the shooter's home; the shooter apparently had shot and killed her the previous day. In total, five people were killed; 14 were wounded, eight from gunshot injuries (including one student) and six from shrapnel injuries (including four students). The shooter committed suicide after being shot and wounded by law enforcement during the pursuit
Aztec High School (Education)	On December 7, 2017, at approximately 8:00 a.m., William Edward Atchison, 21, armed with a handgun, began shooting inside Aztec High School in Aztec, New Mexico. The shooter was a former student. Two students were killed; no one was wounded. The shooter committed suicide at the scene, before police arrived

[a]In A Study of Active Shooter Incidents in the United States Between 2000 and 2013, the FBI identified 11 locations where the public was most at risk during an incident. These location categories include commercial areas (divided into business open to pedestrian traffic, businesses closed to pedestrian traffic, and malls), education environments (divided into schools [prekindergarten through 12th grade] and institutions of higher learning), open spaces, government properties (divided into military and other government properties), residences, houses of worship, and health care facilities. In 2018, the FBI added a new location category, Other Location, to capture incidents that occurred in venues not included in the 11 previously identified locations (Federal Bureau of Investigation 2017). This table only includes educational environments. An entire list of all incidents from 2000 to 2017 at all locations can be found at https://www.fbi.gov/file repository/active-shooter-incidents-2000-2017.pdf/view (Federal Bureau of Investigation 2018)

Prevention means the capabilities necessary to avoid, deter, or stop an imminent crime or threatened/actual mass casualty incident. Prevention is the action schools take to prevent a threatened or actual incident from occurring. *Protection* means the capabilities to secure schools against acts of violence and man-made or natural disasters. Protection focuses on ongoing actions that protect students, teachers, staff, visitors, districts, networks, and property from a threat or hazard. *Mitigation* means the capabilities necessary to eliminate or reduce the loss of life and property damage by lessening the impact of an event or emergency at the school. It also means reducing the likelihood that threats and hazards will happen. *Response* means the school's or school district's capabilities necessary to stabilize an emergency once it has already happened or is certain to happen in an unpreventable way, establish a safe and secure environment, save lives and property, and facilitate the transition to recovery. *Recovery* means the capabilities necessary to assist schools affected by an event or emergency in restoring the learning environment. It also means teaming with community partners to restore educational programming, the physical environment, business operations, and social, emotional, and behavioral health. The majority of Prevention, Protection, and Mitigation activities generally occur before an incident, although these three mission areas do have ongoing activities that can occur throughout an active shooter incident. Response activities occur during an incident, and recovery activities can begin during an incident and occur after an incident (United States Department of Education, Office of Elementary and Secondary Education, Office of Safe and Healthy Students 2013; United States Department of Homeland Security 2018b; United States Department of Homeland Security 2018).

In the *K-12 School Security* guide, the U.S. Department of Homeland Security (DHS) focuses on prevention and protection since the activities and measures associated with them occur prior to an incident (2018). Effective preventative and protective actions decrease the probability that schools (or other facilities) will encounter incidents of gun violence or should an incident occur, it reduces the impact of that incident. The guide emphasizes that the level of security at a facility will be based on hazards relevant to the facility, people, or groups associated with it. It also warns that as new or different threats become apparent, the perception of the relative security changes and insecurity should drive change to reflect the level of confidence of the people of groups associated with the facility. The DHS utilizes a Hometown Security approach that emphasizes the process of Connect, Plan, Train, and Report (CPTR) with the objective to realize effective, collaborative outcomes (United States Department of Homeland Security 2018b).

The initial phase is *Connect* and occurs by a school or district reaching out and developing relationships in the community, including local law enforcement. Having these relationships before an incident or event can help speed up the response when something happens. Each school must begin with identification or development of a security team, group, or organization. This phase also emphasizes outreach, collaboration, and building of a coalition. There should be coalition members from within a school and may include district/school administrators, teachers, aides, facility operations personnel, human resources, administrative, counseling, and student groups. External groups directly related to the school might include boards of education, parent organizations, mental health groups/agencies, and teacher and bus driver unions. External groups indirectly related to the school include all responder organizations such as police and fire departments, sheriff's office, emergency medical services, emergency management, and the local DHS Protective Security Advisor (PSA). Other tangential groups such as volunteer organizations, utility providers, and facilities in close geographic proximity should also be considered. Core and advisory members of the coalition are established. A coalition champion is also identified and is the person who owns the majority of the responsibility for achieving a school's security goals. The champion organizes the coalition as it grows and matures (United States Department of Homeland Security 2018b). The next phase is *Plan*. This will bring the coalition together. *The Guide for Developing High Quality School Emergency Operations Plans* (United States Department of Education, Office of Elementary and Secondary Education, Office of Safe and Healthy Students 2013) is an excellent resource for the coalition. A *School Security Survey for Gun Violence* can be completed and the coalition or user can quickly and effectively determine a facility's security proficiency (United States Department of Homeland Security. 2018). Specific portions of or topics within a school plan should be assigned to individuals, committees, or working groups most qualified to address them. The planning process must be sustainable. The amount of time spent in the planning phase should be commensurate with the amount of effort expended on the other phases (United States Department of Homeland Security 2018b). The next phase of the process is to *Train* on the plan developed by the coalition. Determining who is responsible for what and how it should be done is the basic function of planning. In fact, telling various members of the team what is expected of them and when to do that activity is the function of training. It is vital to utilize the curricula development expertise possessed by the K-12 community. School administrators should take advantage of this skill set and find creative ways to address difficult topics, such as gun violence. It should be carried out in an effective and nontraumatic way. Presenting the training in pieces or steps allows for a more comprehensive learning experience. It is important to validate training through exercises and drills, all of which should include the students. The training event should be followed by the completion and implementation of an after-action improvement plan with adjustment of the CPTR as indicated (United States Department of Homeland Security 2018b). The final phase in the process is *Report*. The reporting phase is arguably the most important of all the phases. Reporting principles underlie the other three phases and have profound prevention and protection impacts by driving forward information. DHS models the reporting phase using the "If You See Something, Say Something®" campaign (U.S. DHS, 2018) and the Nationwide Suspicious Activity Reporting (SAR) Initiative (Nationwide Suspicious Activity Reporting Initiative (NSI) 2019). "If You See Something, Say Something®" focuses on empowering anyone who sees suspicious activity to do something about it by contacting local law enforcement, or if an emergency to call 9–1–1 (United States Department of Homeland Security 2018a). This is a compelling capability when well organized and managed. A good plan for reporting, especially for a K-12 school, involves training staff and students on what is considered suspicious. There are many methods in which schools can employ to facilitate this, such as dedicated telephone numbers, websites for anonymous reporting, email or text messaging, and mobile phone applications. Conducting simple drills for reporters and receivers keeps skills sharp and reinforces the importance of the effort with the goal to save lives. If the plan includes sharing all suspicious activity calls with the local fusion center then the probability of higher fidelity reporting increases (United States Department of Homeland Security 2018b).

When making changes to a school's plans, procedures, and protective measures, it is imperative the needs of individuals with special health care needs be addressed throughout the process. Planning, training, and execution should always consider accessible alert systems for those who are deaf or hard of hearing; students, faculty, and staff who have visual impairments or are blind; individuals with limited mobility; alternative notification measures; people with temporary disabilities; visitors; people with limited English proficiency; sign cards with text- and picture-based emergency messages/symbols; and involving people with disabilities in all planning (United States Department of Homeland Security, Interagency Security Committee 2015).

It is important to understand that no "profile" exists for an active shooter (United States Department of Education, Office of Elementary and Secondary Education, Office of Safe and Healthy Students 2013). However, research indicates there may be signs or indicators. O'Toole (2000) presents an in depth, systematic procedure for school shooter threat assessment and intervention. The model was designed to be used by educators, mental health professionals, and law enforcement agencies. Its fundamental building blocks are the threat assessment standards, which provide a framework for evaluating a spoken, written, and symbolic threat, and the four-pronged assessment approach which provides a logical, methodical process to examine the threatener and assess the risk that the threat will be carried out. Schools should learn the signs of a potentially volatile situation that may develop into an active shooter situation and proactively seek ways to prevent an incident with internal resources, or additional external assistance (United States Department of Education, Office of Elementary and Secondary Education, Office of Safe and Healthy Students 2013). Potential warning signs of a school shooter may include increasingly erratic, unsafe, or aggressive behaviors; hostile feelings of injustice or perceived wrongdoing; drug and alcohol abuse; marginalization or distancing from friends and colleagues; changes in performance at work or school; sudden and dramatic changes in home life or in personality; pending civil or criminal litigation; and observable grievances with threats and plans of retribution (United States Department of Homeland Security 2018b). At a minimum, schools should establish and enforce policies that prohibit, limit, or determine unacceptable behaviors and consequences of weapons possession/use, drug possession/use, alcohol/tobacco possession/use, bullying/harassment, hazing, cyber-bullying/harassment/stalking, sexual assault/misconduct/harassment, bias crimes, social media abuse, and any criminal acts (United States Department of Homeland Security 2018b).

In addition to policies and positive school climates, school districts and administrators should establish dedicated teams to evaluate threats, such as a Threat Assessment Team (TAT). The Team should include mental health professionals (e.g., forensic psychologist, clinical psychologist, and school psychologist) to contribute to the threat assessment process (United States Department of Homeland Security 2018b). It is the responsibility of the TAT to investigate and analyze communications and behaviors to make a determination on whether or not an individual poses a threat to him/herself or others (United States Department of Education, Office of Elementary and Secondary Education, Office of Safe and Healthy Students 2013). As well as TATs, some schools have even opted to establish social media monitoring teams which look for keywords that may indicate bullying or other concerning statements. If a school opts to create such a team, it should work very closely with the TAT to ensure that applicable privacy, civil rights and civil liberties, other federal, state and local laws, and information sharing protocols are followed. Please refer to Chap. 14 for further information.

After an active shooter incident, field triage (e.g., JumpSTART) must commence and the patient must be evaluated by an experienced emergency medicine or trauma surgeon, preferably by a pediatric specialist in those disciplines. If an active shooter incident is coupled with detonation of an explosive device, the child must be screened and decontaminated for radiation exposure ("dirty bomb"). Triage tags are extremely helpful when multiple victims present in a short period of time. Medical response to an active shooter event will focus on control of external hemorrhage along with circulatory stabilization. Operative emergencies will be common and receive the highest priority. Severe extremity injuries may be controlled with tourniquet application or other forms of hemorrhage control. Re-evaluation is paramount to prevent ischemia to distal regions. However, thoracic or abdominal (truncal) injuries will need immediate surgical exploration and intervention. Penetrating trauma will cause more vascular injuries than blunt trauma, and vascular surgical trays may be in short supply at a hospital. Major procedure or surgical trays may become short in supply based on the increased operative demand. Resuscitative blood transfusion therapy may utilize a massive blood transfusion protocol. Since whole blood may be short in supply, some will simply use the 1:1:1 rule (administer one unit of packed cells: one unit of fresh frozen plasma: one unit of platelets). A unit for children may be substituted as an aliquot based on size of the patient (e.g., administer 10 mL/kg of packed cells: 10 mL/kg of fresh frozen plasma: 10 mL/kg of platelets). Calcium must also be replaced when there is a large volume transfusion. Due to extensive blood product utilization, there may be a heavy impact on institutional or regional blood supplies. Plans should be in place to address these problems, including the implementation of allocation of scarce resources. Mental health support and staff debriefs are essential and should be included after an active shooter event (Hick et al. 2016).

5.11 Conclusion

In conclusion, all forms of disasters, whether man-made or natural, impact infants, children, and adolescents throughout the world. Effective and efficient interventions remain the cornerstone of sustaining a child's well-being while reducing untoward complications due to all forms of disasters. Having a deep understanding of pediatric physiology and pathophysiology is crucial to all levels of disaster diagnostics and therapeutics. All nurses and HCPs have an obligation to understand these principles and deliver excellent, compassionate care to the pediatric disaster victim.

References

Adini B, Goldberg A, Cohen R, et al. Evidence-based support for the all-hazards approach to emergency preparedness. Isr J Health Policy Res. 2012;1(1):40. https://doi.org/10.1186/2045-4015-1-40.

Advanced Hazmat Life Support (AHLS). AHLS advanced hazmat life support provider manual. 3rd ed. Tucson, AZ: University of Arizona; 2003.

Advanced Law Enforcement Rapid Response Training (ALERRT) Center, Texas State University and Federal Bureau of Investigation, U.S. Department of Justice. Active shooter incidents in the United States in 2016 and 2017. 2018. https://www.fbi.gov/file-repository/active-shooter-incidents-us-2016-2017.pdf/view. Accessed 29 Jan 2019.

American Academy of Pediatrics (AAP). Radiation Disasters and Children— Committee on Environmental Health. J Am Acad Pediatr. 2003;111:1455–66.

American Academy of Pediatrics and American College of Emergency Physicians. In: Yamamoto L, Fuchs S, editors. APLS: the pediatric emergency medicine resource. 5th ed. Burlington, MA: Jones and Bartlett Learning; 2012.

American Academy of Pediatrics and American Heart Association. In: Weiner GM, Zaichkin J, editors. Textbook of neonatal resuscitation. 7th ed. Elk Grove Village, IL: American Academy of Pediatrics; 2016.

American Academy of Pediatrics, Committee on Pediatric Emergency Medicine, American College of Emergency Physicians, Pediatric Committee, and Emergency Nurses Association Pediatric Committee. Joint policy statement: guidelines for care of children in the emergency department. Pediatrics. 2009;124(4):1233–4.

American College of Surgeons Committee on Trauma, American College of Emergency Physicians, National Association of EMS Physicians, Pediatric Equipment Guidelines Committee Emergency Medical Services for Children (EMSC) Partnership for Children Stakeholder Group, American Academy of Pediatrics. Equipment for ambulances. Pediatrics. 2009;124:e166–71.

American Heart Association. 2015 Handbook of emergency cardiovascular care for healthcare providers. Dallas, TX: American Heart Association; 2015.

American Heart Association. Pediatric advanced life support provider manual. Dallas, TX: American Heart Association; 2016.

Arnold J, Halpern P, Tsai M-C, Smithline H. Mass casualty terrorist bombings: a comparison of outcomes by bombing type. Ann Emerg Med. 2004a;43:263–73.

Markenson D, Reynolds S, American Academy of Pediatrics, Committee on Pediatric Emergency Medicine and Task Force on Terrorism. The pediatrician and disaster preparedness. Pediatrics. 2006;117(2):e340–62. Reaffirmed February 1, 2010.

Arnold J, Halpern P, Tsai M-C, Smithline H. Mass casualty terrorist bombings: a comparison of outcomes by bombing type. Ann Emerg Med. 2004b;43:263–73.

Assistant Secretary for Preparedness and Response, United States Department of Health and Human Services. Strategic National Stockpile. 2018. https://www.phe.gov/about/sns/Pages/default.aspx. Accessed 22 Feb 2019.

Avalon Project—Documents in Law, History and Diplomacy. Avalon Project—The Atomic Bombings of Hiroshima and Nagasaki. n.d.. http://avalon.law.yale.edu/20th_century/mp10.asp. Accessed 22 Nov 2004.

Banks DE, editor. Medical management of chemical casualties handbook. 5th ed. Fort Sam Houston, TX: Borden Institute, US Army Research Institute of Chemical Defense (USAMRICD), Office of the Surgeon General; 2014.

Beigel J, Sandrock C. Intentional and natural outbreaks of infectious disease. In: Geiling J, Burns S, editors. Fundamental disaster management. 3rd ed. Mount Prospect, IL: Society of Critical Care Medicine; 2009. p. 1–5.

Berger RE, Burns EM. Preparedness for acts of nuclear, biological, and chemical terrorism. In: Yamamoto L, Fuchs S, editors. APLS: The Pediatric Emergency Medicine Resource. 5th ed. Burlington, MA: Jones and Bartlett; 2012. Chapter 21 (on-line).

Blair JP, Schweit KW. A study of active shooter incidents, 2000–2013. 2014. https://www.fbi.gov/file-repository/active-shooter-study-2000-2013-1.pdf/view. Accessed 30 Jan 2019.

Born C. Blast trauma: the fourth weapon of mass destruction. Scand J Surg. 2005;94:279–85.

Brabazon F, et al. Intranasal insulin treatment of an experimental model of moderate traumatic brain injury. J Cereb Blood Flow Metab. 2017;37:3203–18.

Burklow T, Yu C, Madsen J. Industrial chemicals: terrorist weapons of opportunity. Pediatr Ann. 2003;32(4):230–4.

Carbone A. Anthrax. In: Keyes D, Brunstein J, Schwartz R, Swienton R, editors. Medical response to terrorism: preparedness and clinical practice. Philadelphia, PA: Lippincott Williams and Wilkins; 2005. p. 56.

Centers for Disease Control and Prevention. Bioterrorism agents/diseases. 2019a. https://emergency.cdc.gov/agent/agentlist-category.asp. Accessed 1 Feb 2019.

Centers for Disease Control and Prevention. Ebola (Ebola virus disease): prevention and vaccine. 2019b. https://www.cdc.gov/vhf/ebola/prevention/index.html. Accessed 7 Feb 2019.

Centers for Disease Control and Prevention. Emergency preparedness and response: information on specific types of emergencies. 2018a. https://emergency.cdc.gov/hazards-specific.asp. Accessed 17 Feb 2019.

Centers for Disease Control and Prevention. Explosions and blast injuries: a primer for clinicians. 2010. http://www.bt.cdc.gov/masscasualties/explosions.asp.

Centers for Disease Control and Prevention. Infection control basics. 2017. https://www.cdc.gov/infectioncontrol/basics/index.html. Accessed 9 Feb, 2019.

Centers for Disease Control and Prevention. Plague: resources for clinicians. 2018b. https://www.cdc.gov/plague/healthcare/clinicians.html. Accessed 10 Feb 2019.

Centre for Research on the Epidemiology of Disasters (CRED). Economic losses, poverty and disasters 1998–2017: CRED/UNISDR Report. Brussels, Belgium: CRED; 2018. https://www.emdat.be/publications. Accessed 15 Feb 2019.

Centre for Research of the Epidemiology of Disasters (CRED). Natural disasters 2017: lower mortality, higher cost. Brussels, Belgium: CRED; 2018. https://www.cred.be/publications. Accessed 15 Feb 2019.

Centre for Research on the Epidemiology of Disasters (CRED). Emergency Events Database (EM-DAT). General Classification of Disasters. 2019. https://www.emdat.be/classification. Accessed 17 Feb 2019.

Centre for Research on the Epidemiology of Disasters (CRED) and United Nations Office for Disaster Risk Reduction (UNISDR). 2018 Review of disaster events: supplementary information. 2019. https://www.cred.be/publications. Accessed 15 Feb 2019.

Cernak I. Understanding blast-induced neurotrauma: how far have we come? Concussion. 2017;2:CNC42.

Cernak I, Wang Z, Jiang J, Bian X, Savic J. Ultrastructural and functional characteristics of blast injury-induced neurotrauma. J Trauma. 2001;50:695–706.

Chai PR, Hayes BD, Erickson TB, et al. Novichok agents: a historical, current, and toxicological perspective. Toxicol Commun. 2018;2(1):45–8.

Cieslak T. Medical management of potential biological casualties: a stepwise approach. In: Bozue J, Cote CK, Glass PJ, editors. Medical aspects of biological warfare. Fort Sam Houston, TX: Borden Institute; 2018. Chapter 5.

Cieslak T, Henretig F. Biologic and chemical terrorism. In: Kliegman RM, Stanton BMD, St. Geme J, Schor NF, editors. Nelson textbook of pediatrics. 20th ed. Philadelphia, PA: Elsevier; 2016. Chapter 723.

Cieslak T, Henretig F. Bioterrorism. Pediatr Ann. 2003;32(3):154–65.

Combs CC. An idea whose time has come? In: Terrorism in the twenty-first century. 8th ed. New York, NY: Routledge; 2018. Chapter 1.

Daniel-Aharonson L, Waisman Y, Dannon Y, Peleg K. Epidemiology of terror-related versus non-terror-related traumatic injury in children. Pediatrics. 2003;112:e280–4.

Dembek ZF, Smith LA, Lebeda FJ, et al. Botulinum toxin. In: Bozue J, Cote CK, Glass PJ, editors. Medical aspects of biological warfare. Fort Sam Houston, TX: Borden Institute; 2018.

DePalma R, Burris D, Champion H, Hodgson M. Blast injuries. N Engl J Med. 2005;352:1335–42.

Departments of the Army, the Navy, and the Air Force, and Commandant, Marine Corps. FM 8–825 Treatment of chemical agent casualties and conventional military chemical injuries. 1995.

Desmond B, Knater RK, Burns J, Barfield WD, Kissoon N, Task Force for Pediatric Emergency Mass Critical Care. Supplies and equipment for pediatric emergency mass critical care. Pediatr Crit Care Med. 2011;12(6):S120–7.

Fagbuyi DB, Schonfeld DJ, American Academy of Pediatrics Disaster Preparedness Advisory Council. Medical countermeasures for children in public health emergencies, disasters, or terrorism. Pediatrics. 2016;137(2):e20154273.

Federal Bureau of Investigation. Quick look: 250 active shooter incidents in the United States from 2000 to 2017. 2017. https://www.fbi.gov/about/partnerships/office-of-partner-engagement/active-shooter-incidents-graphics. Accessed 30 Jan 2019.

Federal Bureau of Investigation. Active shooter incidents in the United States from 2000–2017. 2018. https://www.fbi.gov/file-repository/active-shooter-incidents-2000-2017.pdf/view. Accessed 14 Feb 2019.

Fitzgerald F, Naveed A, Wing K, et al. Ebola virus disease in children, Sierra Leone, 2014-2015. Emerg Infect Dis. 2016;22(10):1769–77. https://doi.org/10.3201/eid2210.160579.

Follman M, Aronsen G, Pan D. U.S. Mass shootings, 1982–2019: data from Mother Jones' Investigation. *Mother Jones.* 2019. https://www.motherjones.com/politics/2012/12/mass-shootings-mother-jones-full-data/. Accessed 30 Jan 2019.

Garth R. Blast injury of the ear. In: Cooper GJ, Dudley HAF, Gann DS, Little RA, Maynard RL, editors. Scientific foundations of trauma. Jordan Hill, Oxford: Butterworth-Heinemann; 1997. p. 225–35.

Gerbatin RDR, et al. Guanosine protects against traumatic brain injury-induced functional impairments and neuronal loss by modulating excitotoxicity, mitochondrial dysfunction, and Inflammation. Mol Neurobiol. 2017;54:7585–96.

Goff AJ, Johnston SC, Kindrachuk J, et al. Smallpox and related othopoxviruses. In: Bozue J, Cote CK, Glass PJ, editors. Medical aspects of biological warfare. Fort Sam Houston, TX: Borden Institute; 2018. Chapter 24.

Goldman A, Perez-Pena R, Fernandez M. Texas church shooting video shows gunman's methodical attack, official says. *The New York Times.* 2017. https://www.nytimes.com/2017/11/08/us/texas-shooting-video-devin-kelley.html. Accessed 29 Jan 2019.

Gonzalez D. Crush syndrome. Crit Care Med. 2005;33:S34–41.

Goodrich JA, Kim JH, Situ R, et al. Neuronal and glial changes in the brain resulting from explosive blast in an experimental model. Acta Neuropathol Commun. 2016;4:124. https://doi.org/10.1186/s40478-016-0395-3.

Greenberg RN, Hay CM, Stapleton JT, et al. A randomized, double-blind, placebo-controlled phase II trial investigating the safety and immunogenicity of Modified Vaccinia Ankara Smallpox Vaccine (MVA-BN®) in 58–80-year-old subjects. PLoS One. 2016;11(6):e0157335. https://doi.org/10.1371/journal.pone.0157335.

Guy R, Kirkman E, Watkins P, Cooper G. Physiologic responses to primary blast. J Trauma. 1998;45:983–7.

Henao-Restrepo AM, Longini IM, Egger M, et al. Efficacy and effectiveness of an rVSV-vectored vaccine expressing Ebola surface glycoprotein: interim results from the Guinea ring vaccination cluster-randomised trial. Lancet. 2015;386:857–66.

Hepburn MJ, Kijek T, Sammons-Jackson W, et al. Tularemia. In: Bozue J, Cote CK, Glass PJ, editors. Medical aspects of biological warfare. Fort Sam Houston, TX: Borden Institute; 2018. Chapter 11.

Hegenbarth MA. Committee on Drugs. Preparing for pediatric emergencies: drugs to consider. Pediatrics. 2008;121(2):433–43.

Hick JL, Hanfling D, Evans B, et al. Health and medical response to active shooter and bombing events: a discussion paper. In: National Academy of medicine perspectives. Washington, DC: National Academy of Medicine; 2016. https://nam.edu/health-and-medical-response-to-active-shooter-and-bombing-events/. Accessed 17 Feb 2019.

Hilmas E, Broselow J, Luten RC, et al. Medical management of chemical toxicity in pediatrics. In: Tuorinsky SD, editor. Medical aspects of chemical warfare. Washington, DC: TMM; 2008. Chapter 21.

Ho AM-H, Ling E. Systemic air embolism after lung trauma. Anesthesiology. 1999;90:564–75.

Hoenig SL. Nerve agents. In: Compendium of chemical warfare agents. New York, NY: Springer Science; 2007. Chapter 5.

Illinois Emergency Medical Services for Children. Caring for non-injured and non-ill children in a disaster: a guide for non-medical professionals and volunteers. 2013. https://www.luriechildrens.org/globalassets/documents/emsc/resourcesguidelines/guidelines-tool-and-other-resources/practice-guidelinestools/caringchildrendisasterbookmay20164.pdf. Accessed 21 Feb 2019.

Illinois Emergency Medical Services for Children. Pediatric disaster preparedness guidelines for hospitals. 3rd ed; 2018. https://www.luriechildrens.org/emsc. Accessed 3 Feb 2019.

Jacobson P, Severin P. Pediatric disaster medicine. In: Nakagawa T, editor. Current concepts of pediatric critical care. Mount Prospect, IL: Society of Critical Care Medicine; 2012.

Johnston WR. Terrorist and criminal attacks targeting children. 2017. http://www.johnstonsarchive.net/terrorism/wrjp39ch.html. Accessed 13 Feb 2019.

Jokanovic M. Pyridinium oximes in the treatment of poisoning with organophosphorus compounds. In: Gupta RC, editor. Handbook of toxicology of chemical warfare agents. 2nd ed. London: Academic Press; 2015. Chapter 71.

Kennedy JS, Greenberg RN. IMVAMUNE®: modified vaccinia Ankara strain as an attenuated smallpox vaccine. Expert Rev Vaccines. 2009;8(1):13–24.

Kluger Y, Peleg K, Daniel-Aharonson L, Mayo A. The special injury pattern in terrorist bombings. J Am Coll Surg. 2004;199:875–9.

Kummerfeldt CE. Raxibacumab: potential role in the treatment of inhalational anthrax. Infect Drug Resist. 2014;7:101–9.

Likhtarev IA, Kovgan LN, Jacob P, Anspaugh LR. Chernobyl accident: retrospective and prospective estimates of external dose of the population of Ukraine. Health Phys. 2002;82:290–303.

Lynch JA, Berman S. Disasters and their effects on the population: key concepts. In: Berman S, editor. Pediatric education in disasters manual. Buenos Aires, Argentina: Service Point S.A; 2009.

Maman M, Yehezkelli Y. Ricin: a possible, noninfectious biological weapon. In: Fong IW, Alibek K, editors. Bioterrorism and infectious agents: a new dilemma for the 21st century. New York, NY: Springer; 2005. Chapter 8.

Markenson D, Redlener I. Pediatric preparedness for disasters and terrorism: National Consensus Conference. National Center for Disaster Preparedness. Mailman School of Public Health, Columbia University. 2007. https://academiccommons.columbia.edu/doi/10.7916/D81R707Q. Accessed 1 Feb 2019.

Martin G. Types of terrorism. In: Dawson M, Kisku DR, Gupta P, Sing JK, Li W, editors. Developing next-generation countermeasures for homeland security threat prevention. Hershey, PA: IGI Global; 2017. Chapter 1.

May P. Novichok: the notorious nerve agent. Molecule of the month. 2018. http://www.chm.bris.ac.uk/motm/novichok/novichokjs.htm. Accessed 9 Feb 2019.

McPhee RB, Leikin JB. Death by Polonium-210: lessons learned from the murder of former Soviet Spy Alexander Litvinenko. Semin Diagn Pathol. 2009;26:61–7.

Merrill E, Ruark C, Gearhart J, et al. Physiologically based pharmacokinetic/pharmacodynamic modeling of countermeasures to nerve agents. In: Gupta RC, editor. Handbook of toxicology of chemical warfare agents. 2nd ed. London: Academic Press; 2015. Chapter 69.

Messele F, Gebremedhin M, Purdon JG, et al. Degradation of pesticides with RSDL® (reactive skin decontamination lotion kit: LC-MS investigation). Toxicol Lett. 2018;293:241–8.

Mettler FA Jr, Voelz GL. Major radiation exposure—what to expect and how to respond. N Engl J Med. 2002;346(20):1554–61.

Migone TS, Subramanian M, Zhong J, et al. Raxibacumab for the treatment of inhalation anthrax. N Engl J Med. 2009;361(2):135–44.

Mirzayanov VS. State secrets: an Insider's chronicle of the Russian chemical weapons program. Denver, CO: Outskirts Press; 2009.

Mitchell C, Decker C. Applying risk-based decision making methods and tools to U.S Navy anti-terrorism capabilities. J Homeland Secur. 2004. http://www.au.af.mil/au/awc/awcgate/ndia/mitchell_rbdm_terr_hls_conf_may04.pdf. Accessed 3 Feb 2019.

Montello MJ, Tarosky M, Pinock L, et al. Dosing cards for treatment of children exposed to weapons of mass destruction. Am J Health Syst Pharm. 2006;63:944–9.

Mytle N, Hopkins RJ, Malkevich NV, et al. Evaluation of intravenous anthrax immune globulin for treatment of inhalation anthrax. Antimicrob Agents Chemother. 2013;57(11):5684–92.

National Council on Radiation Protection (NCRP) & Measurements. Management of terrorist events involving radioactive material. (Report no 138). Author: Bethesda, MD; 2001.

National Council on Radiation Protection (NCRP) & Measurements. Management of persons contaminated with radionuclides: handbook. (Report no 161). Author: Bethesda, MD; 2009.

National Institutes of Health. NIH strategic plan and research agenda for medical countermeasures against chemical threats. 2007. https://www.niaid.nih.gov/sites/default/files/nihstrategic-planchem.pdf. Accessed 1 Feb 2019.

National Institutes of Health. The NIH strategic biomedical research response to the threat of bioterrorism. 2005. https://www.nti.org/media/pdfs/129-NIH.pdf?_=1318522920?_=1318522920. Accessed 1 Feb 2019.

Nationwide Suspicious Activity Reporting Initiative (NSI). National strategy for information sharing. 2019. https://nsi.ncirc.gov/default.aspx. Accessed 31 Jan 2019.

Office for Victims of Crime, Office of Justice Programs, U.S. Department of Justice. Mass casualty shootings. 2019. https://ovc.ncjrs.gov/ncvrw2018/info_flyers/fact_sheets/2018NCVRW_MassCasualty_508_QC.pdf. Accessed 29 Jan 2019.

O'Toole ME. The school shooter: a threat assessment perspective. Quantico, VA: Critical Incident Response Group (CIRG), National Center for the Analysis of Violent Crime, FBI Academy; 2000. p. 1–46. https://permanent.access.gpo.gov/lps54727/school_shooter.pdf. Accessed 31 Jan 2019.

Paran H, Neufeld D, Schwartz I, Kidron D, Susmallian S, Mayo A, Dayan K, Vider I, Sivak G, Freund U. Perforation of the terminal ileum induced by blast injury: delayed diagnosis or delayed perforation? J Trauma. 1996;40:472–5.

Pittman PR, Brown ES, Chambers MS. Medical countermeasures. In: Bozue J, Cote CK, Glass PJ, editors. Medical aspects of biological warfare. Fort Sam Houston, TX: Borden Institute; 2018. Chapter 27.

Place RC, Martin M. Preparedness for pediatric emergencies. In: Yamamoto L, Fuchs S, editors. APLS: the pediatric emergency medicine resource. 5th ed. Burlington, MA: Jones and Bartlett; 2012.

Purcell BK, Cote CK, Worsham PL, et al. Anthrax. In: Bozue J, Cote CK, Glass PJ, editors. Medical aspects of biological warfare. Fort Sam Houston. TX: Borden Institute; 2018. Chapter 6.

Radoshitzky SR, Bavari S, Jahrling PB, et al. Filoviruses. In: Bozue J, Cote CK, Glass PJ, editors. Medical aspects of biological warfare. Fort Sam Houston, TX: Borden Institute; 2018. Chapter 23.

Radiation Emergency Assistance Center/Training Site (REACT/S-CDC). Emergency management of radiation accident victims. REAC/TS—CDC Course. Lecture conducted from Oak Ridge Institute for Science and Education, Oak Ridge, TN; 2006.

Radiation Event Medical Management (REMM) of the U.S. Dept. of Health and Human Services. Decontamination procedures—radiation event medical management & about decontamination of children video. n.d.. http://www.remm.nlm.gov/ext_contamination.htm, http://www.remm.nlm.gov/about_decon_video.htm. Accessed 9 Dec 2009.

Rotenberg J. Cyanide as a weapon of terror. Pediatr Ann. 2003a;32(4):236–40.

Rotenberg J. Diagnosis and management of nerve agent exposure. Pediatr Ann. 2003b;32(4): 242–50.

Rotenberg J, Newmark J. Nerve agent attacks on children: diagnosis and management. Pediatrics. 2003;112:648–58.

Rotz L, Damon I, Cono J. Smallpox. In: Keyes D, Brunstein J, Schwartz R, Swienton R, editors. Medical response to terrorism: preparedness and clinical practice. Philadelphia, PA: Lippincott Williams and Wilkins; 2005. p. 87.

Roxas-Duncan VI, Hale ML, Davis JM, et al. Ricin. In: Bozue J, Cote CK, Glass PJ, editors. Medical aspects of biological warfare. Fort Sam Houston, TX: Borden Institute; 2018. Chapter 16.

Schweit KW. Active shooter incidents in the United States in 2014 and 2015. 2016. https://www. fbi.gov/file-repository/activeshooterincidentsus_2014-2015.pdf/view. Accessed 30 Jan 2019.

Severin P. Pediatric simulation. In: Reuter-Rice K, Bolick B, editors. Pediatric acute care: a guide for interprofessional practice. Burlington, MA: Jones and Bartlett; 2011.

Shah T, Greig J, van der Plas LM, et al. Inpatient signs and symptoms and factors associated with death in children aged 5 years and younger admitted to two Ebola management centres in Sierre Leone, 2014: a retrospective cohort study. Lancet Glob Health. 2016;4(7):e495–501.

Sharpnack D, Johnson A, Phillips Y. The pathology of primary blast injury. In: Bellamy RF, Zajtchuk R, editors. Conventional warfare: ballistic blast and burn injuries. Washington, DC: Office of the Surgeon General; 1991. p. 271–94.

Singer P, Cohen J, Stein M. Conventional terrorism and critical care. Crit Care Med. 2005;33:S61–5.

Sirbaugh PE, DiRocco PJ. Disaster management. In: Yamamoto L, Fuchs S, editors. APLS: the pediatric emergency medicine resource. 5th ed. Burlington, MA: Jones and Bartlett Learning; 2012. Chapter 20 (Online).

Smit MA, Michelow IC, Glavis-Bloom J, et al. Characteristics and outcomes of pediatric patients with ebola virus disease admitted to treatment units in Liberia and Sierra Leone: a retrospective cohort study. Clin Infect Dis. 2017;64(3):243–9.

Stuhmiller J, Phillips Y, Richmond D. The physics and mechanisms of primary blast injury. In: Conventional warfare: ballistic blast and burn injuries. Washington, DC: Office of the Surgeon General; 1991. p. 243–4.

The Medical Letter. *BioThrax* and *Anthrasil* for anthrax. Med Lett Drugs Ther. 2016;58(1494):62.

The Medical Letter. Raxibacumab for anthrax. Med Lett Drugs Ther. 2013;55(1413):27–8.

The Medical Letter. Obiltoxaximab (Anthim) for inhalational anthrax. Med Lett Drugs Ther. 2018;60(1555):150 1.

U.S. Food and Drug Administration. Guidance potassium iodide as a thyroid blocking agent in radiation emergencies. n.d.. w.fda.gov/downloads/Drugs/GuidanceComplianceRegulatory Information/Guidances/ucm080542.pdf. Accessed 27 May 2005.

Timmons R, Carbone A. Botulinum: the most toxic substance known. In: Keyes D, Brunstein J, Schwartz R, Swienton R, editors. Medical response to terrorism: preparedness and clinical practice. Philadelphia, PA: Lippincott Williams and Wilkins; 2005. p. 117.

Traub S. Ricin. In: Keyes D, Brunstein J, Schwartz R, Swienton R, editors. Medical response to terrorism: preparedness and clinical practice. Philadelphia, PA: Lippincott Williams and Wilkins; 2005. p. 134.

United States Army Medical Research Institute of Infectious Diseases (USAMRIID). USAMRIID's medical management of biological casualties handbook. 8th ed. Fort Detrick, MD: Frederick; 2014

United States Department of Education, Office of Elementary and Secondary Education, Office of Safe and Healthy Students. Guide for developing high-quality school emergency operations plans. Washington, DC; 2013. p. 1–67. https://www.fema.gov/media-library-data/20130726-1922-25045-3850/rems_k_12_guide.pdf. Accessed 31 Jan 2019.

U.S. Department of Health and Human Services, Assistant Secretary for Preparedness and Response. 2014–2015 Report of the Children's HHS Interagency Leadership on Disasters (CHILD) Working Group: update on department activities. 2017. https://www.phe.gov/Preparedness/legal/boards/naccd/Pages/default.aspx. Accessed 22 Feb 2019.

U.S. Department of Health and Human Services, Assistant Secretary for Preparedness and Response Biomedical Advanced Research and Development Authority. BARDA Strategic Plan 2011–2016. 2016. https://www.medicalcountermeasures.gov/media/745/bardastrategicplan9-28%2D%2D508.pdf. Accessed 1 Feb 2019.

United States Department of Health and Human Services, Office of the Assistant Secretary for Preparedness and Response, National Library of Medicine. Chemical Hazards Emergency Medical Management (CHEMM). 2019. https://chemm.nlm.nih.gov/index.html. Accessed 17 Feb 2019.

United States Department of Health and Human Services, Chemical Hazards Emergency Medical Management (CHEMM). Fourth generation agents: medical management guidelines. 2019. https://chemm.nlm.nih.gov/nerveagents/FGAMMGPrehospital.htm. Accessed 27 Feb 2019.

United States Department of Health and Human Services. 2017–2018 Public Health Emergency Countermeasures Enterprise (PHEMCE) Strategy and Implementation Plan. 2017. https://www.medicalcountermeasures.gov/BARDA/documents/2017-phemce-sip.pdf. Accessed 1 Feb 2019.

United States Department of Homeland Security. *"If You See Something, Say Something®"*. 2018a. https://www.dhs.gov/see-something-say-something. Accessed 31 Jan 2019.

United States Department of Homeland Security, Interagency Security Committee. Planning and response to an active shooter: an interagency security committee policy and best practices guide. 2nd ed; 2015. https://www.dhs.gov/sites/default/files/publications/isc-planning-response-active-shooter-guide-non-fouo-nov-2015-508.pdf. Accessed 31 Jan 2019.

United States Department of Homeland Security. K-12 school security: a guide for preventing and protecting against gun violence. 2nd ed. Washington, DC: DHS Publications; 2018b. p. 1–28. https://www.dhs.gov/sites/default/files/publications/K12-School-Security-Guide-2nd-Edition-508.pdf. Accessed 30 Jan 2019.

United States Department of Homeland Security. K-12 school security survey. 2018. https://www.dhs.gov/publication/k-12-school-security-guide. Accessed 31 Jan 2019.

United States Department of Homeland Security, Federal Emergency Management Agency. Understanding your risks: identifying hazards and estimating losses. 2001. https://www.fema.gov/media-library-data/20130726-1521-20490-4917/howto2.pdf. Accessed 3 Feb 2019.

United States Department of Homeland Security, Federal Emergency Management Agency. FEMA fact sheet: national planning scenarios. 2019. https://www.fema.gov/national-planning-frameworks. Accessed 5 Mar 2019.

United States Department of Homeland Security. National planning scenarios. Version 21.3 Final Draft. 2006. https://publicintelligence.net/national-planning-scenarios-version-21-3-2006-final-draft/. Accessed 5 Mar 2019.

United States Department of Homeland Security, Office of Inspector General. FEMA's progress in all-hazards mitigation. 2009. https://www.oig.dhs.gov/assets/Mgmt/OIG_10-03_Oct09.pdf. Accessed 14 Feb 2019.

United States Secret Service National Threat Assessment Center. Enhancing school safety using a threat assessment model: an operational guide for preventing targeted school violence. 2018. https://www.dhs.gov/sites/default/files/publications/18_0711_USSS_NTAC-Enhancing-School-Safety-Guide.pdf. Accessed 30 Jan 2019.

Waugh WL. Living with hazards, dealing with disasters: an introduction to emergency management. Armonk, NY: Sharpe Publishers; 2000.

Waugh WL. Terrorism and the all-hazards model. J Emerg Manag. 2005;3(2):8–10.

Wightman J, Gladish S. Explosions and blast injuries. Ann Emerg Med. 2001;37:664–78.

Won E, Carbone A. Viral hemorrhagic fevers. In: Keyes D, Brunstein J, Schwartz R, Swienton R, editors. Medical response to terrorism: preparedness and clinical practice. Philadelphia, PA: Lippincott Williams and Wilkins; 2005. p. 96.

Woo G. Quantitative terrorism risk assessment. J Risk Financ. 2002;4(1):7–14.

Worsham PL, Mcgovern TW, Vietri NJ, et al. Plague. In: Bozue J, Cote CK, Glass PJ, editors. Medical aspects of biological warfare. Fort Sam Houston, TX: Borden Institute; 2018. Chapter 10.

Yu C, Bruklow T, Madsen J. Vesicant agents and children. Pediatr Ann. 2003;32(4):254–7.

Zajtchuk CR, Cerveny TJ, Walker RI. Medical consequences of nuclear warfare (Textbooks of military medicine). Washington, DC: Department of the Army; 1989.

Zhu FC, Wurie AH, Hou LH, et al. Safety and immunogenicity of a recombinant adenovirus type-5 vector-based Ebola vaccine in healthy adults in Sierra Leone: a single-centre, randomised, double-blind, placebo-controlled, phase 2 trial. Lancet. 2017;389:621–8.

General Disaster Preparedness for Families

6

Jessica James and Annaliza Sherry

6.1 Introduction

Modern-day events have awakened an awareness of how vulnerable we are throughout the United States. The attacks of 9/11 and the magnitude of destruction of Hurricane Katrina are prime examples that have eliminated the aura of invincibility of mankind. Each day, organizations work to establish programs and develop plans to prepare for these kinds of events. Many times, disaster planning and management are fragmented and plan for the general population (Ronan et al. 2015). With children comprising nearly 23 percent of the U.S. population in 2016 (Bethesda 2018), they are identified as a vulnerable population (Markenson n.d.).

Historically, disaster preparedness for families and children has been universally low. Prior to 2000, only one study was published exploring disaster preparedness programs for children (Ronan et al. 2015). Although this number is steadily increasing, it is vital that households begin the process of preparation within their homes. The family structure is unique when formulating disaster plans. Each family member's specific needs must be considered, and plans need to prepare for those needs. Families should work together to identify risks and build resiliency while providing motivation, planning, and practice (Ronan et al. 2015). Nurses can play an important role in assisting families with disaster preparations. However, nurses must first ensure that they and their own families are prepared in the event of a disaster.

J. James
Children's Hospital Los Angeles, Los Angeles, CA, USA
e-mail: jejames@chla.usc.edu

A. Sherry (✉)
Ann & Robert H. Lurie Children's Hospital of Chicago, Chicago, IL, USA
e-mail: acamia@luriechildrens.org

© Springer Nature Switzerland AG 2020
C. J. Goodhue, N. Blake (eds.), *Nursing Management of Pediatric Disaster*,
https://doi.org/10.1007/978-3-030-43428-1_6

6.2   Preparing for Disaster

Disasters can happen quickly and without warning. It is of the utmost importance to prepare for disasters in order to ensure the health and well-being of the family members involved. Overall, household disaster preparedness has been consistently low in the U.S. since 2007 (Thomas et al. 2015). The level of disaster preparedness behavior is generally associated with age, income, awareness, and individual health status (Thomas et al. 2015). Although there are many factors associated with disaster preparedness, awareness is the most easily alterable factor. To increase awareness, members of the household should be educated about available resources and strategies.

As nurses, it is important to assess families at all points of interactions. Commonly, the opportunities for assessments would be at office visits and all patient encounters. These are prime times to reinforce the importance of disaster preparedness. Screening and providing anticipatory guidance can help increase family awareness of disasters resulting in more affirmative action to prepare. In addition to educating at offices and clinics, nurses can also encourage the local school systems to train and prepare children and their families on the actions to take prior, during, and after a disaster (Blake 2018). Nurses are key players in the development, design, implementation, and evaluation of disaster preparedness in both health care and the community (Blake 2018). Nurses should take every opportunity to do community education regarding preparedness.

The next step in increasing awareness is to be informed about disaster preparedness. Understanding which disasters are common in the area enables the families to prepare in advance. This includes both advanced warning events such as hurricanes and floods as well as no warning events such as earthquakes or bombings. There are many resources that provide information about common local disasters, such as local emergency management offices or the local American Red Cross chapter. These are two examples of organizations that can provide information about which disasters are common to an area while also providing information about community disaster planning. As a nurse or health care provider (HCP), contact information and informational brochures for these two agencies should be provided to families. In addition, staying current on community response plans, evacuation plans, reunification areas, and emergency shelters can aid in educating families as they prepare their household plans to correlate with existing community plans.

It is also important to understand a community's emergency warning systems. In the U.S., the Emergency Alert System requires all national broadcast and wireless satellites to transmit emergency messages to the public from local authorities all the way to the President. Wireless Emergency Alerts (WEAs) are also utilized to quickly communicate to the public about life-threatening events. WEAs often look like text messages with a unique sound designed to alert the user about the important message (Ready 2019a). Nurses can educate families about this system and assist with locating the alert on their personal communication devices. In addition, it is important for families to be aware that the community is also preparing.

In addition to awareness of the potential hazards in the community, it is important to encourage and educate families to financially safeguard one's home and family. This is a stressor for many households. The more knowledge that can be obtained prior to a disaster, the less it will influence necessary decisions during an event. One of the first components is to know what one owns (AICPA 2015). This includes conducting a household inventory of items that are of both monetary and personal value. For items that are easily mobile, consider establishing a safe deposit box or other secure methods away from the disaster-prone areas (AICPA 2015). This can include important documents, insurance contracts, receipts, and a photographic inventory of valuable items.

Homeowner's insurance and renter's insurance are also going to be contributing factors to ensuring one's family has a well-rounded disaster plan. By well-rounded plan, it is encompassing not only the physical, everyday needs of the family, but also addresses preparing for any financial implications that may arise due to the disaster. This information, used in conjunction with the knowledge of community hazards, is essential. For example, the Federal Emergency Management Agency (FEMA 2004) provides flood maps to convey flood risks to coastal residents. This information influences residents to purchase flood insurance for their homes (Shao et al. 2017). This can be applicable to earthquake-prone regions, areas with high risk for wildfires, and those residing in "tornado alley," to name a few examples. It is essential to be aware of the factors that make one's homeowners or renter's insurance and adding additional components based on the risk factors in one's area. In addition, because of the ever-changing economy, it is imperative that one's home is periodically appraised to ensure that any replacement costs are covered under one's policy (AICPA 2015).

In addition to awareness about home or renter's insurance, nurses should educate families about health insurance. This is a vital piece in constructing a family disaster plan. Public health disasters such as hurricanes, floods, and bioterror incidents such as anthrax, as well as pandemics such as influenza and Ebola have a significant impact on health insurance (Merchant et al. 2015). Health care insurance companies need to be able to rapidly inform their beneficiaries of their level of coverage and what restrictions may be implemented in the event of a disaster. To mitigate this, it is important to emphasize that families discuss the effects of their health insurance should a catastrophic event occur. Families should be knowledgeable of what is covered under their policy as well as the processes that need to be taken to utilize those policy benefits. In addition, does one's family insurance plan include disability insurance? This can be relevant if a family member is injured during a disaster and cannot return to work for a period of time. Unfortunately, life insurance will also play an important role for families during a disaster, and how loved ones are able to manage financially should death occur (AICPA 2015).

6.3   Make a Plan

In the event of disaster, it is vital to have a plan that includes all members of the family. The core of disaster preparedness is education. Families who have knowledge of disaster preparedness were more likely to initiate plans into actions, such as written household disaster plans and disaster kits (Thomas et al. 2015). Creating a household disaster plan consists of three separate parts: discussing types of emergencies, delegating roles and responsibilities, and practicing as many elements as possible (American Red Cross 2019).

Nurses are essential in helping families navigate through this process due to the frequent interaction of nurses and family. The nurse can help the family create a plan by discussing the specific needs of each member of the family and how to prepare. According to the Society of Pediatric Nurses, planning should include "the ability to be self-sustained, including utilities, communication, food, water, and medications for 96 hours" (Blake 2018). Nurses can assist families by providing resources, strategies, and tactics to accomplish these goals.

When educating a family, it is important to outline types of disasters that occur naturally as well as inside the home. Disasters can happen instantly and without warnings, such as an earthquake or fire. Oppositely, there can be ample time to prepare, such as a hurricane. Information regarding disasters that commonly occur in an area can be found through the local American Red Cross or local emergency management office. Nurses should stay current on this information and provide regular education to families during routine clinic visits.

Anticipatory guidance increases preparedness and understanding of what to expect and how to prepare. It is also key to discuss disasters that can occur in the home as well. These include fires and floods. Discussion points should include methods for prevention and plans should these events occur (American Red Cross 2019).

Nurses and HCPs should encourage regular practice and discussion of the many elements. This allows families and children to gain comfort and confidence in their disaster plans. The major components of a disaster plan include but are not limited to: escape routes, reunification, communication, and transportation.

Both a primary and secondary escape or evacuation route should be preestablished when creating a disaster plan. Nurses can assist families in identifying safe pathways and provide resources and examples on visual aids such as a map. Once outside of the house, a reunification point is essential. Multiple possible locations should be predetermined and utilization of well-known landmarks. Examples include but are not limited to parks, friends' homes, and area buildings. It is important to select locations both locally and outside the neighborhood.

Another consideration when establishing reunification points includes care for home pets or animals. Not all shelters have appropriate accommodations for animals, nor may they accept animals. If the family has home pets, consider reunification points that allow animals in their facility. Transportation should also be discussed when selecting locations. Vehicle transportation may not be the most effective mode of transportation, depending on the nature of the event. It is important to identify routes that are feasible on foot. If vehicles are used, education about the importance of a full fuel tank and first-aid kit in the vehicle should be given (Ready 2019b).

There are instances where evacuating one's home is not possible. For instances such as these, it is important to establish a "safe room" in the house should the family need to shelter-in-place. The safe room should have windows and vents that can be sealed off. In addition, doors should be in place that can lock. This room should also contain emergency supplies, such as means to listen to emergency broadcast systems, supplies to seal the room, an emergency kit, food, and water.

It is important to note that family members may not be at home when a disaster occurs. Additional considerations should be made should a family member be in another location such as child care, school, and work. During education sessions with nurses or HCPs, as well as officials from schools, it is important for the family to understand the plans of these external locations and how it will correlate to the family disaster plan (American Red Cross 2019).

Communication is an important element of family disaster planning as well. Families should create and print multiple copies of an emergency contact list of all family members in the household, at least three emergency contacts, and one out of state contact (Fig. 6.1). These emergency lists should contain not only phone numbers but also alternate methods of communication such as email and home address. Cellular communication may not always be available or reliable. In addition to emergency contacts, important contact information for schools and child care should be listed. If there are members of the household with special health care needs that contact information should also be incorporated into the plan. Please see Chap. 8 for further information.

Each able family member should be assigned a role to prepare for a disaster. These roles include maintaining an up-to-date disaster kit, staying informed of local disasters, ensuring that family medical information is up-to-date and accessible, keeping financial information current, and sharing new or revised evacuation plans with the family. Nurses can educate families about these different roles and the importance of each component. Other considerations such as pet care, special medical needs, and the needs of children should also be considered when maintaining an up-to-date plan.

Education should be provided to families to review and exercise their home plans at minimum every 6 months (American Red Cross 2019). If changes are made to the plan, review and exercise should occur more frequently. Exercises should include practicing escape routes, locating meeting spots, practicing communication methods, and reviewing contact information. As a household, it is important to continually discuss disaster plans. The consistent review and practice allow the family to become more familiar with the plan, and increase their confidence levels in response.

6.4   Make a Kit

Families come in all shapes and sizes, and the supplies needed for a disaster are unique to each family (American Academy of Pediatrics 2016). The American Academy of Pediatrics (AAP) and the American Red Cross recommend that families not only create an emergency plan but also develop a family disaster kit (Healthychildren.org 2018). According to the National Center for Disaster Preparedness Periodic survey conducted in 2011, only 50% of American families have a plan and 30% had plans that lacked an essential item such as food or water

EMERGENCY CONTACT LIST (10)

FAMILY NAME and HOME ADDRESS

Family Member Name	Phone Number	Email	Specific Information (medications, school name, special needs, etc.)
PETS			

EMERGENCY CONTACTS:

NAME	PHONE NUMBER	EMAIL ADDRESS

OUT OF STATE CONTACTS

NAME	PHONE NUMBER	EMAIL ADDRESS

MEETING PLACE CLOSE TO HOME

LOCATION NAME	ADDRESS	NEAREST CROSS STREET

MEETING PLACE OUTSIDE OF THE NEIGHBORHOOD

LOCATION NAME	ADDRESS	NEAREST CROSS STREET

OTHER INFORMATION:

Fig. 6.1 Emergency contact list (American Red Cross 2019)

(Bagwell et al. 2016). Nurses and HCPs should provide education and resources related to making a kit. This can be completed at routine clinic visits, community education days, and school events, to name a few.

The contents of a kit can vary depending on the type of family and what hazards are unique to each region. However, each disaster kit should contain items from six major categories: essentials, communication and transportation, food and water, personal needs, medical needs, and miscellaneous items (American Academy of

Pediatrics 2016; Ready 2019c). In addition, family disaster kits should have supplies applicable to infants, children, elderly, and pets. If a family should have a member with special health care needs, their necessities should also be taken into account (see Chap. 8). Lastly, a "grab and go" kit can also be developed to be kept at home, work, and in the car (Table 6.1) (Oberman 2013).

Table 6.1 Family disaster supplies list (Healthychildren.org 2018; Bagwell et al. 2016)

Essentials (paper documents and copies should be kept in a sturdy zip-lock bag)	• Family emergency plan including a fire escape plan
	• List to remind you of what you need to take care of (i.e., get medical equipment, phone charger, and so on)
	• Copies of identifying documents including but not limited to: driver's license, birth certificates, legal documents
	• Family identification photos
	• Credit cards and cash
	• Immunization records
Communication and transportation	• Emergency contact list including phone numbers and addresses (both in state and out of state)
	• Cellular phone and charger
	• Spare set of car keys
	• Map of the area
	• Paper and pencils/pens
	• Hand crank radio
Food and water	• Three-day supply of water (one gallon per day per person)
	• Nonelectrical can opener and utility knife
	• Paper cups, plates, and plastic utensils
	• Ready-to-eat canned food (3-day supply, including pet food)
	• Powdered or single serve drinks
	• Protein bars
	• Water purification method (i.e., bleach or tablets)
Personal needs	• Toiletries (i.e., toothbrush, toothpaste, and hand sanitizer) and toilet paper
	• Garbage bags
	• Plastic bucket with a tight lid
	• Blankets or sleeping bags
	• Infant supplies as needed (i.e., diapers, formula, wipes)
	• Change of clothing
Medical needs	• Emergency Information Form
	• First-aid kit
	• Photocopies of prescriptions
	• Prescription medications (1-month supply recommended)
	– All medications should be clearly labeled and kept separate from other supplies
Miscellaneous items	• Masking or duct tape
	• Disposable gloves
	• Toys or calming devices

After creating a family disaster kit, it will be important to educate the family to store the kit both safely and securely. Taking into account the type of living structure the family resides in, as well as the potential hazards, will play a role in selecting the best storage location that is easily accessible (Oberman 2013). Supplies should be kept in sturdy, waterproof containers, and be clearly labeled. An inventory list of supplies in the kit should also be maintained.

Once a location for the kit is determined, it is vital to develop a regular process to assess supplies in the disaster kit. The AAP recommends checking the kit every 6 months (American Academy of Pediatrics 2016). This includes replacing expired food, replacing items that children may have outgrown such as diapers and clothing, and updating personal and medical records (American Academy of Pediatrics 2016). Although it is important to keep copies of these documents in the disaster kit, instruct families to provide a copy to another trusted individual in another area and save details on a personal communication device, such as a cellular phone, as well.

6.5   Education Specific to Children

Historically, the media has been an avenue to disseminate information on disaster preparedness to communities. However, studies have shown that these methods have not increased disaster preparedness among families and their children (Bagwell et al. 2016). Children have unique needs and considerations during a disaster. They are more susceptible to the detrimental effects due to their physiologic, anatomic, developmental, and psychosocial differences (Blake 2018). In the event of a disaster, children are more at risk of being separated from their families. When separated, depending on age and developmental level, children may not be able to effectively communicate their needs or even their names. Separated children may also experience emotional reactions from disasters. For example, toddlers may exhibit increased temper tantrums or difficulty sleeping or eating. Older children may become withdrawn, anxious, or partake in high-risk behaviors. See Chap. 12 for more details. As nurses, it is important to consider these needs and aid in attending to children's specific developmental and physical needs (Blake 2018). The Centers for Disease Control and Prevention (CDC) recently developed reading material for children specific to disaster preparedness. A CDC book entitled, "Ready Wrigley," can assist with disaster preparedness discussions with children (Center for Disease Control and Prevention n.d.).

6.6   Conclusion

Disaster preparedness for families and children has been universally low. Because of the changing culture of the world, there is an increased awareness for not only nurses and HCPs but also for families and children to ensure that they are prepared. There are many components to being prepared including being knowledgeable, establishing a family plan, and creating emergency kits. Nurses play key roles in this process due to their frequent interaction with families and children. It is important for nurses to emphasize these components as well as provide resources, support, and information. With families and children being at-risk populations, it is paramount that nurses be that first step toward preparedness. With preparedness, families and children will move forward into the future with readiness for high-risk, low-frequency events.

Key Points
Nurses interact with families and children on a regular basis and in a variety of settings, including school, community, and hospital. Education and anticipatory guidance can be provided during every encounter.

- Provide resources to families to assist with identifying hazards within the area.
- Assist families with identifying emergency communication methods both from the community as well as within the family.
- Encourage families to explore insurance options as well as the benefits that are associated with different policies and plans.
- Facilitate families to create a home emergency plan that includes evacuation routes, reunification points, and emergency contact lists.
- Strengthen family plans by encouraging families to participate in community drills to increase awareness, knowledge, and comfort levels.
- Assist families with creating an emergency kit.
- Provide child-friendly education so that children can learn about disaster preparedness and become an active member in their family planning.

References

AICPA. Disasters and financial planning: a guide for preparedness and recovery. 2015. Available from https://www.redcross.org/content/dam/redcross/get-help/pdfs/disasters-and-financial-planning-guide.PDF.

American Academy of Pediatrics. Are you prepared for disasters? Family readiness kit. 2016. https://www.aap.org/en-us/Documents/disasters family readiness kit.pdf. Accessed 19 Apr 2019.

American Red Cross. Disaster preparedness plan. 2019. Available from https://www.redcross.org/get-help/how-to-prepare-for-emergencies/make-a-plan.html.

Bagwell HB, Liggin R, Thompson T, Lyle K, Anthony A, Baltz M, et al. Disaster preparedness in families with children with special health care needs. Clin Pediatr. 2016;55(11):1036–43. https://doi.org/10.1177/0009922816665087.

Bethesda. Child trends: number of children. 2018. Available from https://www.childtrends.org/indicators/number-of-children. Accessed 18 Mar 2018.

Blake, N. SPN position statement: disaster management for children and families. Soc Pediat Nurs. 2018.

Center for Disease Control and Prevention. Center for preparedness and response: books. n.d.. Available from https://www.cdc.gov/cpr/readywrigley/books.htm.

FEMA. Preparing for disaster. 2004. Available from https://www.fema.gov/pdf/library/pfd.pdf.

Goodhue C, Rickenback T, Hays S, Donohoe M. NAPNAP position statement on pediatric-focused advanced practice registered nurses' role in disasters involvement children. J Pediatr Health Care. 2018;33(1):A16–8.

Healthychildren.org. Disaster supplies list for families. 2018. Available from https://www.healthy-children.org/English/safety-prevention/at-home/Page/Family-Disaster0Supplies-List.aspx. Accessed 23 Apr 2019.

Markenson D. Have we forgotten the needs of children? Disaster Med Public Health Preparedness. n.d.;8(3):188–90. https://doi.org/10.1017/dmp.2014.48.

Merchant RM, Finne K, Lardy B, Veselovskiy G, Korba C, Margolis GS, Lurie N. State of emergency preparedness for US health insurance plans. Am J Manag Care. 2015;21(1):65–72.

Oberman, L. Earthquake preparedness: where to store your emergency supplies. Oregon Live. 2013. Available from https://www.oregonlive.com/living/2013/03/earthquake_preparation_where_t.html. Accessed 23 Apr 2019.

Ready. Emergency alerts. 2019a. Available from https://www.ready.gov/alerts.

Ready. Evacuation. 2019b. Available from https://www.ready.gov/evacuating-yourself-and-your-family

Ready. Make a kit. 2019c. Available from https://www.ready.gov/build-a-kit. Accessed 19 Apr 2019.

Ronan K, Alisic E, Towers B, Johnson V, Johnston D. Disaster preparedness for children and families: a critical review. Child Family Disaster Psych. 2015;17(58) https://doi.org/10.1009/s11920-015-0589-6.

Shao W, Xian S, Lin N, Kunreuther H, Jackson N, Goidel K. Understanding the effects of past flood events and perceived and estimated flood risks on individuals' voluntary flood insurance purchase behavior. Water Res. 2017;108:391–400. https://doi.org/10.1016/j.watres.2016.11.021.

Thomas T, Leander-Griffth M, Harp V, Cioffi J. Influences of preparedness knowledge and beliefs on household disaster preparedness. Center Dis Control Prevent. 2015;64(25):965–71.

Physical Development and Disaster Preparedness in Children

7

Lori J. Silao

7.1 Family Theoretical Backgrounds

There are multiple theories of family development, and the body of knowledge for family theory is extensive. Family theory includes the assessment of life cycle stages, emotional and developmental stages, coping strategies, and beliefs of health care that factor heavily into the way a family perceives and reacts to a disaster. For disaster preparedness, the nurse or HCP should be aware of two models for stress and adaptation and attachment: Hill's family stress theory, the ABC-X model, and developmental trauma theory.

7.2 Hill's Family Stress Theory

Hill's ABC-X model is significant to understanding family stress. This model was developed during World War II in response to men leaving families for the war, and Hill examined the responses families had to this sudden change to the family structure. Hill proposed families experienced different stressors or stressor events (factor A) and then examined the ability to meet the demands of the crisis or stressor in the form of coping mechanisms or resources (factor B). The family must then create a definition of the stressor event in order to interact with the stressor (factor C) to create a response or the final outcome (X, crisis or noncrisis) (Hill 1949). Of note, not all families experience crisis in the same way, and families that are considered "functional" typically have a different cognitive appraisal of stress and crisis than "nonfunctional" families. Further research has focused on the factors that influence the postcrisis responses (Friedman et al. 2003).

L. J. Silao (✉)
Azusa Pacific University, Azusa, CA, USA
e-mail: lsilao@apu.edu

© Springer Nature Switzerland AG 2020   209
C. J. Goodhue, N. Blake (eds.), *Nursing Management of Pediatric Disaster*,
https://doi.org/10.1007/978-3-030-43428-1_7

Family stress theory can be applied to any caregiver who works with pediatric patients. The way the caregiver interprets the stressful event as well as how he/she defines the event and responds to the disaster event will affect the way a child views, understands, and responds. According to family stress theory, the X factor ultimately states "there is a crisis" or "there is no crisis." One of the factors that can ease the crisis is the availability of resources (factor B). Resources range from broad community resources including extended family or caregivers, church or spiritual support, to finances, and to basic needs including clothing, shelter, clean water, food, and medications. In the time of emergency, if nurses or HCPs can provide resources to the family, crisis could be averted. The assessment of families in crisis should be a standard protocol in the development of emergency preparedness plans. The education of families to prepare for emergencies will also assist in their understanding and reaction to crisis so that resources are put into place before the arrival of a disaster. The nurse or HCP can continue to support the family by assisting the family in developing coping mechanisms and new ways to respond to crisis.

7.3   Developmental Trauma Theory

The effects of disaster and trauma on the developing child can last a lifetime. The importance of understanding the relationship between trauma and the family system is critical. One of the key developmental stages that all children experience is that of attachment. Trauma and disaster can adversely affect attachment on multiple levels. Traumatic experiences can influence future generations and cannot be underestimated by the nurse or HCP in providing care during a disaster.

Developmental trauma theory proposes that healthy attachment is interrupted by trauma (Heller and LaPierre 2012). Heller and LaPierre (2012) stated that there are specific symptoms that children exhibit as a result of interrupted attachment from trauma. The interference affects connections with others, the ability to self-regulate and recognize physical and emotional needs, the development of trust, the ability to set boundaries, and the ability to develop a sense of love (Heller and LaPierre 2012). The authors also described survival mechanisms that victims develop in order to cope with trauma. Victims may withdraw from or avoid emotional situations, develop a fear of being alone, and may develop a desire for an altered state that can be achieved via drugs or alcohol. Heller and LaPierre (2012) further postulated that the coping strategies in response to trauma also interfere with healthy attachment.

While developmental trauma theory was developed in response to abuse, disasters can also be a significant form of trauma. Disasters do not just go away as there are always sequelae. Many countries have limited access to resources, with the source of trauma prolonged with delayed recovery efforts. Prolonged trauma can negatively impact the family structure and function. If left untreated, children can develop anxiety, feelings of shame, uncontrolled anger, and emotional detachment (Cochlo and Brcen 2019). Physically, children may develop sleep disorders, eating disorders, autoimmune disorders, and even cardiovascular disorders (Coehlo and

Breen 2019). Additionally, children may internalize the perceived threat of danger to their parents and families. The developmental age of the child will influence the child's perception and understanding of emergency situations. Scenarios where families are separated, intermittently or permanently, can lead to extreme stress in the child. The nurse or HCP must focus on consistency and continuity of care, and reunification of families as soon as possible after the crisis has occurred. See Chap. 12 for further information.

7.4 Growth and Development

Children have unique needs throughout their development. These variations should be considered when providing care to children, especially in a disaster situation. There is a common thought that children are just "small adults", and this could not be farther from the truth. Ideally, pediatric patients should have care provided by nurses experienced in pediatric care (Burnweit and Stylianos 2011). Burnweit and Stylianos (2011) recommend that pediatric patients should be separated from other patient groups in a disaster situation. The following section will review normal developmental patterns for children and disaster preparedness concerns for each developmental age group.

7.4.1 Infant: Birth to 12 months

Infants experience rapid growth from birth through the first year of life. Infants change from being completely helpless and dependent on a caregiver to developing early mobility and the ability to point to things that they want as well as respond to simple requests (Centers for Disease Control and Prevention 2018a). The first 3 months are critical to establish a consistent caregiver as the infant begins to develop trust. As the infant forms a relationship with the caregiver, a foundation for future relationship formation is established. The way a parent adjusts to the parenting role is directly related to the establishment of trust in the infant (Franklin and Prows 2017). It is important for parents to learn cues provided by the infant, such as crying, facial expressions, and even temperament.

Physically, infants typically triple their birth weight by 12 months of age (Franklin and Prows 2017). During this time, infants begin to sit unassisted by 6 months of age and infant reflexes disappear by around 6 months. The infant begins to push into a crawling position and can often stand with assistance and starts to babble with sounds. When placed in an infant's hand, a toy almost immediately goes into the infant's mouth in order for the infant to gain a greater understanding of his/her environment. Infants will reach for all things, and especially their caregivers when they enter a room. Infants will lean toward and reach up to the caregiver or parent to signal they wish to be picked up. It is important to note that most infants have a lack of neck muscle strength, especially in proportion to a larger and more heavy head and thus more prone to head injury (Fendya 2006). Infant head and neck support is necessary to help protect the infant from head trauma.

7.4.2   Disaster Preparedness Implications for the Infant

Infants are completely reliant on their caregivers and will generally be immobile. There is the possibility of separation of the infant from its family. Since attachment is a significant developmental foundation in this age group, it is important for the infant to have a consistent caregiver if possible for developmental concerns.

Infants are at higher risk for dehydration and hypovolemia than adults due to thinner skin and lower body volume of fluids due to smaller size (Lozon and Bradin 2018). Infants who are breastfeeding will provide a challenge if breast milk is not available, or if the infant has been separated from its mother. Formula will need to be provided, as well as diapers and blankets. (See Chap. 17 for more information). Infants will need to be assessed for physical injuries, as well as cold exposure and hypothermia. Infants are obligate nose breathers, and exposure to chemicals or toxins in the air supply may complicate the infant's airway and breathing. The nurse or HCP should also keep in mind that the infant's airway is much smaller and more pliable and soft than adults. Simply extending the head too far can block the airway. Equipment used for the infant needs to be sized appropriately, and a pediatric-sized oxygen mask may be inverted in order to fit over the mouth and nose for ventilation.

7.4.3   Toddler: 1–3 Years

The toddler period is one of active change and mobility as motor development grows steadily. There is great exploration of the toddler's environment and language development is rapid during this time. The toddler begins to identify a sense of self and begins to gain some self-control. The ability to say "no" is frequent in the second and third year, often resulting in "temper tantrums" when the caregiver does not acquiesce to the demands of the toddler. Toddlers also may show signs of fear toward strangers and cling to caregivers in new or unfamiliar situations (Centers for Disease Control and Prevention 2019a). Older toddlers, however, separate more easily from parents than younger toddlers and are aware of others' feelings, and may even try to console another friend who is upset.

Toddlers love to play with toys, can begin drawing with crayons, and take part in games. Toddlers understand when it is "their turn" to participate in a game or during play (Centers for Disease Control and Prevention 2019a). Toddlers are easily distracted, and laughter is easily induced between the ages of one and three. It is important to note that toddlers display a wide range of emotions. Those emotions can change very quickly, hence the term "temper tantrums" where 1 min the toddler is quietly playing with toys, and the next minute the toddler is crying.

7.4.4   Disaster Preparedness Implications for the Toddler

Toddlers will need to be assessed for airway patency, hypothermia, injuries, dehydration, and shock. Similar to infants, toddlers may not be able to communicate clearly where their injuries are. Airways are small and pliable in this age group and easily blocked. Emergency equipment size may be difficult in this group as the equipment may be too small (infant sized) or too big (pediatric sized). For the toddler, it may be preferential to use smaller equipment rather than larger size. Toddlers are also still at risk for neck injuries, and neck support will be important. Toddlers should be monitored closely for head injuries due to the weaker neck muscles and often the inability to communicate head or neck pain. Providing warmth, clean water to drink, and food to eat with a familiar caregiver is ideal for the toddler.

Since the toddler may be afraid of strangers and new or unfamiliar situations, it is possible that the toddler may be separated from their caregiver during a disaster. Lozon and Bradin (2018) note that nurses or HCPs may be in protective clothing such as masks, gowns, gloves, and this could be frightening to a toddler. Ways to familiarize a toddler to a routine as well as make medical interventions less frightening should be put into the plan of care. If parents or regular caregivers are present, involve them in the care of the toddler to provide a sense of security. There is a fear among young children that they may lose their loved ones in an emergency (Coehlo and Breen 2019). Simple games and toys may entertain the toddler enough for nurses and health care personnel to provide necessary medical and rescue interventions. Toddlers are easily distracted and the use of medical equipment as a toy may work well in this age group.

7.4.5 Preschool: 3–6 Years

Growth continues steadily during the third to sixth year of life. Average weight gain is 4–5 pounds per year, and height typically increases by 2–3 in. per year (Centers for Disease Control and Prevention 2019a). Most preschoolers sleep for an average of 10–13 h per night, and a daytime nap is usually absent. Preschoolers have significant motor development that includes the ability to run, jump, kick, and catch. The ability to balance on one foot and pedal a tricycle and steer is developed during this time. Preschoolers can draw circles and primitive stick people. They learn to use scissors and can dress themselves with supervision.

Preschoolers begin to understand concepts of time and can begin counting. By the age of 5, most preschoolers know a telephone number and can respond to questions where they are asked "why." For example, "Why is there food spilled on the table?". Usually, preschoolers will respond with answers as their language development progresses rapidly. Of note, some children may develop stuttering at this time, and it is usually related to the fact that many ideas race through their minds faster than their ability to communicate these ideas. Caregivers should be patient and allow the child to have complete attention when the child speaks and not interrupt or comment on the stuttering (Centers for Disease Control and Prevention 2019a).

Costume play and dress up is common in the preschool-age child. Children love to pretend, and they may create elaborate stories with their play. Books and television or the Internet shows factor very heavily into their playtime and are influential in the development of their worldviews. Preschoolers often express interest in the arts at this age, including painting, music, dance, and acting.

7.4.6   Disaster Implications for the Preschooler

Many of the same physiological changes in the toddler apply to the preschooler with primary differences in weight and cognitive appraisal development. Assessment will always need to include airway and breathing since the child's respiratory system is much smaller and more prone to blockage. Cardiovascular status, especially fluid and volume status, is critical for the preschooler due to their smaller size and risk for dehydration, shock, and hypothermia. Children do not usually have cardiac disease as adults do, and thus a child's heart tends to be stronger than their respiratory systems. The heart may be able to overcome the early stages of shock due to its relative health (Fendya 2006). However, injuries, including head injuries, will need to be addressed, especially broken bones and bleeding injuries. Smaller equipment will need to be utilized for the preschooler, and generally, pediatric-sized equipment will fit the preschool child.

Because the preschooler has language development that allows them to express their feelings, it is important for caregivers to acknowledge any fears and to provide comfort during a disaster. Caregivers should limit exposure to the media in times of crisis as preschoolers may not be able to understand repetitive video snippets on the news. They may interpret the news and videos of events as occurring over and over rather than a repeat of a single incident. Preschoolers can begin participating in disaster preparedness such as taking cover under or next to a desk or dialing 9-1-1 on a phone (Federal Emergency Management Agency 2018). Since the preschooler is familiar with costume play, it may assist the emergency personnel when personal protective equipment must be worn. If the caregiver can assist the child in understanding that this "dress up" is necessary, they will be less frightened. Personnel can give the child a mask to draw on and wear themselves to participate in interventions or even during a rescue. Since the preschooler has the ability to memorize a phone number, this information may assist emergency personnel in locating family if separated. Engaging the preschooler in relief efforts in the form of either fantasy play or pretend play will alleviate stress. For example, preschoolers can pretend that they are a fireman, policeman, nurse, or doctor and then pretend to assist the real rescue team in their efforts.

7.4.7   Middle Childhood (School-Age): 6–11 or 12 Years

School-age children have a wide variety of coordination, physical endurance, as well as fine motor skills. Most school-age children have smooth development of muscle coordination. Many children start to play sports during this time, and this may continue through adolescence (and even adulthood!). Height continues to develop, and as many children develop toward age 11 and 12, they may approach their adult height, especially with the onset of puberty. As many families are aware, genetics, nutrition, and family history may play a role in height as well as other developmental factors (Centers for Disease Control and Prevention 2019a). School-age children develop a sense of body image as early as age 6 and frequently compare their own growth and development to other children as well as media images. Secondary sex characteristics begin to develop during this time, with the average onset of puberty around ages 10–14 in girls and ages 12–16 in boys (Centers for Disease Control and Prevention 2019a).

Physiologically, children at this age differ from adults in that they breathe more air per pound of body weight than adults (Beach and Frost 2019). While the older school-age child has a more developed airway, the younger school-age child still has a proportionately small airway that is still somewhat pliable and can block easily. Because they have thinner skin, school-age children are more prone to heat loss and dehydration. Fluid loss is more dramatic in children because they are smaller and have less fluid in their bodies than adults (Centers for Disease Control and Prevention 2018b). One liter of saline loss in a child is proportionately more dramatic than in an adult. Infection is another concern that children at this age are less likely to wash hands consistently, are more likely to put things in their mouths that are not clean, and have a less-developed immune system compared to that of an adult.

7.4.8   Disaster Implications for the School-Age Child

As with all ages, the school-age child will need to be assessed for injuries, hydration status, and mental status. The school-aged child may be very frightened in an emergency, and the first step in evaluating and treating psychological stress is to assure that basic needs are being met such as food, drinking water, shelter, and proper supervision (American Academy of Pediatrics 2019a). School-age children are still developing communication patterns, and it will be important to allow children to express their feelings, including their fears (Centers for Disease Control and Prevention 2017). School-age children may be unaware of what is happening around them, and a loss of control over their environment can be very stressful. The exposure to media following a disaster should be limited due to children's misperception that disaster events are ongoing when, in fact, they were a singular event. Caregivers need to provide reassurance that the child is safe. Children who are aware of what is happening around them tend to cope better, and thus it is important for parents or caregivers to maintain an environment that provides a sense of safety to the child will be very important in their adjustment to an emergency situation (Centers for Disease Control and Prevention 2017). See Chap. 12 for further information.

School-age children are usually very enthusiastic about participating in disaster drills such as earthquake and fire drills and may be helpful in risk reduction. The Centers for Disease Control and Prevention (CDC) (2017) recommends that school-age children plan, practice, and repeat their activities in disaster preparedness. Pfefferbaum et al. (2018) promote the idea that school-age children are ideal to work with older children and adults in preparing for disaster. The authors state that there has been very little research into potential roles for the school-age child in disaster preparedness. For example, school-age children can provide pertinent information about their surrounding communities, potential resources, and needs of their own families and the needs of other families. The potential benefit of including the school-age child in disaster preparedness is that traumatic effects of disaster can be minimized if the child has been involved with adults in planning for response to disaster. Including children in planning for disaster can increase their sense of self-worth and confidence, as well as interpersonal relationships with their local communities (Pfefferbaum et al. 2018).

7.4.9 Adolescence/Later Childhood: 11–19 Years

The adolescent child is one who borders on puberty all the way through young adulthood. Growth is accelerated during this time with the development of secondary sex characteristics. Early adolescents are very egocentric, and most are concerned with their own thoughts (American Academy of Pediatrics 2019b). As adolescence progresses, teens may want more privacy and sexual identity can be confusing for them (American Academy of Pediatrics 2019b). Teens tend to spend less time with their families and more time with their friends. Peer pressure to fit in and conform to their friend groups is very important to teens. It is estimated that one in four teens will experience bouts of depression and anxiety as well as emotional and/or behavioral problems (Duderstadt 2019; Centers for Disease Control and Prevention 2019b). Routine screening for mental disorders is critical, as well as early treatment and support.

Teens may also lack the understanding of risks of activities and can be impulsive, especially when it comes to sexual exploration. Older adolescents are more able to understand the consequences of their actions and may be less impulsive than younger adolescents (American Academy of Pediatrics 2019b). Adolescents are more likely to try new things that are often prohibited without understanding long-term consequences. Teens tend to be very electronic savvy and can easily navigate across the Internet. Video gaming is common, especially in teen boys. Phone use is common, and teens may spend hours on their electronic devices. Parents should be savvy to their child's use of the Internet to make sure the content they are viewing and interacting with is age-appropriate.

7.4.10 Implications for Disaster Preparedness for the Adolescent

Adolescent children are the most likely group to truly participate in disaster preparedness. Their use of the Internet and electronic gadgets may work in their favor during a disaster as they may be able to locate friends and family quickly (assuming that they have access to the Internet). The adolescent uses social media to keep them current on their surroundings as well as to pass on information and photos to their friends. The use of technology can also provide disaster information and instructions. Websites such as YouTube can demonstrate all types of life situations, including how to use a fire extinguisher, how to perform basic CPR, how to dress a wound, and multiple other topics. Cell phones can also be utilized as tracking beacons for emergency responders.

The adolescent may be able to organize groups to provide assistance and to calm younger children, especially in a school setting. Adolescents may also be able to assist in basic first aid and triage, as well as blood donation in the older teen.

Disaster planning should include teen training of basic responses to emergencies. The Federal Emergency Management Agency (FEMA) has joined with the American Red Cross to develop community emergency response training (CERT), and teens who are in the eighth, ninth, tenth, or eleventh grade and who have engaged in community service are encouraged to complete CERT training as a way to enhance a community's response to disaster. Local communities also send youth representatives to Washington, D.C., to participate in a youth preparedness council where they meet with FEMA representatives and develop emergency preparedness projects. Topics such as basic first aid, cardiopulmonary resuscitation, fire safety including home sprinkler management, coping strategies, general preparedness, personal safety, recovery, and resilience are offered (Federal Emergency Management Agency 2016). By engaging youth in disaster preparedness programs, critical thinking skills are developed as well as problem-solving approaches and allows the adolescent to develop strategic planning skills (Pfefferbaum et al. 2018).

The adolescent child will border on adulthood in regard to the assessment of injuries. The pulmonary system should be well developed by adolescence, and the airway develops more cartilage and strength. The adolescent child can have a significant variation in weight and size due to normal growth, and a 13-year-old could be 5 ft. tall or over 6 ft. tall! Basing medication dosages on weight or body surface area is still advisable. Larger adolescents may have similar fluid needs to an adult, and there may be thicker skin and fat layers that can insulate better against hypothermia, but dehydration in a disaster situation must be assessed and treated immediately. Compensatory mechanisms should be recognized, and treatment of underlying conditions should be initiated quickly.

While adolescents can often take charge in many situations, they need to be monitored for unseen psychological trauma that may not be immediately apparent. Nurses and HCPs should recognize signs of stress in teens, especially if they exhibit anxiety, withdraw from stressful situations, and if they begin to over intellectualize a situation and not express emotion (Coehlo and Breen 2019). If the adolescent witnesses the injury or death of a parent or other family member or friend, the risk of post-traumatic stress is increased (Lozon and Bradin 2018). Proper ongoing mental health evaluation is important in this age group, including coping skills training and early intervention (Kolaitis 2017). Please refer to Chap. 12 for more information on mental health.

7.5   Pharmacokinetics and Pharmacodynamics in Pediatric Development

Principles of pharmacokinetics (the movement of a medication from entry to excretion) and pharmacodynamics (the relationship of drug dosing and drug effect) are different in children than adults (Fernandez et al. 2011). Developmental changes influence the bioavailability in a medication, such as total body water, gastrointestinal development, epidermal maturity, body surface area, and kidney and liver maturity. The principles of absorption, volume of distribution, and excretion are also influenced by the physiologic states of the child such as shock, hypoxia, and dehydration.

7.5.1 Absorption

Oral, injection, and intravenous are three main routes of drug administration. Although the most direct delivery of medications is intravenous, the preferred route of medication administration in pediatrics is oral, despite alterations in gut absorption. Injected medications may have erratic absorption due to muscle mass differences, alterations in circulation due to illness, and differences in injection site choices. Unlike intravenous medications, oral medications must undergo absorption in order to reach the systemic circulation (Lu and Rosenbaum 2014). Absorption differs in children in that the gastrointestinal tract is more immature with changes in pH, biliary tract immaturity, and delayed gastric emptying time (Lu and Rosenbaum 2014). Infants have delayed gastric emptying as well as a decreased intestinal absorption area with immature enzymatic activity that can lead to poor gut absorption of medications (Lu and Rosenbaum 2014).

Absorption via percutaneous medication administration can be affected by the thickness of the epidermis and the hydration status of the child. A thinner epidermal layer and increased hydration lead to increased absorption, and thus percutaneous administration can lead to toxicity. Intramuscular absorption is not ideal in pediatrics as absorption is unpredictable due to variations in skeletal muscle blood flow (Lu and Rosenbaum 2014). However, these changes in gut absorption may be favorable for some medications.

7.5.2 Distribution

Once a medication has been absorbed, the medication distributes throughout the body. This distribution is affected by many factors. Infants have an underdeveloped membrane permeability, and thus some medications can cross the blood-brain barrier and cause toxicity (Fernandez et al. 2011). Children have significant changes in the amount of body water and fat as they mature. As they grow, the amount of fat increases and the amount of water decreases. Increased body water may mean more distribution for water-soluble drugs (Fernandez et al. 2011; Lu and Rosenbaum 2014). However, the way medications bind to plasma protein is interrupted. For effective plasma concentrations, medications must bind to plasma proteins. In the neonate, there is decreased plasma protein binding due to decreased plasma proteins in circulation and lower binding capacities of the plasma protein that is present (Fernandez et al. 2011; Lu and Rosenbaum 2014). Additionally, there may be competition for binding at protein sites with certain medications. A common example in the neonate is that of bound acid medications that compete for bilirubin binding sites on albumin, and will actually displace bilirubin that can lead to hyperbilirubinemia (Fernandez et al. 2011; Lu and Rosenbaum 2014).

7.5.3 Excretion

The majority of medications are metabolized by the liver. The rate of metabolism is dependent on several factors such as blood flow, hepatic enzymes and liver function, and the amount of binding with plasma proteins. The goal of liver metabolism is to convert medications into a more water-soluble form to prepare for excretion (Fernandez et al. 2011). Hepatocytes are responsible for this conversion. It would logically reason that if the child has an immature liver, as infants do, this metabolism would be slowed. According to Lu and Rosenbaum (2014), drug metabolizing enzymes within the liver each have their own pattern of development and thus not all drugs will be metabolized equally. In combination with an immature liver, where some of these enzymes have not yet been developed, drug excretion can be varied depending on the child's developmental age as well as any comorbidities that would affect excretion.

Medications are also excreted via the renal system. Excretion is dependent on renal blood flow, glomerular filtration, tubular excretion, and reabsorption (Fernandez et al. 2011; Lu and Rosenbaum 2014). Renal blood flow and cardiac output increase with age in normal child development. By 2 years of age, renal blood flow should be consistent with adult values (Lu and Rosenbaum 2014). Creatinine clearance reaches adult rates by 6 months of age, and renal tubular excretion increases to adult levels by around 7 months of age. Tubular reabsorption is a more gradual process from birth to adolescence, with the main development noted between 1–3 years of age (Lu and Rosenbaum 2014). The main difference in renal excretion of medications is that infants will have a more immature renal system than an adult and thus may not clear medications as quickly as an adult. While children may have similar glomerular filtration rates as adults, their kidneys are still growing and developing and are at risk for nephrotoxic damage from medications.

Pharmacodynamic principles in the pediatric patient have been predominantly extrapolated from pharmacokinetics data. This is due to a general lack of data regarding pharmacodynamics. Each individual medication must be evaluated within the pediatric population to establish what age-related differences occur. While many medications are tested in vitro, studies have shown that in vivo differences exist. In the pediatric patient, there are many developmental variables such as membrane permeability, receptor characteristics, and the existence of active metabolites (Lu and Rosenbaum 2014). Pediatric dosing regimens have been developed utilizing body surface area calculations and principles of pharmacokinetics. The data to support these basic calculations are inconsistent in the pediatric patient, and data on tissue composition (water, protein, and fats) are limited in the pediatric patient (Fernandez et al. 2011). Thus, in terms of disaster preparedness, nurses and HCPs cannot make an assumption that medications used in adults will have the same metabolism and bioavailability in pediatric patients. As advances in pharmacology are made, medication safety profiles will be better developed for the pediatric patient.

7.6   Pharmaceutical Implications

It should be emphasized that in any type of disaster, a pharmacist will most likely not be available, and a pediatric pharmacist even more difficult to find. Based on information available regarding pediatric dosing regimens, it is clear that pediatric pharmacy expertise is necessary in any medication management situation. During a disaster, pediatric medications may be in short supply. In 2016, the American Academy of Pediatrics (AAP) published a policy statement for the management of children in public health emergencies, disasters, or terrorism in which they noted that most emergency medication stockpiles are produced for adults and are not suitable for children (American Academy of Pediatrics 2016). If pediatric dosages of medications are not available, medications will need to be adapted, if possible, for the smaller size of the child. In a disaster situation, the FDA may "authorize emergency use of an unapproved or unlicensed medical product or an unapproved or unlicensed use (such as for a pediatric subpopulation) of an already approved product if certain public health emergency criteria are met or declarations are made" (American Academy of Pediatrics, 2016, p.2). However, all efforts should be made to use appropriate medications that have been FDA approved for children, and appropriate dosages should be calculated based on the child's age and weight.

In the event of a disaster, most pediatric offices are not well-stocked with medical countermeasures for children. One of the main issues is that liquid medications, traditionally used in smaller children, have a short shelf life and, if not used, must be discarded by the expiration date (American Academy of Pediatrics 2016). The cost to maintain a large stockpile of liquid medications is high and prohibitive. The AAP (American Academy of Pediatrics 2016) recommends that an adequate stockpile of medical countermeasures be available for children of all ages, including liquid medications, delivery devices, and instructions for dosing and administration. The AAP disaster policy statement concludes that ongoing research should be conducted for pediatric medical countermeasure medications and that distribution plans and access to medications in an emergency should have a well-developed interagency plan utilizing subject matter experts for best practice.

7.7   Conclusion

Physical development is an important factor for the health care provider to consider when evaluating and assessing needs for disaster preparedness in children. While individual assessment is critical to meet the needs of the pediatric patient, the care provider must also be versed in theoretical foundations of family assessment. Two examples presented in this chapter are Hill's ABC-X model of stress and adaptation, and developmental trauma theory. Both theoretical models provide a framework to understand how children and families respond to disasters and provide a framework for nurses and HCPs to intervene during a crisis mode.

It is evident that children of various developmental ages will have different physical and emotional needs. The nurse or HCP must be adept at recognizing these differences and be able to provide care that is developmentally appropriate. Children, unlike adults, are often not able to fully understand the crisis at hand and can be very uncooperative because of their lack of understanding. Developmentally appropriate interventions will assist the care provider in increased compliance and influence the child's reaction to the crisis. The developmental assessment must also include an understanding of pharmacokinetics and pharmacodynamics in the pediatric patient in order to treat children in a timely and effective manner using best practice. Because developmental assessment directs all care and interventions for the pediatric patient, the nurse or HCP will ultimately be more successful in caring for pediatric patients by utilizing developmentally appropriate interventions and thus will improve outcomes during a disaster.

References

American Academy of Pediatrics. Medical countermeasures for children in public health emergencies, disasters, or terrorism. Pediatrics. 2016;137(2):1–9. https://doi.org/10.1542/peds.2015-4273.

American Academy of Pediatrics. Children and disasters: disaster preparedness to meet children's needs. 2019a. Retrieved from www.aap.org/en-as/advocacy-and-policy/aap-health-initiative/children-and-disasters/pages/default.aspx

American Academy of Pediatrics. Stages of adolescence. 2019b. Retrieved from www.healthychildren.org

Beach M, Frost P. Unique needs of children during disasters and other public health emergencies. In: Veenema T, editor. Disaster nursing and emergency preparedness. 4th ed. New York, NY: Springer Publishing; 2019. p. 179–207.

Burnweit C, Stylianos S. Disaster response in a pediatric field hospital: lessons learned in Haiti. J Pediatr Surg. 2011;46(6):1131–9.

Centers for Disease Control and Prevention. Schools and childcare: Preparing for the unexpected. 2017. Retrieved from www.cdc.gov/features/school-emergency-preparedness/index.html

Centers for Disease Control and Prevention. CDC's developmental milestones. 2018a. Retrieved from www.cdc.gov/ncbddd/actearly/milestones/index.html

Centers for Disease Control and Prevention. How are children different from adults? 2018b. Retrieved from www.cdc.gov/childrenindisasters/differences.html

Centers for Disease Control and Prevention. Child development basics. 2019a. Retrieved from www.cdc.gov/ncbddd/childdevelopment/facts.html

Centers for Disease Control and Prevention. Data and statistics on children's mental health. 2019b. Retrieved from https://www.cdc.gov/childrensmentalhealth/data.html

Coehlo D, Breen H. Trauma and family nursing. In: Kaakinen J, Coehlo D, Steele R, Robinson M, editors. Family health care nursing: theory, practice, and research. 6th ed. Philadelphia, PA: F.A. Davis & Co.; 2019.

Duderstadt K. Pediatric physical examination: an illustrated handbook. 3rd ed. St. Louis, MO: Elsevier; 2019.

Federal Emergency Management Agency. Youth preparedness fact sheet. 2016. Retrieved from www.fema.gov

Federal Emergency Management Agency. Earthquake safety at school. 2018. Retrieved from www.fema.gov/earthquake-safety-school

Fendya D. When disaster strikes: Care considerations for pediatric patients. J Trauma Nurs. 2006;13(4):161–5.

Fernandez E, Perez R, Hernandez A, Tejada P, Arteta M, Ramos J. Factors and mechanisms for pharmacokinetic differences between pediatric population and adults. Pharmaceutics. 2011;3(1):53–72. https://doi.org/10.3390/pharmaceutics3010053.

Franklin Q, Prows C. Developmental and genetic influences on child health promotion. In: Hockenberry M, Wilson D, Rodgers C, editors. Wong's essentials of pediatric nursing. 10th ed. Amsterdam: Elsevier; 2017.

Friedman M, Bowden V, Jones E. Family nursing: research, theory, and practice. 5th ed. Upper Saddle River, NJ: Prentice Hall; 2003.

Heller L, LaPierre A. Healing developmental trauma: how early trauma affects self-regulation, self-image, and the capacity for relationship. Berkeley, CA: North Atlantic Books; 2012.

Hill R. Families under stress. New York, NY: Harper & Row; 1949.

Kolaitis G. Trauma and post-traumatic stress disorder in children and adolescents. Eur J Psychotraumatol. 2017;8(suppl 4):1–2. https://doi.org/10.1080/20008198.2017.1351198.

Lozon M, Bradin S. Pediatric disaster preparedness. Pediatr Clin N Am. 2018;65(2018):1205–20. https://doi.org/10.1016/j.pcl.2018.07.015.

Lu H, Rosenbaum S. Developmental pharmocokinetics in pediatric populations. J Pediatr Pharmacol Ther. 2014;19(4):262–76.

Pfefferbaum B, Pfefferbaum R, Van Horn R. Involving children in disaster risk reduction: the importance of participation. Eur J Psychotraumatol. 2018;9(2):1–6. https://doi.org/10.1080/20008198.2018.1425577.

Children with Special Health Care Needs and Disasters

8

John S. Murray

8.1 Introduction

Emerging science shows that with a rapidly changing climate, the frequency and magnitude of extreme weather events will continue to increase in years to come (Ronoh et al. 2015a; Bagwell et al. 2016; Dyregrov et al. 2018; American Academy of Pediatrics 2019). There is also growing concern among pediatric nurses and HCPs that man-made disasters are occurring with increasing frequency and causing unprecedented destruction (American Academy of Pediatrics 2019). Currently, it is estimated that as many as 175 million children worldwide will be impacted annually by disasters related to climate change (Dyregrov et al. 2018; Codreanu et al. 2014; Philipsborn and Chan 2018). While it is important for all individuals to be prepared for future disasters, this is especially true for vulnerable populations such as children with special health care needs (CSHCN), which includes over ten million (or 15%) of all children in the United States (U.S.) (Bagwell et al. 2016; United States Department of Health and Human Services, Health Resources and Services Administration 2019) and over 93 million youth worldwide (United Nations Children's Fund 2018).

8.2 Children with Special Health Care Needs Defined

The U.S. Department of Health and Human Services, Health Resources and Services Administration (HRSA), defines CSHCN as children 18 years of age and younger who have been diagnosed with, or are at increased risk for, chronic conditions that are physical, developmental, behavioral, or emotional in nature. These children may have developmental delays, learning disabilities, autism, as well as problems with

J. S. Murray (✉)
Bouvé College of Health Sciences, Northeastern University, Boston, MA, USA

© Springer Nature Switzerland AG 2020
C. J. Goodhue, N. Blake (eds.), *Nursing Management of Pediatric Disaster*,
https://doi.org/10.1007/978-3-030-43428-1_8

hearing, vision, or mobility as just a few examples (Toor et al. 2018). CSHCN also have requirements for health care services that are above and beyond what is typically required by the pediatric population in general. Additionally, CSHCN and their caretakers frequently require provisions from a number of community agencies such as social services, public health, and education (United States Department of Health and Human Services, Health Resources and Services Administration 2019). For purposes in this textbook, the term CSHCN will also include children with functional and access needs.

8.3 Vulnerabilities of Children with Special Health Care Needs in Disasters

Over the past decade, nurses and HCPs have emphasized that children have very different needs than adults during disasters (Zagory et al. 2016; Murray 2010; Murray 2011; Murray and Monteiro 2012). A number of factors related to anatomy and physiology, as well as social and emotional development, make the pediatric population more susceptible to risk. The younger the child's age, the greater the vulnerability (Zagory et al. 2016; Murray 2010; Murray 2011). However, during disasters, CSHCN have several additional factors (e.g., physical, sensory, developmental, cognitive, emotional, special medical accommodations, geography, and poverty) that can increase their susceptibility to adverse outcomes (Zagory et al. 2016).

8.3.1 Physical and Sensory Factors

There is a paucity of literature available on how physical and sensory factors (e.g., blindness, hearing impairments, a combination of both [dual sensory loss], etc.) affect children in disasters (Murray 2010; Wolf-Fordham et al. 2015; Stough et al. 2017). Most empirical evidence is based on findings from research on adults with physical and sensory deficits. For example, adults with mobility limitations may experience challenges during the evacuation process such as residing in temporary shelters that may not be handicap accessible (Stough et al. 2017; Brodie et al. 2006). This was an important lesson learned with Hurricane Katrina in 2005 (Brodie et al. 2006). More recently, the 2010 and 2011 earthquakes in Christchurch, New Zealand, demonstrated how CSHCN are particularly susceptible to adversity during disasters. The magnitude 7.1 earthquake in 2010 caused widespread damage to communities. Office buildings, hospitals, schools, places of worship, etc., were reduced to rubble (Fig. 8.1). The following year, a magnitude 6.3 earthquake struck the same location causing even further destruction as well as 185 fatalities (Ronoh et al. 2015a; Potter et al. 2015). The population most adversely affected was CSHCN. Temporary shelters were not adapted to accommodate children in wheelchairs nor did they have the capacity for specialized medical equipment requiring a power source (Ronoh et al. 2015a, b).

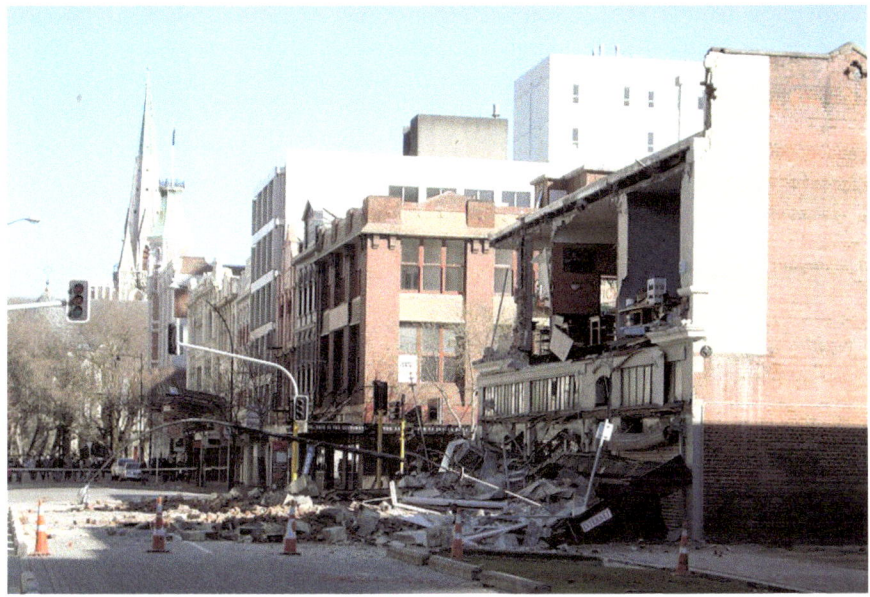

Fig. 8.1 Christchurch, Canterbury Earthquake, 4 Sept 2010. (Courtesy of Wikipedia)

CSHCN, such as those with an autism spectrum disorder (ASD), have increased vulnerability in disasters because of difficulties with sensory integration. Children with ASD are highly sensitive to unusually loud noises (e.g., emergency alert systems, rescue vehicle sirens, falling debris, breaking glass, calls for help, etc.), unexpected stimuli (e.g., bright lights or poor lighting, burning smells, etc.), environmental sensations (e.g., ground shaking, high winds, etc.), and/or touch or contact by strangers during disasters (Ronoh et al. 2015a; Baker and Cormier 2013; Boon et al. 2011).

8.3.2   Developmental, Cognitive, and Emotional Factors

While all young children may not be able to communicate effectively because of age, exchange of information in disasters is even more challenging for those with developmental delays (Zagory et al. 2016; Wolf-Fordham et al. 2015; Stough et al. 2017). Most CSHCN rely on a caregiver for some level of support. However, this is especially so for children with cognitive impairment. Some cognitively impaired children rely heavily on a caregiver to communicate their needs. If separated from caregivers in a disaster, children with a cognitive impairment may not be able to communicate who they are, the name of someone to contact, special medical needs, and/or any injuries experienced (Stough et al. 2017). Emotional behavioral disorders also place CSHCN at greater risk in disasters. For example, children with neurobehavioral disorders such as attention-deficit/hyperactivity disorder (ADHD) may place themselves at greater risk because they are less capable of paying attention to instructions and controlling impulsive behaviors (Stough et al. 2017). Children with ADHD may engage in risk-taking behavior and demonstrate poor judgment as defiance toward authority figures such as disaster response personnel (Mattson 2013; Ghandour et al. 2018). Please see Chap. 7 for more details on developmental issues.

8.3.3 Special Medical Accommodation Factors

From 2001 until 2010, the U.S. HRSA Maternal and Child Health Bureau allocated funding on three occasions to conduct the National Survey of CSHCN. The purpose of this survey was to examine at the state and national level the requirements of CSHCN when it comes to access to health care, utilization of services, quality of assistance provided, and the most common requests of family members as well as communities where the child resided (Ghandour et al. 2018). Results of one survey showed that almost 50% of CSHCN had a requirement for a minimum of five or more dedicated health care services and/or specialized medical equipment needs (National Survey of Children with Special Healthcare Needs (NC-CSHCN) 2016). The most frequently identified equipment needs are for CSHCN with a gastrostomy tube or requiring supplemental oxygen (Hipper et al. 2018). Any disruption in the availability of electrical power, limited access to clean water, or inaccessibility to required medications and/or sources of nutrition (e.g., enteral, parenteral, etc.) could have life-threatening consequences during disasters (Toor et al. 2018; Zagory et al. 2016; Hipper et al. 2018; Goodhue et al. 2016).

8.3.4 Geographic Factors

Disasters can result in the complete devastation of cities as happened in October 2018 when Hurricane Michael struck the Florida (FL) panhandle causing catastrophic and widespread damage to Mexico Beach and Panama City (Fig. 8.2). Hurricane Michael was a powerful Category 5 storm—the strongest and most destructive hurricane to make landfall in the northwestern part of FL. The disaster resulted in the deaths of 49 people and $25 billion in damage (United States Department of Commerce, National Oceanic and Atmospheric Administration, National Hurricane Center 2019). When disasters hit rural settings, the impact is even greater than in metropolitan areas. Unlike urban settings, where municipal governments are fully equipped to return major systems (e.g., transit, water, power, sewer, etc.) back to being operational, rural areas do not have the additional capability and resources required to respond to disasters in the same manner (Cutter et al. 2016).

Residing in rural communities poses significant challenges for CSHCN during a disaster because of their distinctive needs for sheltering-in-place, transportation, evacuation to safety, communication, and health care (Baker and Cormier 2013;

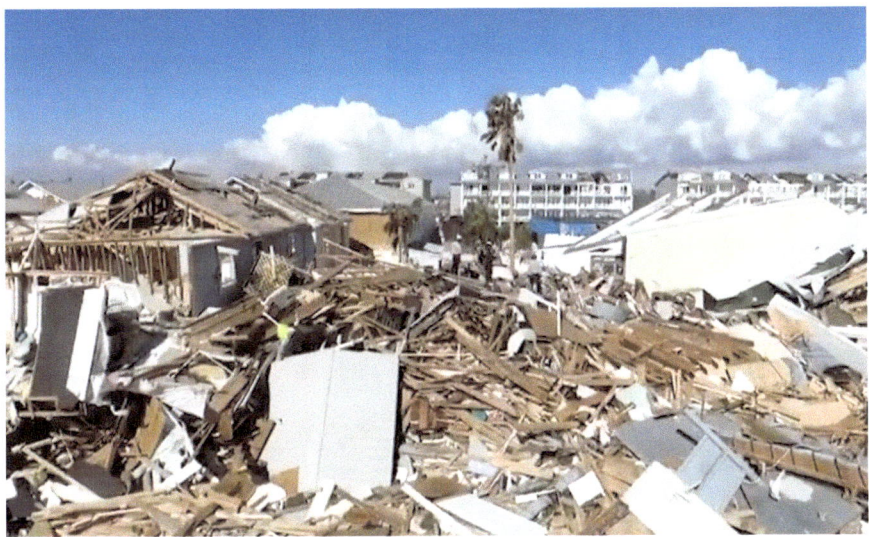

Fig. 8.2 Hurricane Michael damage. (Courtesy of Wikimedia Commons)

Hipper et al. 2018; Ashida et al. 2016; Cohen et al. 2011). These requirements also pose additional challenges for caretakers, as well as disaster response providers, in communities located outside of cities where public health systems may not have adequate resources to care for CSHCN (Ashida et al. 2016; Cohen et al. 2011). During disasters, rural communities are frequently already operating at or near full capacity because they oftentimes have limited resources and personnel to respond to the needs of residents (Toor et al. 2018; Hamann et al. 2016; Ashida et al. 2016; Cohen et al. 2011). When impacted by disaster, if the existing infrastructure of a rural community cannot adequately address the needs of the general population, it is most likely they will not be capable of meeting the unique and complex requirements of CSHCN (Hamann et al. 2016; Ashida et al. 2016; Cohen et al. 2011).

8.3.5   Poverty

CSHCN living in poverty are significantly more susceptible to the negative physical effects of disasters. Individuals living in poverty frequently reside in poorly constructed, below standard housing and buildings that are more susceptible to widespread damage and collapse in disasters (Ronoh et al. 2015a; Murray and Monteiro 2012; Daoud et al. 2016). A poignant example of this is the 2008 magnitude 8.0 earthquake that struck Sichuan, China. This disaster resulted in approximately 70,000 deaths including over 5300 schoolchildren who died while attending school. During the earthquake, over 80% of buildings collapsed as a result of poor construction. Over 7000 schoolrooms in carelessly built schools, mainly in rural areas of south-central China, collapsed during the earthquake (Fig. 8.3) (Yang et al. 2014;

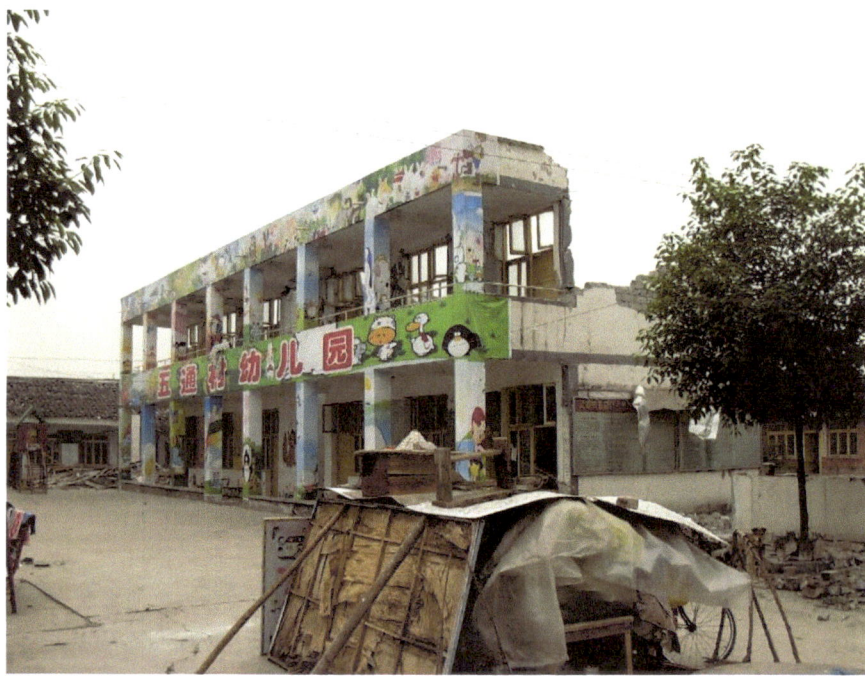

Fig. 8.3 This kindergarten was one of the many schools badly damaged, 2008 Sichuan earthquake. (Courtesy of Wikimedia Commons)

Chan et al. 2019). Families with CSHCN living in poverty also do not have the financial resources to evacuate when disasters strike (Ronoh et al. 2015a; Murray and Monteiro 2012; The Brookings Institution 2017).

8.4 Disaster Survival

As noted throughout the chapter, there are a number of factors that place CSHCN at increased risk for adversity in disasters. As such, it is vitally important that every effort is taken to keep CSHCN safe, and their specific health care needs met, as much as possible during disasters. Nationally and internationally recognized agencies such as the National Association of Pediatric Nurse Practitioners, American Academy of Pediatrics, Centers for Disease Control and Prevention, National Center for Disaster Preparedness, Children's Health Fund, and others are united in their goal to communicate the critical importance of planning in advance of disasters for all children, but especially CSHCN (Wolf-Fordham et al. 2015; Centers for Disease Control and Prevention 2019a). These organizations also stress the importance of caretakers of CSHCN being proactive with anticipating and planning for any potential disruptions in the delivery of care to their child in the event of power outages, water shortage, limited or no mobile phone capacity hindering communication, environmental damage preventing travel, etc. (Wolf-Fordham et al. 2015; Marchigiani et al. 2013).

8.4.1 Basic Needs

Most agencies providing guidance on emergency preparedness kits for disasters recommend having available enough supplies (e.g., nonperishable food, water for drinking and sanitation, prescription and nonprescription medications, etc.) to last at least 3 days (American Academy of Pediatrics 2019; The American Red Cross 2019). For CSHCN, it is recommended that families have enough supplies for 5–7 days (Trento and Allen 2014). For families where there is not a member with a significant health problem, adaptation in disaster is possible. For example, loss of electricity may mean preparing foods differently, completing as many activities as needed during the day when there is natural light, altering hygienic practices, etc. However, for families with a CSHCN, adaptation in disasters is much more complicated (The American Red Cross 2019; Trento and Allen 2014).

8.4.2 Power

For families with a CSHCN, loss of power is more dangerous because many aspects of the child's care depend on the availability of electricity. The loss of power oftentimes means seeking care at a local hospital. However, in disasters, roads may be impassable, public transportation at a standstill, or even the hospital closed due to damage (Sakashita et al. 2013). Battery backups are critically needed for CSHCN who may use critical equipment such as mechanical ventilators or oxygen concentrators (Sakashita et al. 2013; Sterni et al. 2016). However, most battery backups last for only 3–9 h before needing to be recharged (Gregoretti et al. 2013; Nakayama et al. 2014). Additional backup can be achieved through the use of a car battery that requires a proper inverter device and an adequate amount of gasoline in the vehicle (Sakashita et al. 2013). It is important that the automobile is run in an area that is appropriately ventilated. Electric garage doors will not be operational in a power outage. As such, the garage door will require being opened manually (Sakashita et al. 2013). Additionally, the auxiliary power outlet in an automobile can be used in disasters to charge cellular telephones with the proper adapter (Sakashita et al. 2013).

Another method for supporting power to life-saving equipment, which can be costly especially for families living in poverty, is by producing electricity using a home generator. This can be done using both gasoline and diesel fuel. The challenge with gasoline is that it cannot be stored for extended periods of time either in the generator or a storage container. If gasoline is left in the generator for too long, it degrades leaving the equipment inoperable. Additionally, gas-fueled generators require proper ventilation to prevent carbon monoxide (CO) poisoning (Sakashita et al. 2013). If gas-fueled generators are used, it is recommended that homes have working battery-operated CO detectors. Batteries for the CO detectors must be changed every 6 months to ensure proper functioning. The CO detectors themselves have a lifetime of only 5–7 years and so require periodic replacement (Centers for Disease Control and Prevention 2019b). Energy experts recommend the use of diesel fuel versus gasoline for home generators. Diesel fuel is less expensive, safer to store, burns cleaner, and the hazard for combustion is lower than with gasoline. It is important that diesel-fueled generators are well maintained. Annually, all filters must be replaced, and the oil changed using a specially formulated brand, to ensure efficient and safe operation (Sakashita et al. 2013; Ericson and Olis 2019). Backup power generators should be capable of supporting lifesaving equipment for at least 24 h until CSHCN can be safely transported to a higher level of care (Nakayama et al. 2014). Regardless of the type of generator used, all families with CSHCN requiring ventilator support should have available at all times a self-inflating bag and mask to decrease the occurrence of a life-threatening situation in the event of loss of power (Sakashita et al. 2013; Sterni et al. 2016). Likewise, an emergency action plan for the loss of power should be readily available (Wolf-Fordham et al. 2015; Sakashita et al. 2013). During the 2011 Japan earthquake and ensuing tsunami, 24 children requiring power for the proper functioning of home medical equipment were admitted to the hospital as a result of the long-lasting blackout period and the absence of backup power generators (Nakayama et al. 2014).

8.4.3 Supplies

Another aspect of care that must be considered for CSHCN is the availability of a sufficient quantity of supplies for disasters. For example, CSHCN who are dependent on home parenteral and enteral nutrition (HPEN) have a significant need for an adequate amount of readily available supplies required for ample hydration and nutrition (Toor et al. 2018; Trento and Allen 2014; Adams et al. 2014). In addition to electrical power and a source of clean water, CSHCN receiving HPEN require sufficient amounts of enteral formula, parenteral solution, as well as supplies to administer the nutrition and maintain feeding tube functioning (e.g., delivery sets, extensions, adapters, tape, etc.) and venous catheter access (e.g., infusion pumps, tubing, syringes, etc.) for up to 7 days (Toor et al. 2018; Trento and Allen 2014; Dibb and Simon 2017). It is important that caretakers of CSHCN inspect expiration dates on all supplies regularly using a checklist as needed (Toor et al. 2018; Trento and Allen 2014). While feeding pumps should be routinely charged, in the event of a power outage, this may not be possible. Either battery packs, a backup generator, and/or enteral gravity bags should be available (Toor et al. 2018). Additionally, parents should be provided with an instruction sheet regarding enteral gravity infusion (Trento and Allen 2014). For CSHCN requiring total parenteral nutrition (TPN), without electrical power or batteries, IV hydration will be required using 10% dextrose solution, Lactated Ringer's, and/or sodium chloride 0.9% solution (Toor et al. 2018). TPN as well as additives, such as vitamins, require refrigeration. Once the bag is spiked, TPN is only stable at room temperature for 24 h (Toor et al. 2018; Trento and Allen 2014). An alternative plan for fluids should be developed for the family by HCPs managing the nutrition support of the CSHCN. The appropriate administration supplies will also be needed (Toor et al. 2018; Trento and Allen

2014). TPN clinic HCPs should make available to families letters for insurance companies authorizing the storing of necessary emergency supplies and fluids (Trento and Allen 2014). Regardless of the supply requirements of CSHCN, caretakers are encouraged to have disaster kits with the essentials in the event of a disaster (Toor et al. 2018).

8.4.4   Emergency Information Form

During disasters, it is possible that CSHCN will require care delivered by professionals and busy health care facilities not familiar with the child. CSHCN have extensive medical records that may not be accessible in a disaster. Even if available, the records are usually too lengthy to review in an emergency situation (American Academy of Pediatrics, Committee on Pediatric Emergency Medicine and Council on Clinical Information Technology, American College of Emergency Physicians, Pediatric Emergency Medicine Committee 2010). As such, caretakers are encouraged to complete, and have available, an Emergency Information Form (EIF) (Bagwell et al. 2016; American Academy of Pediatrics 2019; Zagory et al. 2016; Murray 2010). The EIF is two pages in length and includes important names and telephone numbers for family members, emergency contacts, HCPs, as well as where the child receives medical care when needed (e.g., clinic, hospital, subspecialists office, etc.). The EIF also lists past medical procedures, current medications prescribed, allergies, immunizations, recommended treatments for specific health issues, and more (Toor et al. 2018; American Academy of Pediatrics, Committee on Pediatric Emergency Medicine and Council on Clinical Information Technology, American College of Emergency Physicians, Pediatric Emergency Medicine Committee 2010; Copper et al. 2018). Pediatric health care experts recommend that the EIF be succinct without excessive information in order to permit the expeditious retrieval of the most significant information (Copper et al. 2018). The EIF plays a critical role in ensuring CSHCN receive emergency care in a timely and efficient manner (American Academy of Pediatrics, Committee on Pediatric Emergency Medicine and Council on Clinical Information Technology, American College of Emergency Physicians, Pediatric Emergency Medicine Committee 2010; Copper et al. 2018; Dudley et al. 2015). Caretakers of CSHCN are also encouraged to have the EIF available in different formats such as on a waterproof flash drive or phone application. A hard copy of the EIF should also be available and stored in a waterproof sealed bag (Toor et al. 2018; American Academy of Pediatrics, Committee on Pediatric Emergency Medicine and Council on Clinical Information Technology, American College of Emergency Physicians, Pediatric Emergency Medicine Committee 2010; Copper et al. 2018; Dudley et al. 2015; Abraham et al. 2016). The EIF should be updated every 2 years or more frequently with the growth of the child as well as when the condition, treatment plan, medications, and/or HCPs of the CSHCN change (American Academy of Pediatrics, Committee on Pediatric Emergency Medicine and Council on Clinical Information Technology, American College of Emergency Physicians, Pediatric

Emergency Medicine Committee 2010). In a disaster, it is possible that the CSHCN will become separated from caretakers. CSHCN may not be able to communicate with unfamiliar people, including HCPs, because of fear or cognitive inability. As such, the EIF should be accessible in more than one location (e.g., homes of the CSHCN, relatives, neighbors, etc.) (American Academy of Pediatrics, Committee on Pediatric Emergency Medicine and Council on Clinical Information Technology, American College of Emergency Physicians, Pediatric Emergency Medicine Committee 2010; Copper et al. 2018; Abraham et al. 2016). The EIF can be located at https://www.acep.org/by-medical-focus/pediatrics/medical-forms/emergency-information-form-for-children-with-special-health-care-needs/ (American College of Emergency Physicians 2019).

Emerging evidence has helped considerably to clarify what parents of CSHCN find helpful with preparing for a disaster. Parents have described the need for education and training related to filling out the EIF, developing an emergency plan, preparing a disaster kit, etc. (Wolf-Fordham et al. 2015; Hipper et al. 2018). Caretakers of CSHCN shared that it would be of immense value to receive in-person or online training from emergency responders in advance of a disaster (Wolf-Fordham et al. 2015; Hipper et al. 2018). Receiving education using a personal, one-to-one format in particular has been shown to increase disaster preparedness in families of CSHCN (Baker et al. 2012). Additionally, speaking with emergency responders regarding community resources (e.g., shelter sites, emergency notification systems, evacuation procedures, etc.) available in disasters would be of immense help (Wolf-Fordham et al. 2015). Families of CSHCN living in rural areas also identified the importance of receiving support from other caretakers in a similar situation and community networks. This support is associated with improved disaster planning and preparedness (Hipper et al. 2018; Hamann et al. 2016).

8.5   Conclusion

CSHCN are especially vulnerable during disasters, yet a paucity of evidence related to their needs endures when it comes to preparedness (Baker and Cormier 2013). In the event of a disaster, caretakers of CSHCN must have available the resources and support needed, as well as an emergency plan to provide the level of specialized care required by the child. For this to happen, emergency responders, nurses, and HCPs in the community where the child resides should be provided with the education and resources needed to meet the essentials of the CSHCN for the optimal delivery of care in a disaster (Murray 2010; Wolf-Fordham et al. 2015; American Academy of Pediatrics, Committee on Pediatric Emergency Medicine and Council on Clinical Information Technology, American College of Emergency Physicians, Pediatric Emergency Medicine Committee 2010; Abraham et al. 2016; American College of Emergency Physicians 2019). Appropriately preparing families of CSHCN, emergency responders, nurses, and HCPs will contribute to ensuring that the child's unique needs are met in the event of a disaster.

References

Abraham G, Fehr J, Ahmad F, Jeffe DB, Cooper T, Yu F, et al. Emergency Information Forms for children with medical complexity: a simulation study. Pediatrics. 2016;138(2):e1–6. https://doi.org/10.1542/peds.2016-0847.

Adams RC, Elias ER, Council on Children with Disabilities. Nonoral feeding for children and youth with developmental or acquired disabilities. Pediatrics. 2014;134(6):e1745–62. https://doi.org/10.1542/peds.2014-2829.

American Academy of Pediatrics. Children & disasters. Disaster preparedness to meet children's needs. 2019. https://www.aap.org/en-us/advocacy-and-policy/aap-health-initiatives/Children-and-Disasters/Pages/default.aspx. Accessed 12 Sep 2019.

American Academy of Pediatrics, Committee on Pediatric Emergency Medicine and Council on Clinical Information Technology, American College of Emergency Physicians, Pediatric Emergency Medicine Committee. Policy statement—Emergency Information Forms and emergency preparedness for children with special health care needs. Pediatrics. 2010;125(4):829–37. https://doi.org/10.1542/peds.2010-0186.

American College of Emergency Physicians. Emergency Information Form for children with special health care needs. 2019. https://www.acep.org/by-medical-focus/pediatrics/medical-forms/emergency-information-form-for-children-with-special-health-care-needs/. Accessed 2 Oct 2019.

Ashida S, Robinson EL, Gay J, Ramirez M. Motivating rural older residents to prepare for disasters: moving beyond personal benefits. Ageing Soc. 2016;36(10):2117–40. https://doi.org/10.1017/S0144686X15000914.

Bagwell HB, Liggin R, Thompson T, Lyle K, Anthony A, Baltz M, et al. Disaster preparedness in families with children with special health care needs. Clin Pediatr. 2016;55(11):1036–43. https://doi.org/10.1177/0009922816665087.

Baker LR, Cormier LA. Disaster preparedness and families of children with special needs: a geographic comparison. J Commun Health. 2013;38(1):106–12. https://doi.org/10.1007/s10900-012-9587-3.

Baker M, Baker L, Flagg LA. Preparing families of children with special health care needs for disasters: an education intervention. Soc Work Health Care. 2012;51(5):417–29. https://doi.org/10.1080/00981389.2012.659837.

Boon HJ, Brown LH, Tsey K, Speare R, Pagliano P, Usher K, et al. School disaster planning for children with disabilities: a critical review of the literature. Int J Spec Educ. 2011;26(3):223–37.

Brodie M, Weltzien E, Altman D, Blendon RJ, Benson JM. Experiences of Hurricane Katrina evacuees in Houston shelters: implications for future planning. Am J Public Health. 2006;96(8):1402–8. https://doi.org/10.2105/AJPH.2005.084475.

Centers for Disease Control and Prevention. Children and youth with special needs. 2019a. https://www.aap.org/en-us/advocacy-and-policy/aap-health-initiatives/Children-and-Disasters/Pages/CYWSN.aspx. Accessed 25 Sep 2019.

Centers for Disease Control and Prevention. Carbon monoxide (CO) poisoning prevention. 2019b. https://www.cdc.gov/features/copoisoning/index.html. Accessed 26 Sep 2019.

Chan EYY, Man AYT, Lam HCY. Scientific evidence on natural disasters and health emergency and disaster risk management in Asian rural-based area. Br Med Bull. 2019;129(1):91–105. https://doi.org/10.1093/bmb/ldz002.

Codreanu TA, Celenza A, Jacobs I. Does disaster education of teenagers translate into better survival knowledge, knowledge of skills, and adaptive behavioral change? A systematic literature review. Prehosp Disaster Med. 2014;29(6):629–42. https://doi.org/10.1017/S1049023X14001083.

Cohen E, Kuo DZ, Agrawal R, Berry JG, Bhagat SK, Simon TD, et al. Children with medical complexity: an emerging population for clinical and research initiatives. Pediatrics. 2011;127(3):529–38. https://doi.org/10.1542/peds.2010-0910.

Copper TC, Jeffe DB, Ahmad FA, Abraham G, Yu F, Hickey B, et al. Emergency Information Forms for children with medical complexity: A Qualitative Study. Pediatr Emerg Care. 2018;1–6. Advance online publication. https://doi.org/10.1097/PEC.0000000000001443.

Cutter SL, Ash KD, Emrich CT. Urban–rural differences in disaster resilience. Ann Assoc Am Geogr. 2016;106(6):1236–52. https://doi.org/10.1080/24694452.2016.1194740.

Daoud A, Halleröd B, Guha-Sapir D. What is the association between absolute child poverty, poor governance, and natural disasters? A global comparison of some of the realities of climate change. PLoS One. 2016;11(4):1–20. https://doi.org/10.1371/journal.pone.0153296.

Dibb M, Simon L. Home parenteral nutrition: vascular access and related complications. Nutr Clin Pract. 2017;32(6):769–76. https://doi.org/10.1177/0884533617734788.

Dudley N, Ackerman A, Brown KM, Snow SK, American Academy of Pediatrics Committee on Pediatric Emergency Medicine, American College of Emergency Physicians Pediatric Emergency Medicine Committee, et al. Patient-and family-centered care of children in the emergency department. Pediatrics. 2015;135(1):e255–72. https://doi.org/10.1542/peds.2014-3424.

Dyregrov A, Yule W, Olff M. Children and natural disasters. Eur J Psychotraumatol. 2018;9(Suppl 2):1–3. https://doi.org/10.1080/20008198.2018.1500823.

Ericson S, Olis D. A comparison of fuel choice for backup generators. 2019. https://www.nrel.gov/docs/fy19osti/72509.pdf. Accessed 26 Sep 2019.

Ghandour RM, Jones JR, Lebrun-Harris LA, Minnaert J, Blumberg SJ, Fields J, et al. The design and implementation of the 2016 National Survey of Children's Health. Matern Child Health J. 2018;22(8):1093–102. https://doi.org/10.1007/s10995-018-2526-x.

Goodhue CJ, Demeter NE, Burke RV, Toor KT, Upperman JS, Merritt RJ. Mixed-methods pilot study: disaster preparedness of families with children followed in an intestinal rehabilitation clinic. Nutr Clin Pract. 2016;31(2):257–65. https://doi.org/10.1177/0884533615605828.

Gregoretti C, Navalesi P, Ghannadian S, Carlucci A, Pelosi P. Choosing a ventilator for home mechanical ventilation. Breathe. 2013;9(5):394–409. https://doi.org/10.1183/20734735.042312.

Hamann CJ, Mello E, Wu H, Yang J, Waldron D, Ramirez M. Disaster preparedness in rural families of children with special health care needs. Disaster Med Public Health Preparedness. 2016;10(2):225–32. https://doi.org/10.1017/dmp.2015.159.

Hipper TJ, Davis R, Massey PM, Turchi RM, Lubell KM, Pechta LE, et al. The disaster information needs of families of children with special healthcare needs: a scoping review. Health Security. 2018;16(3):178–92. https://doi.org/10.1089/hs.2018.0007.

Marchigiani R, Gordy S, Cipolla J, Adams RC, Evans DC, Stehly C, et al. Wind disasters: a comprehensive review of current management strategies. Int J Crit Illn Inj Sci. 2013;3(2):130–42. https://doi.org/10.4103/2229-5151.114273.

Mattson ME. Emergency department visits involving attention deficit/hyperactivity disorder stimulant medications. 2013. https://www.ncbi.nlm.nih.gov/books/NBK384678/. Accessed 22 Sep 2019.

Murray JS. Disaster preparedness for children with special healthcare needs and disabilities. Crit Care Nurs Clin N Am. 2010;22(2010):481–91. https://doi.org/10.1016/j.ccell.2010.09.002.

Murray JS. Disaster preparedness for children with special health care needs and disabilities. J Spec Pediatr Nurs. 2011;16(2011):226–32. https://doi.org/10.1111/j.1744-6155.2011.00293.x.

Murray JS, Monteiro S. Disaster risk and children. Part I: why poverty-stricken populations are impacted most. J Spec Pediatr Nurs. 2012;17(2):168–70. https://doi.org/10.1111/j.1744-6155.2011.00317.x.

Nakayama T, Tanaka S, Uematsu M, Kikuchi A, Hino-Fukuyo N, Morimoto T, et al. Effect of a blackout in pediatric patients with home medical devices during the 2011 eastern Japan earthquake. Brain Dev. 2014;36(2):143–7. https://doi.org/10.1016/j.braindev.2013.02.001.

National Survey of Children with Special Healthcare Needs (NC-CSHCN). Child and adolescent health measurement initiative. 2016. https://www.childhealthdata.org/old-(pre-july-2018)/learn/NS-CSHCN. Accessed 22 Sep 2019.

Philipsborn RP, Chan K. Climate change and global child health. Pediatrics. 2018;141(6):1–7. https://doi.org/10.1542/peds.2017-3774.

Potter SH, Becker JS, Johnston DM, Rossiter KP. An overview of the impacts of the 2010-2011 Canterbury earthquakes. Int J Disast Risk Re. 2015;14(2015):6–14. https://doi.org/10.1016/j.ijdrr.2015.01.014.

Ronoh S, Gaillard JC, Marlowe J. Children with disabilities and disaster risk reduction: a review. Int J Disaster Risk Sci. 2015a;6(2):38–48. https://doi.org/10.1007/s13753-015-0042-9.

Ronoh S, Gaillard JC, Marlowe J. Children with disabilities and disaster preparedness: a case study of Christchurch, Kōtuitui: New Zealand. J Soc Sci. 2015b;10(2):91–102. https://doi.org/10.1080/1177083x.2015.1068185.

Sakashita K, Matthews WJ, Yamamoto LG. Disaster preparedness for technology and electricity-dependent children and youth with special health care needs. Clin Pediatr. 2013;52(6):549–56. https://doi.org/10.1177/0009922813482762.

Sterni LM, Collaco JM, Baker CD, Carroll JL, Sharma GD, Brozek JL, et al. An official American Thoracic Society clinical practice guideline: pediatric chronic home invasive ventilation. Am J Respir Crit Care Med. 2016;193(8):e16–35. https://doi.org/10.1164/rccm.201602-0276ST.

Stough LM, Ducy EM, Kang D. Addressing the needs of children with disabilities experiencing disaster or terrorism. Curr Psychiatry Rep. 2017;19(4):1–10. https://doi.org/10.1007/s11920-017-0776-8.

The American Red Cross. Survival kit supplies. 2019. https://www.redcross.org/get-help/how-to-prepare-for-emergencies/survival-kit-supplies.html. Accessed 25 Sep 2019.

The Brookings Institution. Hurricanes hit the poor the hardest. 2017. https://www.brookings.edu/blog/social-mobility-memos/2017/09/18/hurricanes-hit-the-poor-the-hardest/. Accessed 25 Sep 2019.

Toor KT, Burke RV, Demeter NE, Upperman JS, Merritt RJ, Wee CP, et al. Improving disaster preparedness of families with a parenteral nutrition-dependent child. J Pediatr Gastroenterol Nutr. 2018;67(2):237–41. https://doi.org/10.1097/mpg.0000000000002048.

Trento L, Allen S. Hurricane Sandy: nutrition support during disasters. Nutr Clin Pract. 2014;29(5):576–84. https://doi.org/10.1177/0884533614536927.

United Nations Children's Fund. Introduction—children with disabilities. 2018. https://www.unicef.org/disabilities/. Accessed 13 Sep 2019.

United States Department of Commerce, National Oceanic and Atmospheric Administration, National Hurricane Center. Hurricane Michael. 2019. https://www.nhc.noaa.gov/data/tcr/AL142018_Michael.pdf. Accessed 25 Sep 2019.

United States Department of Health and Human Services, Health Resources and Services Administration. Children with special health care needs. 2019. https://mchb.hrsa.gov/maternal-child-health-topics/children-and-youth-special-health-needs#ref1. Accessed 13 Sep 2019

Wolf-Fordham S, Curtin C, Maslin M, Bandini L, Hamad CD. Emergency preparedness of families of children with developmental disabilities: what public health and safety emergency planners need to know. J Emerg Manag. 2015;13(1):7–18. https://doi.org/10.5055/jem.2015.0213.

Yang J, Chen J, Liu H, Zheng J. Comparison of two large earthquakes in China: the 2008 Sichuan Wenchuan Earthquake and the 2013 Sichuan Lushan Earthquake. Nat Hazards. 2014;73(2):1127–36. https://doi.org/10.1007/s11069-014-1121-8.

Zagory JA, Jensen JR, Burke RV, Upperman JS. Planning for the pediatric patient during a disaster. Curr Trauma Rep. 2016;2(4):216–21. https://doi.org/10.1007/s40719-016-0064-9.

Decontamination

9

Katherine Meyer

9.1   Introduction

On 9/11, the first patient who presented to the New York Veterans Administration Medical Center was a 5-month-old infant transported from the World Trade Center and was covered in gray ash. This facility did not have pediatric facilities but was able to provide staff who had training in pediatric emergencies to care for this infant. The infant was transported to a pediatric facility and had a positive outcome (Freyberg et al. 2008; Authority 2014). In the aftermath of the 9/11 attacks, there has been greater emphasis on health care facilities to take on the role of the first receiver and become the primary source of decontamination, especially for the pediatric population.

Many of the principles of pediatric decontamination are congruent to those of adult decontamination; however, the application is much more challenging, especially with younger children. Children have unique needs that require careful planning and implementation. Proper plans, training, and supplies must be in place in order for the medical care system to remain effective (Heon and Foltin 2009) and properly care for the pediatric population during a HAZMAT event. Pediatric decontamination must be thorough, safe, and expedient.

Regulatory agencies such as The Joint Commission (TJC) require hospitals to have Emergency Operations Plans that describe how they will care for radioactive, biological, and chemical isolation along with proper decontamination procedures (TJC Standard EM.02.02.02.02) (Freyberg et al. 2008). The Occupational Health and Safety Administration (OSHA) further outlines specific protocols with regard to protecting hospital staff from exposure and contamination, the proper training, and the utilization of personal protective equipment (PPE) (Occupational Health and

K. Meyer (✉)
Department of Bioterrorism, Children's Hospital Los Angeles, Los Angeles, CA, USA
e-mail: kmeyer@chla.usc.edu

© Springer Nature Switzerland AG 2020   237
C. J. Goodhue, N. Blake (eds.), *Nursing Management of Pediatric Disaster*,
https://doi.org/10.1007/978-3-030-43428-1_9

238 K. Meyer

Safety Administration 2005). In addition to regulatory guidance, pediatric considerations should be implemented into the hospital's decontamination plan as they make up approximately one-quarter of the US population.

9.2 Decontamination

Decontamination of the pediatric patient is utilized in response to exposure to hazardous chemicals, biological agents, or radiation, causing the individual to become contaminated. Biological, radiological, or chemical materials that cause an adverse reaction to an individual is termed hazardous materials or HAZMAT (Holland and Cawthon 2015). Once the patient has become contaminated, the process of decontamination should be executed expeditiously. Decontamination is used to mitigate and prevent adverse health effects to the victim by removing or reducing the contaminant on the victim's body to an acceptable level, which prevents further patient exposure and subsequent morbidity and mortality (Foresman-Capuzzi and Eckenrode 2012). The objective of decontamination is to ensure the removal or reduction of harmful substance from the victim's body, prevention of further inhalation or absorption of the substance to the patient, or exposure to first responders, health workers, and secondary victims. Theoretically, patients should be decontaminated on the scene of the incident and then transported to the hospital for further care and medical evaluation. This was shown not to be the reality when 85% of exposed patients self-transported to hospitals during the sarin gas attacks in Tokyo, Japan (Okumura et al. 1996). Further confirmation of patients self-presenting directly to hospitals was evident in the Alfred Murrah federal building bombing in Oklahoma City (Teague 2004) and in Washington, DC, and New York City during the 9/11 terror attacks. Many patients, including pediatric patients, presented to hospitals in lower Manhattan covered in an unknown substance of gray ash. Hospitals at that time were unprepared to deal with the scope of decontamination that was presented to them (Hick et al. 2003a). Following the attacks on 9/11, the federal government released funds to support and establish methods of providing decontamination to patients outside of hospitals. These methods included decontamination showers, decontamination supplies and equipment, and training of decontamination teams to support these efforts.

The National Disaster Recovery Framework that was put forth in response to a presidential declaration outlines the expectations of disaster recovery in the U.S. This document specifies that children require special considerations that need to be implemented in response to efforts and core capabilities (United States Department of Health and Human Services Security 2016). Furthermore, the health benefits of decontamination can mitigate adverse health effects of the victim, prevent further exposure to the contaminant for both the victim and health care worker, streamline access to medical care, and protect the infrastructure of the health care facility. All of these benefits warrant decontamination as a medical countermeasure and should be incorporated into the larger application of medical countermeasure utilization (Cibulsky et al. 2014). Decontamination training programs specific to hospital first receivers are evolving compared to many established protocols and mass decontamination guidance for first responders (Freyberg et al. 2008). These protocols do not include or are limited in the inclusion of pediatric-specific response and procedures.

Further events such as the organophosphate chemical attack on populations in Syria in 2013 revealed the need for immediate recognition of the clinical presentations of nerve agents even without standard detection equipment, proper utilization of PPE for hospital and clinic staff, expedient decontamination, timely treatment, and long-term follow-up (Eisenkraft et al. 2014). Proper training in decontamination practice is essential to hospitals to decrease the risk of secondary contamination and improve the outcome of the exposed victim.

9.3 Personal Protective Equipment

Personal protective equipment, or PPE, is designed to provide protection from HAZMAT incidents. The first priority for managing HAZMAT events is to prevent secondary contamination that can lead to adverse health effects in staff treating victims and contamination of the health care facility and equipment. Secondary contamination can cause significant delays to emergency care for victims and the community (Horton et al. 2003). Health care facilities must meet OSHA requirements for proper PPE utilization in response to HAZMAT incidents, as contaminated patients may present directly to the facility without undergoing decontamination at the scene. The health care facility must perform a hazard vulnerability assessment to plan for possible HAZMAT scenarios and identify, obtain, and provide an appropriate type and amount of PPE needed to ensure an adequate decontamination response. Under OSHA guidelines, staff who will respond to a HAZMAT incident must be trained on the appropriate PPE necessary for the incident; procedures to properly don, doff, adjust, and wear the PPE; limitations of PPE; proper care and maintenance; and must be able to demonstrate the proper wear and usage of PPE.

OSHA specifies that hospitals must provide Hazardous Waste Operations and Emergency Response Standard (HAZWOPER) training or the equivalent for first receivers who are expected to provide triage, treatment, or decontaminate victims during a HAZMAT event. The Occupational Health and Safety Administration standard 29 CFR 1910.120(q)(6)(ii) puts forth first responder training requirements that include hazard recognition, decontamination procedures, and selection of PPE (Occupational Health and Safety Administration 2005). Staff must demonstrate competency levels and maintain annual refresher training. All personnel who may be required to don PPE as part of their duties for decontamination should be medically screened to determine if the staff member is fit to work in PPE. Additionally, prior to any HAZMAT event, staff should complete a medical form, documenting a set of vital signs to prevent any adverse reactions for the health care worker while working in PPE.

There are four classes of PPE (Table 9.1) that have been identified by OSHA (Occupational Health and Safety Administration 2005) for utilization against a contaminant listed below:

Early identification of the hazardous chemical is critical to providing the proper level of PPE to protect health care workers during an incident. In the event that the contaminant is unknown, the safety officer will determine the appropriate level of PPE that should be utilized. OSHA regulations for health care workers caring for contaminated patients exposed to an unknown substance include chemical resistant,

Table 9.1 PPE classification (Heon and Foltin 2009)

OSHA classification	Level A	Level B	Level C	Level D
Level of protection	Maximum for skin, eye, and respiratory protection	Maximum respiratory protection. Lower level of skin and eye protection	Lower level of respiratory and skin protection	Minimal
Elements	Fully encapsulated suit with self-contained breathing apparatus	Encapsulated suit with sealed seams and a self-contained breathing apparatus located outside of the suit or supplied air respirator	Powered air purifying respirator (PAPR) Chemical resistant, waterproof suit	Work clothes Gowns Gloves
Indications	Toxic gases Liquids Vapors Aerosols Solids Radiation	Toxic solids Liquids that may contain toxic gases	Vapors Gases Aerosols Liquid Solid Radiation	Solids
Type of responder	First responders in the hot zone in an oxygen poor environment	First responders in prehospital warm zone	First responders or first receivers	First receivers working in the cold zone or post-decontamination area
Advantages/ disadvantages	High training requirements, physical demands, poor mobility and dexterity, and limited air supply (Heon and Foltin 2009)	Expensive, fit testing requirements, high training requirements, physical demands, poor mobility and dexterity, dependent on limited air supply (Heon and Foltin 2009)	High level of protection, improved mobility, lower physical demands, is less expensive, and no fit testing is needed (Heon and Foltin 2009)	Full mobility and requires low training level and is less expensive (Heon and Foltin 2009)

waterproof suit that works with a PAPR, or Level C protection (Occupational Health and Safety Administration 2005). Health care workers should be aware of the location of the PPE, manufacturer recommendations, proper sequence of donning and doffing the PPE, decontamination event activation procedures, and proper inspection of PPE.

9.4   Zones of Protection

9.4.1   Hot Zone

The hot zone is where the incident occurred or immediately adjacent to the location. The hot zone poses the greatest risk of exposure to harmful toxins. The triage and medical care should be kept at a minimum only employing immediate lifesaving procedures or hemorrhage control. Unless the incident takes place at the health care facility, the hot zone is generally located off-site (Hick et al. 2003a). All staff are in the highest level of PPE for the incident in the hot zone depending on the incident and the priority to quickly evacuate patients out of the hot zone to stop exposure and transport to an area for decontamination. Special consideration should be made for children in the hot zone as children may not recognize there is danger and may not be able to evacuate themselves or follow instructions to shelter-in-place. Children may also be scared of the situation and may not cooperate with rescuers. Children are also closer to the ground and will breathe in a higher density of gases at a higher minute volume than adults (Heon and Foltin 2009).

9.4.2   Warm Zone

The warm zone is the area where decontamination of victims and equipment takes place. All attempts for the warm zone should be made to locate it uphill, upwind, and at least 300 ft. away from the scene of the incident. In the prehospital setting, fire and EMS personnel may stage for transport and gross decontamination in the warm zone. At health care facilities, the warm zone is where the contaminated victims arrive and rapid triage takes place. In both settings, treatment should be limited to hemorrhage control as the priority is to disrobe and decontaminate the patients expeditiously. Special considerations for children should be made to keep families together and provide appropriate supervision and areas for children, especially unaccompanied minors. All staff must wear appropriate PPE in the warm zone to prevent secondary contamination (Cibulsky et al. 2014).

9.4.3   Cold Zone

The cold zone is the location patients enter post-decontamination. Victims in the cold zone enter into a more thorough triage assessment and treatment area. This area is considered to be free of contaminants and also referred to as the clean zone. All staff members and patients who enter into the cold zone must have undergone decontamination (Cibulsky et al. 2014). Patients, especially young children, should be warmed and clothed immediately when entering the clean zone to prevent hypothermia. The cold zone should have a pediatric safe area, with proper supervision and cribs or playpens to place infants and toddlers. All efforts should be made to ensure families remain together unless immediate care needs to be rendered to parents or guardians. If children are unaccompanied, all characteristics should be documented and placed and reported to the family information center.

Zones of protection at the health care facility should have clear demarcated areas with controlled access to each area. There should be a singular point of entry with security staff directing traffic and providing security measures to protect the zones. When the health care facility is notified that they are receiving contaminated victims, it is recommended the facility activates a lockdown procedure or shelter-in-place plan to protect the building from secondary contamination.

9.5   Decontamination Risk for Children

There are approximately 69 million children under the age of 18 in the U.S., comprising one-quarter of the population. As terrorism and industrial accidents become an increasingly real threat, children pose a risk for decontamination for a variety of HAZMAT events (Falkenrath et al. 1998). Children may be targeted or become victims of a larger event. Since children tend to congregate together at schools, camps, parks, and other locations, HAZMAT incidents can potentially target large groups of children who may not be with their caregivers. Facilities that accommodate a large density of children can also pose potential targets for terrorists.

9.5.1   Chemical Events

Early decontamination after chemical exposure is vital in the approach to chemical casualty management (USAMRIID 2011). On November 17, 2005, a school bus full of children sustained a chemical exposure to n-butyl mercaptan from a release of a child's personal protective device and required decontamination. Patients arrived at Cincinnati Children's Hospital Medical Center with symptoms of vomiting, coughing, shortness of breath, and choking at the scene. The hospital successfully decontaminated, treated, and discharged 53 children and 3 adults within 2 and a half hours mitigating any further adverse health conditions (Timm and Reeves 2007).

In chemical exposure, clothing should be removed expeditiously to prevent further exposure due to off-gassing of the agent and to prevent secondary contamination to the rescuers and other victims. Washing with soap and water is the preferred method of washing if chemical deactivation agents such as alkaline hypochlorite are not available. Chemical agents have a low solubility in water; hydrolyzing agents or alkaline soaps can slowly break down and dilute the chemical. If chemical burns are present, early decontamination with a copious amount of water has shown to reduce the severity (Veenema 2019). Chemical agents can produce symptoms as soon as a few seconds after exposure further warranting the immediate need for decontamination.

There are several types of chemical agents:

1. Nerve agents are extremely toxic with a rapid onset of symptoms. They can inhibit the activation of acetylcholinesterase (AChE), which results in overstimulation of the exocrine glands, skeletal and smooth muscles, and the central nervous system causing seizures, apnea, loss of consciousness, and death. Examples include sarin and VX. MARK 1 Kits, that include atropine and 2-PAMCI along with the administration of diazepam, is the antidote of choice; however, they are not formulated for children. Depending on the size of the child, antidotal medications may have to be drawn up to separately, which can be time-consuming (Novak and Gill 2018). The Strategic National Stockpile has distributed chempacks to many hospitals around the U.S. that include nerve agent antidotes for immediate deployment.
2. Blood agents or cyanides are absorbed into the blood causing tissue hypoxia. Exposure induces anxiety, hyperventilation, hypoxia, seizures, and death. Cyanide kits that include sodium nitrite, amyl nitrite, and sodium thiosulfate are used in antidotal therapy for cyanide poisoning (Novak and Gill 2018).
3. Vesicants produce large fluid-filled blisters on the skin, eyes, and respiratory tract on contact. Vesicant exposure is painful when it comes in contact with the skin, so pain management should be considered. The most common vesicants include mustard, sulfur, and lewisite. Antidotal therapy includes decontamination with soap and water and British anti-Lewisite for Lewisite (Novak and Gill 2018).
4. Pulmonary agents cause severe irritation or swelling of the eyes and respiratory tract causing life-threatening pulmonary edema. Symptoms are often delayed, and antidotal therapy includes oxygen and supportive therapy. Examples include ammonia, chlorine, and sulfuryl fluoride.
5. Riot control agents have an acute onset and cause stimulation of the lacrimal glands, which produce irritation of the eyes, nose, mouth, respiratory tract and induce vomiting. Common agents include oleoresin capsicum (pepper spray) and Adamsite (tear gas). Decontamination with soap and water is the primary treatment; however, it may initially increase the burning sensation (Siegel et al. 2014).

9.5.2 Radiological Events

Radiological events such as exposure to a dirty bomb or a nuclear spill such as the one in Japan will need to employ decontamination after external exposure. Nuclear bombs may spread a layer of dust and solid debris over the victims. External radiation exposure is generally contained to the victim, and irradiation stops once the victim is removed from the source. Radiation exposure can be detected by using a device such as a Geiger counter or the collection of body fluid swabs that are sent to the lab. Decontamination of radiological contaminants will remove external sources the victim may have sustained.

Decontamination will not alleviate internal radiation as a result of inhalation, ingestion, direct absorption, or penetration; however, it will alleviate further exposure mitigating further internal radiation. Staff must be cautious while decontaminating as not to spread further radiation to unaffected areas of the body, open wounds, and into orifices.

9.5.3 Biological Events

The role of decontamination for biological events is rare. Patients contaminated with biological pathogens generally will not present to a health care facility until days after the attack when decontamination is unnecessary. The incubation period of bio-agents makes it unlikely that patients will present to Emergency Departments until days after exposure. There are exceptions such as aerosolized anthrax exposure that will require decontamination to remove active spores on the patient (USAMRIID 2011).

Although the vulnerabilities of the pediatric population have been identified, the standard protocols for the decontamination of children are emerging. In 2014, evidence-based practice guidelines for mass decontamination were released by the US Department of Health and Human Services (HHS) Office of the Assistant Secretary for Preparedness and Response (ASPR) and the US Department of Homeland Security (DHS) Office of Health Affairs. This guidance lays out planning and response plans that address unintentional chemical release, terrorism incidents, mass casualty, external decontamination, and decontamination guidelines. General recommendations for the pediatric population are described, but further specific protocols are lacking and still need to be developed (Cibulsky et al. 2014). At present, HHS and DHS are developing companion guidance focusing on the decontamination of pediatric patients (American Academy of Pediatrics 2019).

The pediatric population is more susceptible to adverse environmental effects of decontamination when compared to adults (Cibulsky et al. 2014), specifically aerosolized biologic or chemical agents. Children have a higher respiratory rate and less blood volume when compared to adults, which exposes them to larger doses in the same time period. Children also have thinner skin and a larger skin surface-to-body mass ratio, which increases absorption of agents that act on skin surfaces (American Academy of Pediatrics 2019).

Young children and children who are nonverbal are unable to provide a reliable medical history or communicate symptoms during pre-decontamination triage (Freyberg et al. 2008); therefore, exposure to contaminants may be unknown or assumed. Triage staff is dependent on the history obtained by caregivers or emergency medical services (EMS) personnel.

9.6 Pediatric Decontamination in the Emergency Department

Pediatric patients may present to the Emergency Department (ED) following exposure to a contaminant as a result of a singular or mass casualty incident. Pediatric patients do not have the ability to self-transport and will be dependent on caregivers or EMS for transportation. Decontamination and JumpSTART triage methods should be performed outside the ED to avoid secondary decontamination and to expedite the care of the patient.

During decontamination events, children may present alone or with their family or caregivers, who also require decontamination. All attempts should be made to keep children with their caregivers through the decontamination process. Keeping children with their caregivers can help streamline the decontamination process with communication and preventing separation anxiety for children. Children can become distressed if separated from their caregivers, which can pose challenges both during the decontamination process and after (Gurwitch et al. 2004). If caregivers are unavailable, dedicated staff should be assigned to children throughout the decontamination process. Child life specialists and staff trained in pediatric triage and decontamination are preferable as they have specialized training in developmental methods and can recognize the decompensation of the patient.

9.7   Communication

Effective communication can greatly influence the efficiency of the decontamination process. There are communication challenges during decontamination, especially when decontaminating children. During mass casualty incidents, environmental factors further hinder effective communication with noise from multiple patients, sirens, and powered air-purifying respirator (PAPR) noises. Staff wearing PAPRs have to rely on shouting instructions through the mask, bullhorns, electronic device, hand signals, or signs. Children may be frightened by the distorted sound of voices or by the appearance of PAPRs, which may exacerbate the situation. Infants and toddlers will be unable to follow instructions and communicate challenges and will be completely dependent on others for the decontamination process. Predeployed videos or signs with step-by-step illustrations may be utilized and will work well for children unable to read or who have language barriers. Preschoolers and school-age children have the ability to undress and assist in the decontamination process when given short, specific instructions. Caregivers may be able to assist in communicating instructions to children (Freyberg et al. 2008).

9.8   Decontamination Triage

When potentially contaminated patient(s) present to the health care facility, determining the appropriate response to the incident will require decisions to be made based on victim estimates and suspected agents involved. Decontamination triage is the process of determining which victims have the need for decontamination and which do not. Separating those victims who do not need decontamination can significantly reduce time and resources in mass casualty incidents. Evaluating the need for decontamination takes into account a variety of factors to determine if decontamination is necessary. These include a verbal report from rescuers, proximity of the patient to the release, visible evidence of contamination, signs and symptoms of exposure, verified contaminant on detection technology, known chemical identity, and request by the patient or family for decontamination. The status of contamination may be obtained from the scene of the incident or by signs and symptoms presenting as a recognized toxidrome, which is a group of symptoms associated with an exposure to a given toxin or hazardous material (Toxidrome n.d.) (see Chap. 5 for further details). Decontamination triage in young children is more challenging as they are unable to communicate symptoms, and history is based on guardian or caretaker testimony. Victims who do not need decontamination should be directed to a safe refuge area or the medical triage area. Unaccompanied minors not in need of triage should be escorted to family resource centers or medical triage areas that have designated supervisory capacities.

Pediatric patients should be triaged according to nonambulatory and ambulatory groups. Nonambulatory patients should be disrobed by either the "hot zone" staff or by their caregiver in preparation for decontamination. Nonambulatory patients include infants and young toddlers in addition to injured patients and children with special health care needs. Nonambulatory patients are not always injured as the inability to walk may be baseline in cases of infants and children in wheelchairs or other functional needs. Ambulatory patients should be categorized by age group and by gender for modesty issues. Toddlers, preschoolers, and younger school-age children will likely need assistance with disrobing and will need supervision throughout the decontamination process. Caregivers should be utilized to assist with the decontamination process if at all possible. This age group will often need extra time to disrobe and will need extra time and convincing to enter the shower even if their caregiver is present. Older school-age children (8 and older) to adolescents should be able to disrobe themselves and independently move through the decontamination process (Heon and Foltin 2009). Older children to adolescents may also be uncomfortable disrobing in front of strangers (Zhao et al. 2016). Considerations should be made to protect the patient's privacy if at all possible.

Children, especially young children, should be prioritized prior to adults when classified in the same decontamination triage category. Children do not always recognize the danger and may not flee or be able to rescue themselves during a HAZMAT event. This combined with their increased respiratory rate, low blood volume, permeable skin, and stature being closer to the ground may increase their exposure. Physiologic responses such as vomiting, salivation, lacrimation, or sweating due to exposure to toxins can result in rapid dehydration. Children have less fluid reserves than adults and may progress to hypovolemic shock more rapidly than adults (Lynch and Thomas 2004). Since children cannot always communicate symptoms and have sophisticated compensation systems, they may decompensate rapidly with little warning or change in vital signs. Children should be hemodynamically monitored, and fluid resuscitation should be considered in accordance with pediatric advanced life support (PALS) guidelines. Expectant victims should not be decontaminated until all other victims have been treated and should be placed in an alternate location (Heon and Foltin 2009).

9.9 The Process of Decontamination

Decontamination may vary from gross decontamination that the pediatric patient receives at the scene from fire personnel or EMS responders to technical decontamination at the health care facility. Typically, decontamination at the scene of the incident is gross decontamination and does not address the specific needs of the pediatric patients (Freyberg et al. 2008).

Prior to decontamination, unaccompanied minors should be photographed if possible. Documentation should consist of clothing the patient arrived in and method of transportation to the hospital (EMS, self-transport, and caregiver). This information assists reunification efforts especially if the child can only give limited or no information as to their identity or the identity of their family or caregivers. Decontamination efforts and care should not be delayed due to photographing. If the need for decontamination is confirmed, staff will triage the patient into expectant, immediate, delayed, and minor categories. Patients in the immediate category will be prioritized to rapidly expedite medical care. If adverse weather conditions are present, consideration should be made to protect patients from the elements.

9.9.1 Gross Decontamination

Gross decontamination uses standard equipment to provide a decontamination process for a large number of victims prior to obtaining specialized decontamination equipment. The most common method is the Ladder Pipe System (Fig. 9.1). This

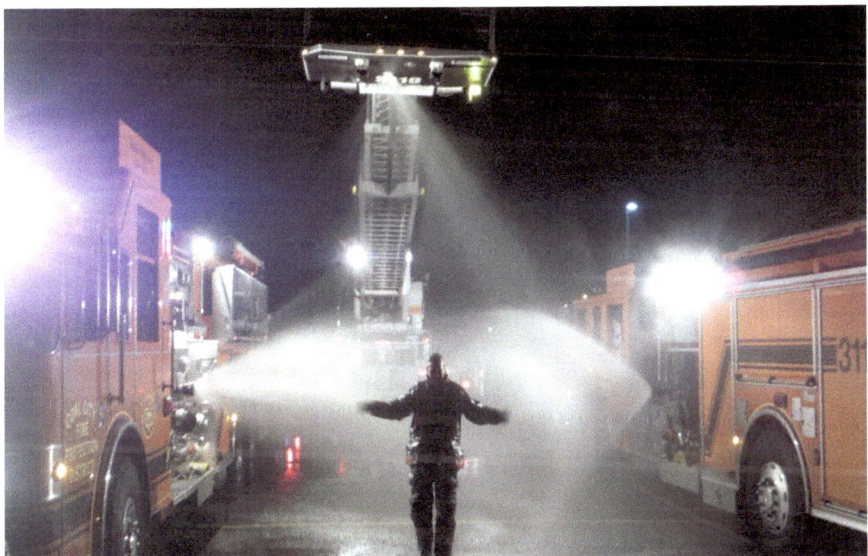

Fig. 9.1 Ladder pipe system (Fire Department Mass Decon [Internet] 2011)

system stages fire pumps parallel to each other to create a high-volume and low-pressure corridor. This corridor is designed for victims to pass-through (with their head tilted back, raising their arms, spreading their legs and turning 90° to 360°). New evidence suggests the duration of showering should not exceed 90 s and that soap or mild detergent solutions may be used. Gross decontamination is most effective if casualties can actively wash themselves. This method can be utilized with older children; however, younger children will need assistance. Gross decontamination may not be appropriate for younger children as it will depend on caregivers or emergency personnel to take them through the corridor. Other disadvantages include the inability to control the pressure and temperature of the water, lack of specialized equipment, and dependence the victims to provide self-decontamination (Chilcott et al. 2019).

9.9.2   Technical Decontamination

The objective of technical decontamination is to provide a complete and thorough reduction or elimination of the contaminant to the lowest level possible. This may be performed after gross decontamination at the scene or as patients self-present at the facility and includes a more concerted effort with specialized equipment, staff, and dedicated facilities. Technical decontamination is more appropriate for young children as gross decontamination relies on self-contamination or cooperation from the victims.

9.9.3   Disrobing

Disrobing the patient is an extremely essential and effective decontamination technique that should be performed at the earliest opportunity preferably within minutes of exposure (Chilcott et al. 2019). Since clothing can provide a protective barrier between the skin and contaminant, disrobing can reduce the level of contamination by up to 90%. Disrobing is also an effective strategy if wet or dry decontamination is not immediately available. Additionally, contaminants can transfer from clothing to the patient's skin surface if decontamination is performed on victims who have not disrobed. Disrobing should be completed expeditiously following the exposure to prevent the transfer of the contaminant to the skin and to prevent secondary contamination via off-gassing from the clothing. This concept should be emphasized in young children as they have increased skin permeability and absorption. Ideally, clothing should be removed utilizing the cut out procedure to prevent the contaminant from coming into contact with the victim's face. If cutting the patient's clothing is not possible, victims should be instructed to hold their breath when removing the victim's clothing over their heads. The rationale of disrobing should be explained to all victims to help them understand the necessity of disrobing. The developmentally appropriate explanation should be employed (Chilcott et al. 2019). All attempts to provide privacy, keep the caregiver with the patient, and utilizing a hospital worker of the same gender (Lynch and Thomas 2004) should be made during the disrobing process to make the child feel more comfortable and to streamline the process. Cultural considerations should also be taken into account for older children, and caregivers also undressing for decontamination in providing privacy and same-gender hospital workers (Chur-Hansen 2002). Providing privacy tents or having separated shower stalls for males and females should be considered during the disrobing process, through the showers, and into the cold zone. Victim's clothing and any valuables or medical devices that cannot undergo (hearing aids, insulin pumps) the decontamination process should be placed in bags and labeled so they can be returned if contamination is not found to be dangerous or to hand over to law enforcement for evidentiary purposes if the contamination is the result of a crime.

If victims are refusing to disrobe or having difficulty due to their age, they should stand aside until they can receive help with disrobing to prevent any delay of cooperative victims. If patients refuse to disrobe due to modesty issues, all efforts should be made to communicate the importance of disrobing to the patient and the risks associated with undergoing decontamination while clothed (Chilcott et al. 2019).

9.9.4 Dry Decontamination

Dry decontamination should be used if the contaminant is a non-caustic liquid or water-reactive chemical compound. Dry methods will also be considered in cold environments without warming elements or when water is not available. Dry decontamination methods include paper towels, wipes, and certain powders (baking powder). Dry decontamination methods should be employed when adequate water is unavailable, the agent is liquid and not caustic, or environmental conditions are adverse, such as freezing weather and heat is unavailable. Various guidance documents suggest either blotting or wiping exposed skin surfaces from the face and neck down to the rest of the body. The skin should be either blotted or wiped using absorbent material to avoid spreading the contaminant. Dry methods are not appropriate when the contaminating agent is caustic, and victims exhibit signs of itching or burning.

9.9.5 Wet Decontamination

Wet decontamination is of particular importance if the agent is particulate or caustic in nature. Wet decontamination employs water and is generally the standard method of decontamination. Special consideration should be made to keep families together, if possible, through the decontamination shower. Younger children and those who are immobile or have special health care needs will need to be escorted through in secure devices such as stretchers or laundry baskets with drainage capabilities. Proper airway position must be maintained manually with careful monitoring as children can be at risk of drowning during showering. If the patient is unable to walk, they should be placed on their side to reduce the risk of aspiration. Staff along with caregivers should use a rinse–wipe–rinse method with concentration on the scalp, hair, face, neck, hands, and arms. Previously, it was recommended to shower victims for 5 min; however, new evidence now suggests that an ideal decontamination time is around 90 s (Chilcott et al. 2019). This may take longer if children are scared or hesitant to go in the shower (Foresman-Capuzzi and Eckenrode 2012). Staff should wash victims using soap or mild detergent, with washcloths, sponges, or soft bristled brushes. Careful consideration should be made, especially for younger children, as rubbing and scrubbing with too much force may enhance contaminant absorption and damage the skin. Pediatric skin, especially in the younger ages, is thinner and more permeable, which can lead to increased absorption of the contaminant to the child.

Water connections in the decontamination area should be compatible with the facility's water lines, with the availability to control the water pressure and temperature. If the decontamination shower is within or adjacent to the facility, then it is recommended that the area be under negative pressure, which may need to be tested prior to decontaminating the victims to ensure the contaminant is not recirculated into the hospital's heating ventilation and air-conditioning (HVAC) system. The decontamination area also needs the ability to collect and contain large quantities of water as contaminated runoff has to be disposed of separately according to state and local regulations. The area should have adequate lighting, connection to electricity, adequate space for families, decontamination staff for nonambulatory patients, and curtains or separated areas to maintain patient privacy. Water pressure and temperature should be monitored and adapted as the pediatric patient has sensitive skin and is at greater risk for hypothermia. Water pressure should be maintained at approximately 60 psi. Handheld adjustable sprayers are ideal for adjusting pressure. Water temperature must be at a minimum 98 °F or 36.0 °C to prevent hypothermia. If cutaneous injuries are present, they can exacerbate hypothermia. Decontamination should be performed primarily with water. A low-alkaline mild soap may be useful, but alcohol or bleach-based cleansers are not recommended due to the potential of systemic intoxication.

9.9.6 Drying

Distance from the shower to the drying area should be kept to a minimum to avoid hypothermia. After the patient has completed decontamination in the shower, actively drying the patient should be completed. Active drying of the skin post wet decontamination is a vital step in removing contaminants from the patient using a towel or other suitable absorbent material. This will prevent further spread of contaminants and prevent hypothermia. Although all victims will benefit from active drying, it is especially beneficial to younger children to avoid hypothermia (Chilcott et al. 2019). Young children should be carefully monitored so they do not develop hypothermia. Children should be placed in warm blankets or foil-type blankets, and their temperatures should be monitored (Jorgensen et al. 2010). Children should be provided with appropriate clothing or gowns as well as diapers if needed. Used towels should be considered contaminated waste, and the drying stage should be maintained within the warm zone (Chilcott et al. 2019).

9.9.7 Evaluating the Effectiveness of Decontamination

Evaluating the effectiveness of decontamination centers around whether the contamination has been eliminated or reduced to a safe level. There are both subjective and objective indicators that include visualization of the elimination of contaminant from the skin and hair, improvement in signs and symptoms, and results from detection equipment such as Geiger counters or chemical paper. Effective decontamination standards have not been effectively established (Raber et al. 2004); however, the overall goal is to improve the patient's health outcomes and avoid secondary contamination. In the chemical decontamination event at Cincinnati Children's Hospital Medical Center, one fifth-grade girl exposed to n-butyl mercaptan required additional decontamination because when evaluated she still had the smell of the chemical in her braided hair (Timm and Reeves 2007). Ultimately, a combination of the above indicators can give a comprehensive picture of effective decontamination.

9.9.8 Post-decontamination

Once the decontamination process is determined to be effective, children should immediately be re-triaged and warmed with blankets and size-appropriate re-dress kits. Warming devices such as warm blankets, foil blankets, clothing, hats, and warmers can be used to regulate the victim's temperature. The patient's vital signs should be carefully monitored to prevent hyper- or hypothermia. Diapers in a variety of sizes and safe childproof areas including cribs and bassinets as well as adequate supervisory staff should be available for children who are waiting for or receiving medical care after decontamination. Proper identification of the child that ideally corresponds with the caregiver should be issued and placed via a wristband. Medical monitoring and treatment including antidotes and supportive therapy are initiated after the patient is triaged. It is important to note that an actual or estimated weight should be taken as antidotes and supportive medication dosages can vary in dosages and routes and are calculated based on the patient's weight. The Broselow tape can be used to easily estimate a child's weight if scales or time is limited. Processes should be in place for evaluation of psychological trauma after the incident and decontamination procedure. If caregivers are not present, and no further medical care is deemed necessary by providers, a family resource center can be activated and can help care for children and locate parents and guardians. See Chap. 11 for further information on reunification.

9.9.9 Decontaminating Equipment

There are generalized cleanup considerations to make depending on the type, scope, and size of the contaminant and incident. If it is a known contaminant and can be safely cleaned up with existing resources, then staff properly trained in HAZMAT procedures can dispose of the contaminant in accordance with local, state, and federal regulations. Equipment that is not able to be decontaminated or single-use items should be disposed of properly. If victims arrived in a vehicle or ambulance, the vehicle will need to be decontaminated. Health care facilities should establish and maintain contracts or memorandums of understanding (MOU) for any vendors that have been contracted to provide cleanup and disposal services.

9.10 Developmental and Age-Based Recommendations

9.10.1 Physiological Considerations

Children have unique physical needs to be taken into account when undergoing decontamination. Vital signs (Table 9.2), medication dosages, and physical needs are dependent on age and weight. Pediatric skin, especially in the younger ages is thinner and more permeable, which can lead to increased absorption of the contaminant of the child. Children have a smaller airway, so substances that cause airway constriction can have an increased severity in younger children. Since children have a higher respiratory rate, off-gassing of substances can be inhaled at a greater rate. Dense gasses stay lower to the ground, in the path of younger children. Pediatric medications and fluids are dependent on the patient's weight and age. Children are more susceptible to dehydration and the effects of contaminants because they have less blood volume, and minimal blood should be taken when needed (Heon and Foltin 2009).

Table 9.2 Pediatric vital signs (Novak and Gill 2018)

	Temperature	Heart rate	Respirations	Blood pressure
Infants	97.8–99.7 °F 35.5–37.5 °C	100–190 bpm	30–53 bpm	Systolic: 72–92 Diastolic: 37–56
Toddlers	97.8–99.7 °F 35.5–37.5 °C	98–140 bpm	22–37 bpm	Systolic: 86–106 Diastolic: 42–63
Preschoolers	97.8–99.7 °F 35.5–37.5 °C	80–120 bpm	20–28 bpm	Systolic: 89–112 Diastolic: 46–72
School-age (5–9 years)	97.8–99.7 °F 35.5–37.5 °C	75–118 bpm	18–25 bpm	Systolic: 97–115 Diastolic: 57–76
Preadolescent (10–11 years)	97.8–99.7 °F 35.5–37.5 °C	75–118 bpm	18–25 bpm	Systolic: 102–120Diastolic: 61–80
Adolescents	97.8–99.7 °F 35.5–37.5 °C	60–100 bpm	12–20 bpm	Systolic: 100–131 Diastolic: 64–83

Source: adapted from http://pedscases.com/pediatric-vital-signs-reference-chart

9.10.2 Developmental Considerations

The pediatric population has unique needs based on their developmental level and age group (see Chap. 7 for further information on developmental levels). Special considerations must be made during the decontamination process as children have unique physical, cognitive, and emotional needs and may not have the developmental understanding of the situation. Children may become fearful, uncooperative, combative, or not have the ability to assist health care workers in the decontamination process. If possible, all efforts should be made to allow families to remain together, as it may reduce emotional and psychological anxiety. Space and privacy accommodations should be provided to incorporate keeping families together while still maintaining privacy. For younger children, parents or caregivers should participate in the decontamination of the child if they are unable to self-decontaminate. When decontaminating families together, caregivers may need help caring for the child while the parent is undergoing disrobing or decontamination themselves. Child safe spaces, appropriate apparatuses to place infants or toddler, and staff should be available to accommodate the child. If parents or caregivers are unavailable, patients should have adequate supervision and assistance through the decontamination process.

The following are a list of developmental and age-based recommendations during the decontamination process:

9.10.3 Infants (0–12 months)

Infants require great caution when undergoing decontamination. Infants are the most vulnerable of the age groups and are unable to verbalize or assist in the decontamination process. The infant must be disrobed in the hot or warm zone by their caregiver or staff. If caregivers are present during the decontamination process, they will still require assistance or a safe environment to place the infant as they cannot disrobe themselves and the infant at the same time. History, contamination exposure, and symptoms are based on visual observation and parent or caregiver testimony. Infants are slippery when they are wet and require great caution during showering as there is a risk of trauma due to an accidental fall or dropping the infant. Infants should be placed in a secure device for decontamination that has drainage capabilities such as an infant bathtub, laundry basket, bassinet, or stretcher. Ideally, caregivers should not carry the infant through the decontamination shower to prevent injury or accidentally dropping the infant. Infant's airway position must be maintained manually and carefully observed due to their large occiput and developing muscle control. Signs of compromised airway, asphyxia, respiratory distress, and decompensation can be subtle and should be monitored by staff who have training in caring for infants. Children also differ in their ability to secrete toxins as their immune system is immature, and their organs are at various levels of development and differentiation (Zhao et al. 2016). Post-decontamination the infant should be dried immediately and undergo warming measures to prevent hypothermia. The infant's temperature should be monitored frequently and warming measures applied as necessary. Post-decontamination supplies such as infant-sized clothing and diapers should be available. Identification such as a bracelet should be placed on the infant that corresponds with their parent or guardian if possible. If possible, infants should remain in the care of their parent, guardian, or assigned to a staff member if the infant is unaccompanied. The facility should have safe cribs or bassinets to place the infants post-decontamination (Heon and Foltin 2009).

9.10.3.1 Holding Infants

Although it is preferred for families to decontaminate together, they still will require assistance. It will be difficult for a parent to undress themselves and their children at the same time, especially if they are injured. Experience with newborns has shown that "they are difficult to hold when wet." This problem is exacerbated further by the reduced dexterity of hospital personnel wearing chemically resistant gloves and suits. It is recommended that two people handle any transfer of children in the shower and that the child be held tightly and securely, close to the body of the chaperone. Infant handling positions and procedures where the head is supported in the palm and the body straddles the arm of the provider while tucked under the opposite arm can be used while in the shower. This is controversial, and many find it difficult to perform. Thus, the recommendation was made that infants can be placed and secured on a stretcher and decontaminated to decrease the risk of being dropped (Heon and Foltin 2009).

Other characteristics of infants to consider during decontamination include:

- Thermoregulation becomes more efficient as the infant matures.
- Infants are obligate nasal breathers until 2–4 months old.
- No bowel or bladder control; dependent on diapers.
- The infant has a protruding abdomen due to immature abdominal musculature and a high rib cage.
- Fears unfamiliar situations and separation from parents/caregivers at 8–12 months of age.
- Calculate medication/fluids to an infant's weight and age.
- Draw minimum volume blood samples.
- Encourage parents to be present and to assist in decontamination, as appropriate.
- Provide and encourage touch and cuddling, especially after a procedure.
- Utilize appropriate-sized equipment for care (bathtubs, BP cuffs).
- Be aware that elevated blood pressure, heart rate, respirations, and fussiness may be indications of pain.
- Limit the number of strangers caring for the infant.
- Keep infant warm.
- Avoid loud noises, bright lights, and sudden environmental changes.
- Skin integrity is fragile and scrubbing and water temperature should be monitored.
- Provide frequent repositioning.
- Explain procedures, care, and care practices to the parents/caregivers.
- Use simple directions when communicating with the infant.

- Keep the side rails up on cribs and carts at all time.
- Keep small objects, medications, and potential poisons out of the infant's reach.
- Do not leave the infant unsupervised in potentially hazardous situations.
- Provide tactile stimulation and motor skill development with age-appropriate and safe toys.
- Evaluate toys for choking hazard (Bowden and Greenberg 2010).

9.10.4 Toddlers (12–36 months)

Although toddlers undergo great growth in cognitive, communication, and physical maturation, they do not have the ability to provide self-contamination and can cause great disruption in the flow of decontamination. Disrobing toddlers can be particularly challenging even with the assistance of a caregiver (Freyberg et al. 2008). Toddlers need supervision at all times, and they should not be left unsupervised in potentially hazardous situations. If caregivers are not present or have to participate in the self-decontamination process, staff should be assigned to supervise the toddler during the duration of the decontamination process. Allow the toddler to play with medical equipment when possible and allow them to also hold the scrub brush or washcloth if possible. The showering process may upset them, and although they have increased head control, the airway requires monitoring. Toddlers prefer consistency with routine, and a decontamination event can cause great disruption. Small objects, medication, and other potentially dangerous items should be kept from the toddler's reach.

Other characteristics of toddlers to consider during decontamination include:

- Responds to light, sound, and temperature—may be overwhelmed by the situation.
- Gains fine motor coordination.
- Progresses to walking independently, may be mobile.
- Runs, jumps, and climbs, maintain anti-slip surfaces in shower.
- Able to talk about the past and may remember the incident.
- Increasingly curious and will ask "why" questions.
- Likes routines.
- Requires supervision due to impulsive behavior and inability to recognize dangers.
- Short attention span.
- Understands and uses what, who, and where questions.
- Associates experience with their world and draws conclusions.
- Learns through imitation, exploration/play, and trial and error.
- Fears being alone and stranger danger.
- Asserts self-independence.
- Seeks attention and approval.
- Frequent temper tantrums due to poor behavior control.
- Keep small objects, medications, and potentially dangerous items out of reach (Bowden and Greenberg 2010).

9.10.5 Preschoolers (3–6 years)

Preschoolers have a limited ability to provide self-care during a decontamination event. Family members are the most important people to preschoolers, and they can experience separation anxiety, stranger anxiety, and avoidance of situations. It is important to involve their families or caregivers in the decontamination process and keep them together throughout the decontamination process. Preschoolers may experience fear of the staff in PPE along with the distortion of voices. Preschoolers may not want to help rescuers and may cause a delay in the flow of victims. Play is of particular importance and can be incorporated into the decontamination process. Psychological trauma can present through repetitive play or reenactment of the incident. Any procedures that could scare or traumatize a preschooler should be explained just prior to administration.

Other characteristics of a preschooler to consider during decontamination include:

- Increased skills and coordination.
- Improved balance and muscular strength.
- Can dress self with little supervision.
- Learns by imitation.
- Increased attention span.
- Logical reasoning emerges, but still lacks understanding of cause and effect.
- May have a distorted understanding of body which may affect decontamination.
- May believe they have to undergo decontamination and treatment because they did something wrong.
- Clear rules and boundaries promote a sense of security (Bowden and Greenberg 2010).

9.10.6 School-Age (6–12 years)

School-age children can provide certain self-care activities during decontamination as coordination improves especially at the age of 8 (Heon and Foltin 2009). School-age children start to prefer friends and develop a need for modesty and may want to decontaminate without their family especially in the preadolescent stage (ages 10–11). School-age children begin to understand cause and effect, so explanations and clear instructions will aid in the self-contamination methods. It is important to assure the child that any procedures and treatments they receive are not punishments or as a result of something they did. School-age children need to be supervised but can be directed through the shower independently (Heon and Foltin 2009).

Other characteristics of school-age/preadolescents include:

- Logical reasoning and understanding of cause and effect.
- Increase in gross and fine motor abilities and coordination.
- Greater muscular strength.

- Maturing perspectives.
- Can move focus from present to also understand past and future.
- Acquiring reading skills.
- Able to describe pain and symptoms in some detail.
- Hospitalization enhances fears of the unknown, bodily harm, separation, and death.
- Starts to prefer friends to family.
- Develops a need to fit in with peers.
- Begins taking on more responsibility.
- Provide privacy.
- Explain process of decontamination and equipment in terms the child can understand.
- Involve the family and child in care.
- Encourage the child to talk about their feelings and ask questions.
- Provide the child opportunities for decision-making (Bowden and Greenberg 2010).

9.10.7 Adolescent (12–19 years)

Privacy and modesty issues are imperative when decontaminating adolescents. Due to their maturing developmental level and need for privacy, decontamination along with family members may not appropriate; however, providing gender-specific shower stalls with curtains in stalls is important. They are independent and can participate in self-decontamination with proper instructions. Accidents are a threat to that age group and the leading cause of death. They are susceptible to peer pressure without regard for consequences. This may result in exposure to HAZMAT substances such as succumbing to a riot control agent or experimenting with explosive devices. Although smaller adolescents may still need weight-based dosages, generally adult dosages are acceptable.

Other characteristics to consider with adolescents include:

- Abstract and logical thinking.
- Choices and decision-making are desired. Hypothetically thinks through situations and can understand disease processes.
- Abstract thinking improves the ability to understand the cause and effect of treatment.
- Reluctant to admit not understanding something.
- May not ask for adult support even if needed.
- Sense of control, parents go from authority figure to peers, but still has an underlying need to please adults.
- Authority is meant to be challenged.
- Bodily changes, appearance, and acceptance are a concern.
- Privacy is important.
- Peer separation is difficult.

- Pregnancy precautions for female patients.
- Parents/guardians may not know their location or involvement in the incident.
- Adult consent is needed (Bowden and Greenberg 2010).

9.11   Children with Special Health Care Needs

Decontaminating children with special health care needs pose additional challenges. Children who are dependent on equipment such as ventilators, insulin pumps, and hearing aids pose additional considerations because these devices can be damaged with excessive contact with water. Careful attention to triaging these patients as to the need for decontamination should be performed, as the consequences of being without these devices will incur greater care and staffing needs for these patients. If it is determined that the patient does need decontamination, dry decontamination can be considered if appropriate. The patient device should also be inspected for contaminants such as solid or liquid foreign bodies. If no contamination is found on the devices, then it can be safe to use. If any contamination is found, the device should be left in the hot zone if there are no methods to decontaminate the device. Some devices are able to withstand wet decontamination like prosthetic limbs or eye glasses. These devices should be washed in the shower with the patients (Heon and Foltin 2009). Patients who arrive with service animals can be decontaminated together, and hospital plans should address how they will decontaminate service animals.

9.12   Psychological Considerations

Psychological considerations in children vary depending on the developmental level, cognitive understanding, and limited coping strategies. Psychological reactions in children differ than those of adults following an incident and are underestimated both in intensity and duration of stress and coping reactions by caregivers and professionals (Kar 2009).

Self-care during a decontamination incident has been shown to positively impact the psychological outcome during an event; however, many young children have limited or no ability to perform these actions. Providing kits to support self-care decontamination and allowing families to remain together can prevent psychological stress.

Children may have difficulty understanding and coping with the situation. Psychological support services for unaccompanied minors should be accessible in the family resource center with staff who has had training to meet the psychological needs of children. Child life specialists, social workers, and music and art therapists can help children with psychological support. Other services to consider are the use of pet therapy and play therapy.

There are known long-term psychological consequences for children who experience a traumatic event. Studies show that children who have not received treatment from traumatic events have increased hospital visits over their life span. Children have a limited ability to seek help for themselves and are dependent on caregivers and providers to seek proper care and resources. Assessment tools such as Psychological Simple Triage and Rapid Treatment (PsySTART) can be utilized to evaluate psychological risk and to make appropriate referrals to mitigate long-term mental health disorders (Schreiber 2010). Follow-up and continued monitoring of the child may help ensure that the child gets the appropriate support that they need. Please refer to Chap. 12 for further information.

9.13 Hospital Incident Command Structure

Depending on the size and scope of the incident, incorporating the Hospital Incident Command System (HICS) and the National Incident Management System (NIMS) guidelines into the decontamination response will enable a more organized and efficient response in managing the event. Small, isolated events generally will not require a full activation; however, a response may require the activation of additional resources to successfully manage the incident. The Operations Section has oversight responsibility over all hospital operations during incident activation (Schreiber 2010) and reports to the Incident Commander. The Safety Officer can support the operation and mitigate any potential safety hazards. Specialized positions (Fig. 9.2) that manage a HAZMAT incident include the following (Authority 2014):

Fig. 9.2 HICS HAZMAT branch director hierarchy (Authority 2014). (Source: Adapted from https://emsa.ca.gov/hospital-incident-command-system-job-action-sheets-2014)

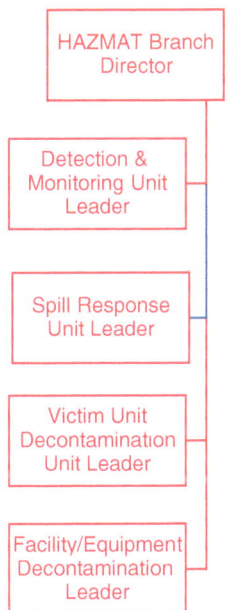

- HAZMAT Branch Director organizes and directs hazardous material (HAZMAT) incident response activities including detection and monitoring, spill response, victim, decontamination, hospital, and equipment decontamination.
- Detection and Monitoring Unit Leader coordinates all the detection and monitoring activities related to a HAZMAT incident response.
- Spill Response Unit Leader coordinates activities related to the implementation of the hospital's internal HAZMAT Spill Response Plan and established perimeter of the incident.
- Victim Decontamination Unit Leader coordinates the hospital's patient decontamination activities related to the HAZMAT incident response.
- Facility/Equipment Decontamination Leader Coordinate the on-site hospital and equipment decontamination activities related to HAZMAT incident response.

Additional HICS sections and roles can be activated to support HAZMAT incidents. As the size and scope of the incident grow, certain HICS roles are recommended to support the incident. Within the Operations Section, the Patient Family Assistance Branch Director can be activated if there are unaccompanied minors present. Command Section roles to activate include the Public Information Officer, Liaison Officer, and Medical–Technical Specialist (chemical). Additional Operations Section roles include the Section Chief, Medical Care Branch Director, Security Branch Director, and Infrastructure Branch Director. Planning Section roles include the Section Chief, Resources Unit Leader, Situation Unit Leader. Logistics Section roles would include the Section Chief, Support Branch Director, and the Labor Pool and Credentialing Unit if needed. Further descriptions of actions within the HICS structure that can support a Chemical Incident are listed under the HICS Incident Response Guide (Authority 2014). More about HICS can be found in Chap. 4.

9.14   Planning for Health Care Facilities

Advanced planning for health care facilities can optimize the decontamination process and improve overall response and health outcomes of patients. A written decontamination/hazardous materials plan should be a component within the Emergency Operations Plan. Plans and procedures should be reviewed and updated with staff as needed and annually. The decontamination plan should incorporate the needs of children and is scalable to small or large incidents. Plans should include a method of activation and include points of contact for all team members, vendors, subject matter experts, and governmental agencies. Family resource center plans should also be incorporated to support any unaccompanied minors. The facility should obtain all necessary equipment and maintain an inventory of fully charged, routinely tested PAPRs. Facilities should maintain a separate cache of PPE that is designated for training purposes and is clearly labeled to keep the integrity and stock of PPE that is needed in a real event (Harvard School of Public Health 2014).

Preestablished MOUs and any available vendor information can be placed in the decontamination plan to ensure accessibility. Please refer to Chap. 13 for further information on hospital preparedness.

9.15   Recommended Training

Staff tasked with supporting the decontamination response require specialized training to successfully manage contaminated victims and prevent secondary contamination. The Occupational Safety and Health Administration require hospital personnel to undergo annual Hazardous Materials (HAZWOPER) Training in accordance with 29 CFR 1910 OSHA standards. HAZWOPER elements include organizational structure, comprehensive work plan, safety and health plan, and medical surveillance training (Occupational Health and Safety Administration 2005).

Staff should receive training on the vulnerabilities of children and how to address these during a decontamination event in addition to cut out procedures, START, and JumpSTART triage. Ensure that the Emergency Department staff is familiar with the hospital's decontamination plan and basic HAZMAT response. This includes the recognition of contaminated victims, proper activation procedures, and appropriate use of PPE, detection and monitoring procedures, and the activation and utilization of all equipment (Table 9.3).

During a singular or small-scale event, when a hospital does not activate their emergency operations plan, Emergency Department staff may be able to successfully provide decontamination and follow-up for victims. However, any event that requires the decontamination of more than a few isolated victims or is part of a larger activation should activate the Hospital HAZMAT or decontamination team that is made up of members outside of the Emergency Department. Larger events require Emergency Department staff to provide triage, immediate care, and medical for victims post-decontamination (Harvard School of Public Health 2014).

The employer must document the training of each employee required to wear or use PPE by preparing a certification containing the name of each employee trained, the date of training, and clear identification of the subject of the certification. Emergency Department personnel should receive training or have access to documents that provide the signs and symptoms of various contaminants and isolation procedures.

The facility should have just-in-time training material for support personnel that includes the type of contaminant, anticipated duties, detection equipment, and the appropriate use of PPE that can be deployed during a large event or if decontamination team members are unavailable. Health care facilities should conduct at least one decontamination drill/exercise annually that tests the decontamination plan. Drills and exercises that incorporate children of all ages into the scenario can verify pediatric decontamination capabilities and readiness. Specific elements of the plan should be evaluated including activation of the plan/team, ability to set up and functionality of decontamination equipment, staff competency in doffing/donning

Table 9.3 Recommended equipment (Heon and Foltin 2009; Zhao et al. 2016; Lynch and Thomas 2004; Allen et al. 2007)

Pre-decontamination
- Biohazard bags/sealable drums for disposal or storage of patient belongings.
- Equipment to take vital signs and temperature.
- Illustrated signage.
- Megaphone or amplified devices for verbal instruction.
- Photo capability.
- Plastic chairs.
- PPE and method for taking vital signs.
- Self-care decontamination kits.
- Small and large sealable plastic bags.
- Tape/tarps or rope to clearly demarcate lanes and zones of protection.
- Tents, dividers.
- Waterproof triage and Identification tags.
- Waterproof labels.
- Wax pens/permanent markers (Bowden and Greenberg 2010).

During decontamination
- Adjustable pressure nozzle or handheld nozzle.
- Anti-slip surfaces.
- Mild soap.
- Soft bristle brushes, wash cloths, or sponges.
- Sterile saline for wound irrigation.
- Sterile sponges/sterile gauze.
- Transportation or method to secure infants, young children, and nonambulatory patients (infant bath tubs, laundry baskets, and gurneys).
- Warm water .

Post-decontamination
- Cribs/cots.
- Diapers in a variety of sizes.
- Identification bands.
- Re-dress kits in a variety of sizes.
- Towels for drying.
- Warm blankets/foil kits.

procedures, patient throughput, and communication/coordination of coalition partners and vendors. Plans and training methods should be evaluated and updated based on any deficiencies (Harvard School of Public Health 2014).

9.16   Conclusion

Pediatric HAZMAT incidents create unique challenges for hospitals. Decontamination plans should be a part of each facility's emergency preparedness plan and implement considerations for the pediatric population. Plans should be evaluated and tested on a regular basis and updated regarding the effectiveness of the plan. Proper equipment, antidotes, communication procedures, and training are essential to a successful decontamination program. Decontamination in hospitals lends itself to a multidisciplinary approach and may include both internal and external partners. Having established prior communication and training with external agencies such as the fire department, EMS, social services, subject matter experts, and mutual aid partners (Table 9.4) can prevent potential problems when a real-life

Table 9.4 Hospital sources and hotlines for CBRNE incidents

American Association of Poison Control Centers
1–800–222-1222 (24 h)
Information on poison substances/exposures and antidotes. Online support available.
https://www.poison.org/
ASPCA National Animal Poison Control Center
1–888–426-4435 (24 h)
*fee may be charged
Information on poison substances/exposures and antidotes for animals.
Centers for Disease Control and Prevention
1–770-7100 Public Response Hotline (CDC)
1–800-CDC-INFO
888–232-6348 (TTY)
Information and resources on responding to public health emergencies including biological agents.
https://www.cdc.gov
CHEMTREC
1–800–424-9300
(24 h) public service hotline for emergency responders. CHEMTREC® is part of the American Chemistry Council.
https://www.chemtrec.com/
Domestic Preparedness Chemical/Biological Help Line
1–800–368-6498
Federal Bureau of Investigation (FBI)
1–202–324-3000 (Headquarters)
Resources for preparing for and respond to a terrorist event, including victim assistance, training, incident reporting, and understanding threat levels.
Federal Emergency Management Agency (FEMA)
1–800-621-FEMA
Contains chemical emergency-related information for households and communities, including preparation, and what to during and after an emergency event.
National Response Center (USCG)
1–800–424-8802 (24 hours)
http://nrc.uscg.mil/
Federal point of contact for reporting oil and chemical spills; hotline for chemical & biological weapons of mass destruction incidents.
Nuclear Regulatory Commission Operations Center
Phone: 301–816-5100 (accepts collect calls),
NRC's Toll-Free Safety Hotline: (800) 695–7403
https://www.nrc.gov/
Accept reports involving nuclear facilities or radioactive accidents

event occurs. Having security involved in providing lockdown procedures is essential in maintaining the integrity of the hot, warm, and cold zones as well as crowd management. Decontamination must be expedient, safe, and thorough to properly care for victims of HAZMAT incidents, especially pediatric victims.

References

Allen GM, et al. Principles of disaster planning for the pediatric population. Prehospital Disast Med. 2007;22(6):537–40.
American Academy of Pediatrics. Children and disasters: disaster preparedness to meet children's needs. 2019. Available from https://www.aap.org/en-us/advocacy-and-policy/aap-health-initiatives/Children-and-Disasters/Pages/Decontamination.aspx. Accessed 11 May 2019.
Authority C.E.M.S. Hospital incident command system—job action sheets 2014.
Bowden VR, Greenberg CS. Children and their families: the continuum of care. Philadelphia, PA: Lippincott Williams & Wilkins; 2010.
Chilcott RP, et al. Evaluation of US Federal Guidelines (Primary Response Incident Scene Management [PRISM]) for mass decontamination of casualties during the initial operational response to a chemical incident. Ann Emerg Med. 2019;73(6):671–84.
Chur-Hansen A. Preferences for female and male nurses: the role of age, gender and previous experience–year 2000 compared with 1984. J Adv Nurs. 2002;37(2):192–8.
Cibulsky S, et al. Patient decontamination in a mass chemical exposure incident: National Planning Guidance for Communities. Washington, DC: US Department of Homeland Security and US Department of Health and Human Services; 2014.
Eisenkraft A, et al. What can we learn on medical preparedness from the use of chemical agents against civilians in Syria? Am J Emerg Med. 2014;32(2):186.
Falkenrath RA, Newman RD, Thayer BA. America's Achilles' heel: nuclear, biological, and chemical terrorism and covert attack. Cambridge, MA: MIT Press; 1998.
Fire Department Mass Decon. [Internet]. 2011. Available from https://www.foap.com/photos/fire-department-mass-decon-dd4a29f2-46db-4173-856c-d5fbb01a9308. Accessed 30 Sept 2019.
Foresman-Capuzzi J, Eckenrode P. When Mr Yuck meets Mr Bubble: a primer on pediatric decontamination. J Emerg Nursing. 2012;38(5):490–2.
Freyberg CW, et al. Disaster preparedness: hospital decontamination and the pediatric patient—guidelines for hospitals and emergency planners. Prehosp Disaster Med. 2008;23(2):166–73.
Gurwitch RH, et al. When disaster strikes: responding to the needs of children. Prehosp Disast Med. 2004;19(1):21–8.
Harvard School of Public Health. Hospital decontamination self-assessment tool. Commonwealth of Massachusetts Department of Public Health—Office of Emergency Preparedness and Emergency Management. Boston, MA: Harvard School of Public Health; 2014.
Heon D, Foltin GL. Principles of pediatric decontamination. Clin Pediat Emerg Med. 2009;10(3):186–94.
Hick JL, et al. Protective equipment for health care facility decontamination personnel: regulations, risks, and recommendations. Ann Emerg Med. 2003a;42(3):370–80.
Holland MG, Cawthon D. Personal protective equipment and decontamination of adults and children. Emergency Medicine Clinics. 2015;33(1):51–68.
Horton DK, Berkowitz Z, Kaye WE. Secondary contamination of ED personnel from hazardous materials events, 1995–2001. Am J Emerg Med. 2003;21(3):199–204.
Jorgensen AM, Mendoza GJ, Henderson JL. Emergency preparedness and disaster response core competency set for perinatal and neonatal nurses. J Obst Gynecol Neonat Nurs. 2010;39(4):450–67.
Kar N. Psychological impact of disasters on children: review of assessment and interventions. World J Pediatr. 2009;5(1):5–11.

Lynch EL, Thomas TL. Pediatric considerations in chemical exposures: are we prepared? Pediat Emerg Care. 2004;20(3):198–208.

Novak C, Gill P. Pediatric vital signs reference sheet. 2018. Available from http://pedscases.com/pediatric-vital-signs-reference-chart. Accessed 31 May 2019.

Occupational Health and Safety Administration. OSHA best practices for hospital-based first receivers of victims from mass casualty incidents involving the release of hazardous substances. Washington, DC: Occupational Health and Safety Administration; 2005.

Okumura T, et al. Report on 640 victims of the Tokyo subway sarin attack. Ann Emerg Med. 1996;28(2):129–35.

Raber E, et al. How clean is clean enough? Recent developments in response to threats posed by chemical and biological warfare agents. Int J Environ Health Res. 2004;14(1):31–41.

Schreiber M. The PsySTART rapid mental health triage and incident management system. Irvine: Center for Disaster Medical Sciences, University of California; 2010.

Siegel D, Strauss-Riggs K, Needle S. Prioritization of pediatric chemical, biological, radiologic, nuclear, and explosive disaster preparedness education and training needs. Clin Pediatr Emerg Med. 2014;15(4):309–17.

Teague DC. Mass casualties in the Oklahoma City bombing. Clin Orthop Relat Res. 2004;422:77–81.

Timm N, Reeves S. A mass casualty incident involving children and chemical decontamination. Disast Manag Resp. 2007;5(2):49–55.

Toxidrome. (n.d.) Mosby's medical dictionary 2009.

United States Department of Health and Human Services Security. National disaster recovery framework. 2nd ed. Washington, DC: United States Department of Health and Human Services Security; 2016.

USAMRIID. Medical management of biological casualties handbook. 7th ed. Fort Detrick, MD: USAMRIID; 2011.

Veenema TG, editor. Disaster nursing and emergency preparedness. 4th ed. New York, NY: Springer Publishing Company, LLC; 2019.

Zhao X, Dughly O, Simpson J. Decontamination of the pediatric patient. Curr Opin Pediatr. 2016;28(3):305–9.

Marian K. Nowak

10.1 Shelter Setup

Mass care shelters provide for the basic needs of displaced individuals. They provide disaster victims with water, food, over-the-counter medication, personal care facilities, and a place to stay. Although shelters attempt to provide for the basic needs of daily living, families should plan to take some personal care and child-friendly items with them. Mass care sheltering can involve living with many people in a confined space, so bringing familiar items to shelters can offer comfort in times of evacuation (Shelter Ready 2018). Suggested items include medications, formula, diapers, games, favorite toy, toothbrush, and important phone numbers (Federal Emergency Management Agency 2018). Some shelters also provide care for animals; thus, house pets often are accommodated in shelters.

At a minimum, each location needs to include capacity for temporary housing, bathrooms, showers, American Disabilities Act (ADA) accessibility, and floor plans (American Disabilities Act 2018). In addition, the facilities should have a place for diversional activities (e.g., movies, arts and crafts, playroom, and games). The staffing of the shelters depends on the size and anticipated length of shelter operation.

State law sets the responsibility for emergency care and shelter at the local level. Mass shelters are located at predetermined locations that are screened for the ability to house large numbers of people. Examples of predesignated locations include (1) public and private schools, school gymnasiums and large multipurpose rooms, (2) city-owned facilities such as community centers, senior centers, recreational facilities, or auditoriums, and (3) congregation centers such as churches, temples, synagogues, or other privately owned facilities.

M. K. Nowak (✉)
QSEN International Task Force, Cleveland, OH, USA
e-mail: mnowak@cse.edu

© Springer Nature Switzerland AG 2020

267

C. J. Goodhue, N. Blake (eds.), *Nursing Management of Pediatric Disaster*,
https://doi.org/10.1007/978-3-030-43428-1_10

10.1.1 Sanitation and Hygiene

Sanitation practices are paramount to prevent the spread of contagious diseases. Both residents and staff are encouraged to follow the basic tenets of personal hygiene. Methods for preventing the spread of contagious diseases include development of a cleaning plan for the shelter, encouraging clients to cover their mouths when coughing and sneezing, encouraging frequent hand washing, and use of hand sanitizer, as well as avoiding close contact with sick people, disinfecting toys after use, and prompt reporting of illnesses or other medical concerns to shelter staff (Federal Emergency Management Agency and American Red Cross 2015).

Should any contagious disease outbreak occur, shelter staff must isolate those who are ill. If individual rooms are not available, designate a separate area for isolation precautions. In addition, shelter staff takes the following precautions: promote personal hygiene measures and report any outbreak to the local public health department and the shelter agency. Staff may request medical assistance as necessary. Increasing the distance between people can assist with infection control. Cleanup staff may be asked to perform additional environmental cleaning when necessary. Parents and caregivers are encouraged to monitor children for symptoms of illness and report immediately to shelter staff. Cleaning of toys is performed with a focus on items that are more likely to have frequent contact with the hands, mouths, or body fluids of children. Many shelters have hand sanitizers available at several locations to assist with personal hygiene.

Food preparation staff follows the following practices: use of gloves, proper hand washing prior to food preparation, and serving food in a timely manner. These practices help ensure the prevention of infection originating from food sources. Cafeteria-style service is preferred over self-service, buffet-style, or family-style. Food handlers should also use fresh water for food preparation, separate raw and cooked foods, cook food thoroughly, and ensure that food is kept within the temperature safety zone (above 140 °F or below 40 °F). Food handlers also ensure that food preparation and serving surfaces and equipment are sanitized properly (Federal Emergency Management Agency and American Red Cross 2015).

Box 10.1 How to Locate a Shelter
To locate shelters in any US locations, text SHELTER and a Zip Code *to* 43362. Ex: Shelter 01234 (standard rates apply), visit: http://www.disasterassistance.gov/, call your local Red Cross or Department of Health.

10.1.2 Staffing Shelters

The shelter staff generally includes a shelter manager who deals with the day-to-day logistics of all shelter operations, registration staff who signs in the clients, food services staff, security staff, dormitory managers (monitor sleeping arrangements), day care workers, spiritual counselors, mental health counselors, animal services, and communication services. Shelters should be designed to meet children's needs

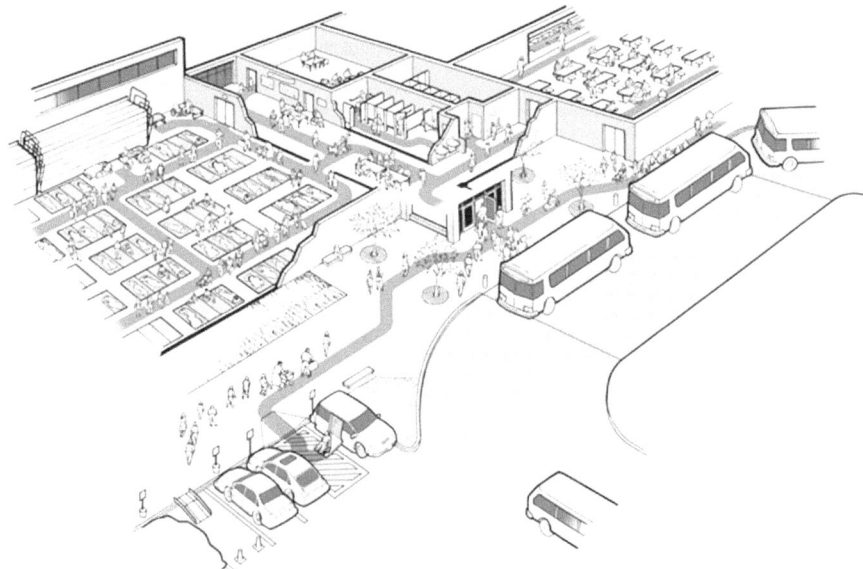

Fig. 10.1 Mass shelter diagram. Retrieved from https://www.ada.gov/pcatoolkit/chap7shelterchk.htm

for activities of daily living. Client services include, but are not limited to, socialization, spiritual, psychological, nutrition, resting, privacy, and personal hygiene needs. Shelter managers will designate spaces to meet these functional needs (Federal Emergency Management Agency 2017b).

A typical shelter layout has many separate sections to meet client needs. Although the setup of the various sections of the shelter depends on the location and building space, Fig. 10.1 depicts a commonly used setup.

This diagram shows a typical shelter setup. It includes an entry point where clients are registered, general sleeping area (cot rooms), and special sleeping room for families or special health care needs individuals as well as rooms to provide food, entertainment, and nursing care. Most shelters also have rooms for volunteers to discuss shelter management debriefing, as well as areas for child-focused activities, spiritual, and mental health care (not shown in this diagram).

10.1.3 Shelter Services

Upon entering shelters, clients are received by the registration staff. The information collected includes family name, total number of family members, predisaster address, phone numbers and email addresses, method of transportation to the shelter, primary language and name(s) of family member(s) who speak English, and information on individual members (e.g., name, age, gender, and arrival date) (Federal Emergency Management Agency and American Red Cross 2015). The clients are generally given a card or wristband for identification. After registration is complete, shelter workers will give tours of various areas of the shelter (Federal Emergency Management Agency and American Red Cross 2015). These areas include the following:

- Parking and drop-off
- Registration (near the facility's main entrance)
- Cot/dorm (sleeping area)
- Nursing and first aid
- Food services
- Diversional activity.

Specifications for sleeping (cot/dorm rooms) are designed to provide secure restful locations. It is recommended that 20 sq. ft. per person be made available for short-term, or "evacuation," sheltering, and up to 40 sq. ft. per person for "long-term" sheltering. "Long-term sheltering" is generally defined as any period longer than 72 h. Typical American Red Cross (ARC) or military surplus cots require about 21 sq. ft. (7 ft. × 3 ft.) of floor space, as shown in Fig. 10.1. By allowing space for maneuverability around the cot, expanding the assigned space to approximately 4 ft. × 10 ft., one can arrive at the recommended floor space of 40 sq. ft. per occupant. The relatively narrow, long space allotment allows for the storage of belongings at the foot of each cot. Figure 10.2 shows an operating shelter with roughly 4 ft. × 10 ft. space allotments per person (Federal Emergency Management Agency and American Red Cross 2015).

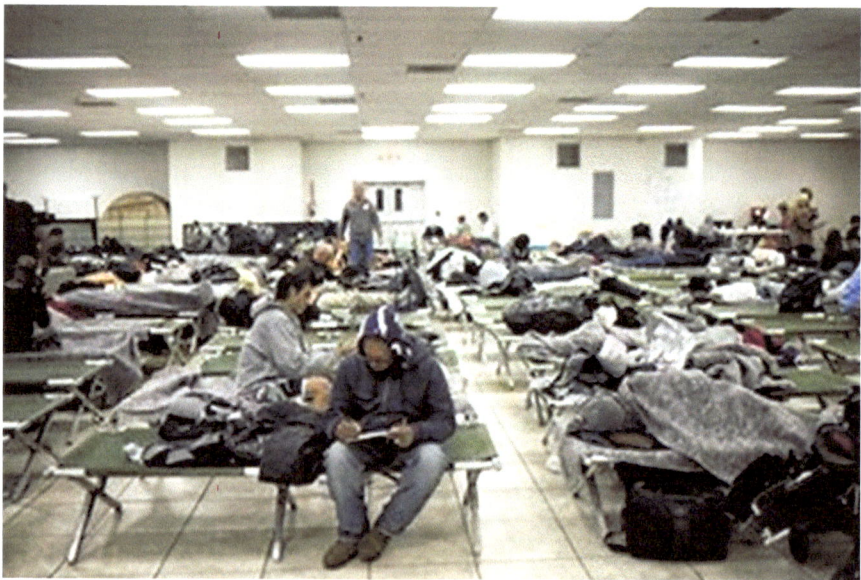

Fig. 10.2 Picture found in: Daily Breeze. April 16, 2018. LA mayor unveiling $20 million emergency shelter plan to tackle homelessness crisis. Retrieved from: https://www.dailybreeze.com/2018/04/16/la-mayor-to-unveil-20-million-emergency-shelter-plan-to-tackle-homelessness-crisis/

10.1.4 Staffing Shelters

According to Schonfeld and Demaria (Schonfeld et al. 2015), approximately 14% of U.S. children between the ages of 2–17 years have been exposed to disaster incidents. Children are vulnerable to traumatic events due to the lack of life experience and the development of coping mechanisms (Schonfeld et al. 2015). Please refer to Chap. 12 for more detailed information.

Appropriate staffing considerations can ensure that children's needs are met. Security and safety needs are generally met through police stationed at the shelter or by other designated volunteer members with specialized training. First aid and medical care are generally provided by registered nurses with training in shelter care. Nurses aid client care in accordance with their licensing regulations dictated by each state board of nursing (Nowak et al. 2015).

10.1.5 Special Needs of Families

When setting up shelters, families with children should be given special consideration. This may include the common needs of children based on their developmental level. Mental, social, physical, and spiritual needs are different based on the developmental stage. The 2013 Pandemic and All Hazards Preparedness Reauthorization Act defines special needs and high-risk individuals as children, older adults, pregnant women, and individuals needing assistance (Pandemic and All Hazard Preparedness Reauthorization Act 2018). At-risk individuals may also include, but are not limited to, those with disabilities, from diverse cultures, who have limited English proficiency or are non-English speaking, who are homeless, who have chronic medical disorders, and who have pharmacological dependency. At-risk individuals may have a number of additional needs that must be considered in planning for mass shelters. A check list for shelters for accommodations for those with disabilities can be found at https://www.ada.gov/pcatoolkit/chap7shelterchk.htm.

Children with physical or mental impairments often need special accommodations for activities of daily living (ADL). Age-appropriate considerations for ADL include diapers, seats that adapt, wheelchairs, cribs, baby formula, breast feeding location, and food. Temporary child care in a supervised area is often provided (Nowak and Adams 2014). A recommended approach for integrating the access and functional needs of these individuals is found in the guidelines published in the CMIST Framework (communications, medical, independence, supervision, and transportation) (United States Department of Health and Human Service 2018). The CMIST Framework is available at https://www.phe.gov/Preparedness/planning/abc/Pages/at-risk.aspx. More information can be found in Chap. 8.

10.1.6 Nursing and First Aid

Disaster response agencies deploy nurse and paraprofessional volunteers. Health services personnel include those with first aid, nursing, or medically related backgrounds. Nurse volunteers who engage in disaster incidents have many legal protections. Immunities allow protection for public health emergency care workers under certain circumstances. The National Fire Protection Agency and post-9/11 federal law has created new standards that apply to all emergency management personnel since the availability of federal funds for emergency management is contingent on having defined criteria for state and local emergency management performance (US Legal 2014).

The Good Samaritan Rule refers to someone who renders aid on a voluntary basis in an emergency to an injured person and applies to nurses who volunteer to serve (US Legal 2014). Shelter personnel must plan to have basic first aid assistance available at the shelter as health care issues often arise during sheltering. People who are displaced commonly complain of headaches, stomach aches, muscle aches, and stress-related issues. The role of nurses is outlined by scope and standards of nursing (Bickford et al. 2015). Nursing services provided while serving in shelters should be consistent with the Scope of Practice; clinical knowledge regarding disease pathophysiology and epidemiology in conjunction with basic assessment skills can serve a crucial role in emergency shelters. The Scope of Practice describes the actions a nurse is permitted to undertake in keeping with the terms of their professional license. Nurses practice in mass shelters to the extent allowable by licensing regulations in their state and to the extent of their training for disaster response. If a medical emergency occurs, nurses will call upon local paramedics or coordinate with other local medical operations units. Clients who have serious injuries, or anyone who is very sick, are transported to a local hospital. Please refer to Chap. 18 for more details on volunteering for disaster relief.

Agencies available for specialized training for disaster response nurses are included in Table 10.1.

Prescription drug management considers medication regimes that cannot be interrupted without consequences. If an individual arrives at a shelter without their prescription medications, every effort is made to retrieve the medication from their home or to replace them within the parameters of the shelter system policies. Shelter planning personnel should establish vendor agreements with local pharmacies and clarify how to obtain medications postdisaster (e.g., with a current prescription, with a prescription phoned in by a licensed physician, with a prescription validated by another pharmacy, or with a prescription bottle). Nurses also plan for the storage of medications to provide secure locations and in some instances, refrigeration if required. All the services provided by health personnel are documented on medical records.

The nurse should be aware of common reactions in children and how they may influence nursing assessments. Children in shelters often experience reoccurrence or new health-related symptoms. Table 10.2 outlines some common reactions. Please refer to Chaps. 7 and 12 for more detailed information.

Table 10.1 Training resources for nurses

Agency list
ARC introduction to disaster. http://www.redcross.org/flash/course01_v01/
Community emergency response teams. https://www.fema.gov/community-emergency-response-teams
FEMA independent study program: IS-22 are you ready? An in-depth guide to citizen preparedness. http://training.fema.gov/EMIWeb/IS/is22.asp
Introduction to the Incident Command System for Healthcare/Hospitals Command System (HICS). https://training.fema.gov/is/courseoverview.aspx?code=is-100.hcb
Introduction to mental health preparedness for disasters. http://sph.unc.edu/nciph/mental-health-prep/
Medical Reserve Corp. http://www.medicalreservecorps.gov/volunteerFldr/AboutVolunteering
Psychological first aid: field operations guide (MRC). http://www.medicalreservecorps.gov/File/MRC_Resources/ MRC_PFA.doc
Ready.Gov. http://www.ready.gov//business

Adapted from: *Nowak M., Ashton, K., Sayers, P. (2015).* Frontline nurses: ethical and legal considerations of disaster preparedness. The Journal of Legal Nurse Consulting, 26(3), p. 28

Table 10.2 Common reactions in children and adolescents

Sleep problems	• Difficulty falling or staying asleep • Difficulty waking up in the morning • Bedwetting or nightmares
Eating problems	• Loss of appetite • Increased appetite
School performance	• Missed days • Academic success falls • Concentration impaired • Difficulty retaining new information
Mood changes	• Sadness or depression • Anger • Fears • Worries
Substance abuse	• Onset of substance abuse • Exacerbation of substance use
Somatization	• Increased physical symptoms • Increased complaints of stomach aches, headaches, other physical symptoms, or pain

Source: Adapted from Schonfeld & Demaria, The Disaster Preparedness Advisory Council & Committee on Psychosocial Aspects of Child Family Health. (2015). Providing psychosocial support to children and families in the aftermath of disasters and crisis. *Pediatrics, 136*(4): e-1120–1130

10.2 Children with Special Health Care Needs

Research indicates that children with disabilities are especially vulnerable in disaster situations. It is recommended that a written national disaster preparedness standard be mandated for all facilities caring for children (Soulliere 2017). In addition to special needs of physically handicapped children, language barriers may also provide a barrier to care.

Children with special needs may need special accommodations for sleeping, nutrition, toileting, and communications. Families should be in a separate location from the general shelter "cot room" and grouped together for safety and security needs during sleeping. Some shelters have side rooms to place children in a quiet location. When a child is using a using a motorized wheelchair, he or she should be placed to accommodate power needs within the shelter. While many motorized wheelchairs can go several days between charges, sudden disasters may bring people whose chairs may need immediate charging, and as days wear on, nearly all people relying on wheelchairs will need to charge them (Nowak et al. 2015).

When working with families of diverse backgrounds, nurses may experience communication challenges. Children are sometimes asked to interpret for their parents and relatives who may not speak English. This responsibility may require the child to function beyond their developmental stage. The stress of the incident and demands on the activities of daily living often cause children to reach out to the nurse with stress-related symptoms. The nurse can relieve the child of this responsibility by seeking out adult interpreters for the family (Federal Emergency Management Agency 2017b). In addition, cellular telephone applications such as Google Translate may be useful in communicating with clients of different languages; however, they are not as accurate as medically approved interpreters. Google Translate has only 57.7% accuracy when used for medical translations and should not be trusted for important medical communications (Davies 2014). However, it remains the most easily available, free mode of communication between a provider and patient when language is a barrier. Although caution is needed when providing lifesaving communications, it can be useful to use Google Translate when professional translation services are not available (Davies 2014). More about children with special health care needs can be found in Chap. 8.

10.2.1 Agency Support

In times of disaster, disaster response programs by various governmental and nongovernmental agencies (NGOs) can supplement the response of local jurisdictions for various health-related needs. Nurses may contact these agencies directly for assistance in meeting the needs of families—see Table 10.3.

10.3   Unaccompanied Minors

Minors entering shelters must be accompanied by adults. In cases where minors are found at shelters without adult accompaniment, child protective authorities should be notified. Issuing identification (e.g., wristbands, cards, and quick response [QR] codes) to shelter residents and staff assists in the identification and accounting of those individuals present in shelter areas. If a disaster occurs in the middle of a workweek, when children are either at school or in child care, or if a disaster causes

Table 10.3 Disaster response programs

Agency	Services
The County Health Care Services Agency	A variety of services such as: • Making public health nursing services available • Addressing food and water safety • Addressing sanitation issues in shelters • Medical care • Behavioral care • Public health and environmental health • Sanitation • Communicable disease control • Disaster-related illness • Monitoring, assessing, and reporting the community disaster health status
Emergency Medical Services (EMS)	Services include: • Emergency medical dispatch • Emergency ambulance services • Nonemergency ambulance services
Behavioral Health Care	• Assesses stress issues • Provides activities to support • Makes counselors available to shelters • Provides referral to mental health services • Ensures the continuation of care • Assists with treatment and housing (for those clients in the mental health system)
Social Services Agencies	• Area Agency on Aging (seniors and people with disabilities). • Adult Protective Services (services to adults with developmental disabilities, including mentally disabled adults and elderly persons) • Child Abuse and Children's Protective Services (services for children who are victims of neglect or care) • In-Home Supportive Services (home care services to low-income elderly, blind, and disabled)
Salvation Army	• Mass care feeding • Mobile kitchen units • Sheltering • Clothing distribution • Counseling • Assistance in home cleanup (for seniors and people with disability (Headquarters, 916-563-3700, or available at www.salvationarmydeloro.org)
FEMA	Postincident recovery services Academic community resources available at https://www.dhs.gov/topic/academic-engagement

children to become separated from their lost, injured, or deceased caregivers, shelters are required to provide a safe place and a system for reunification. An example of tracking logs and tracking forms are available at the National Center for Missing & Exploited Children (www.missingkids.org/home). The National Center for Missing & Exploited Children is the agency responsible for locating missing individuals in a disaster.

To identify next of kin, school directory information, such as basic contact information, may be disclosed to emergency management officials to assist in locating legal guardians (United States Department of Education 2010). The disclosure is strictly limited to the time of the emergency and must be documented in the educational records to whom, what threat, and when the information was disclosed. The Family Educational Rights and Privacy Act (FERPA) is a Federal law that protects the privacy of student education records. In emergency situations, school administrators may disclose nondirectory information to those disaster officials charged with protecting the safety of children (United States Department of Education 2010). In a disaster, HIPAA is waived for the purposes of family reunification.

The American Red Cross (ARC) provides tracing and messaging services to assist families to reunite. TRACES can be initiated when the location of a loved one is unknown. The TRACE program seeks to reunite families who may be separated by a disaster. It is an online repository of information relating to victims. The ARC caseworker will gather the available information, and then the ARC will work with its international Red Cross and Red Crescent partners to try to locate the sought person. The American Red Cross also provides Red Cross Messaging services. Red Cross messages can be used to facilitate communication internationally in instances where the sought person's location is known, but regular means of communication are unavailable. A Red Cross "Safe and Well Service" will provide tracking of shelter residents during a crisis to see if a family member has registered to access these services through the Red Cross (American Red Cross 2018). For more information, please refer to Chap. 11 on reunification.

In 2010, a Working Group was created to comprehensively integrate the activities related to the needs of children across all Health and Human Services (HHS) inter- and intragovernmental disaster planning operations (Department of Health and Human Services 2011). Co-led by the Administration for Children and Families (ACF) and the Assistant Secretary for Preparedness and Response (ASPR), the Group then developed recommendations for how HHS can deliver care to children impacted by disasters. The working group divided itself into four subcommittees: (1) Mental and Behavioral Health, (2) Medical Countermeasures, (3) Child Physical Health, Emergency Medical Services, and Pediatric Transport, and (4) Child Care and Child Welfare. A summation of their findings can be found at https://www.phe.gov/Preparedness/planning/abc/Documents/2011-children-disasters.pdf (Department of Health and Human Services 2011).

10.3.1 Day Care Centers in Shelters

Day care or child-focused activities are often offered at shelters. Volunteers who work with children are preapproved for service in these roles. The Office of Children and Family Services provides support for people and organizations interested in providing child day care programs in their communities. FEMA (2017a) includes several recommendations for protecting children in child care and early education settings that can be applied to shelter management. Recommendations include state child care regulatory agencies to provide training and exercising requirements enabling the safety of children.

The U.S. Department of Justice's statistics show that sexual assault is the most commonly reported violent crime against children. Children are the victims in 70% of all reported sexual assaults. Several state-regulated facilities and programs are designed to safeguard the public's health and welfare and to protect the state's most vulnerable populations, such as children in child care, foster care, and schools. Criminal background checks are required for licensed, certified, and authorized child care providers, foster care providers, and school employees. State laws and agency administrative rules prohibit people who have committed certain crimes from living or working in schools and homes where children are in care (Sonntag 2012).

10.3.2 Security Measures

Providing for the safety and well-being of children in shelters is an important aspect of shelter operations. A shelter security plan should consider 24-h coverage. The following factors are considered when planning for security: age of residents, number of residents, number of individuals with disabilities, number of children, and the physical layout (e.g., lighting, number of rooms, and access). Security needs are coordinated with law enforcement and, at times, a security services agency. If individuals with a documented history of child abuse are noted, those individuals should be placed in a shelter sleeping location separate from or distanced from child sleeping dorms. In addition, the shelter staff will be notified to monitor the activity of these individuals while in the shelter (Federal Emergency Management Agency and American Red Cross 2015).

To avoid conflicts in a stressful situation, it is important to cooperate with shelter managers and others assisting them. Keep in mind that alcoholic beverages and weapons are forbidden in emergency shelters and smoking is restricted (Shelter Ready 2018). It is important for the shelter management team to be realistic about the security risks and to constantly monitor for signs of developing situations. It is vital to seek local law enforcement's advice and technical support.

Special security measures that may need to be instituted at a shelter include issuing shelter identification (wristbands, cards, etc.), identification checks at all doors, limiting the number of public entrances and exits, monitoring the doors to the dormitory and children's recreation area, searching packages at doors, monitoring bathrooms, establishing "off limits" areas, and instituting roving external patrols of the immediate area around the shelter (Shelter Ready 2018). Safety of children and families at shelters is paramount.

10.3.3 Activities to Aid with Normalcy

Children sense parental anxiety and stress. For most children, life in shelters is a new and sometimes scary experience filled with uncertainty. During shelter stay, nurses can offer alternative activities as part of the overall treatment plan for children. As a nurse serving in shelters, offering links to community-based, developmentally appropriate activities can help restore their sense of safety and address the child's developmental needs (Kostelny and Wessells 2005). Some activities may include dance, exercise, viewing pleasant videos or movies, playing games, playing cards, arts and crafts, playing drums (guided by a music teacher), singing, and practicing deep breathing for relaxation response.

The Agency for the National Commission on Children and Disasters recommends the integration of mental and behavioral health activities for children into disaster management activities (Institute of Medicine 2014). To this end, disaster response agencies offer pediatric disaster mental health training. Even nurses who are not able to be on location may assist children. In these instances, nurses may engage in remote nursing services (e.g., case management or counseling services). For example, during Hurricane Irma, a team of nursing students developed a nursing intervention dubbed "Nurse Line for Kids" whereby they offered emotional support via prearranged phone contacts with children in shelters. These students, under the direction of a Red Cross nurse, developed a relay phone system whereby they offered information to children via scheduled phone sessions. This intervention addressed the children's anxiety, reinforced available shelter activities, gave verbal support, and enabled children to practice deep breathing and relaxation exercises from a remote location (Cassidy 2018).

10.4 Conclusion

During a disaster, children and families may be displaced from their homes. They may need to take refuge at a mass shelter. It is imperative that shelters provide a safe and secure area for not only children and families but also for unaccompanied minors. Systems must be in place in order to create a safe haven for those affected by a disaster.

References

American Disabilities Act. Home page. 2018. Available from https://www.ada.gov/2010_regs.htm
American Red Cross. Reconnecting families. Home page. 2018. Available from https://www.red-cross.org/faq.html#Reconnecting-Families
Bickford C, Marion L, Gazaway S. ANA nursing: scope and standards of practice. 2015. Available from https://www.augusta.edu/nursing/cnr/documents/seminar-files/pp8.28.pdf
Cassidy K. Rowan University professor and NACN-USA member serves in disaster relief efforts. NACN-USA Newslett. 2018, Spring. Available from https://nacn-usa.org
Davies P. Use of Google Translate in medical communication: evaluation of accuracy. Br Med J. 2014;349:g7392. https://doi.org/10.1136/bmj.g7392.
Department of Health and Human Services. Update on children and disasters: summary of recommendations and implementation efforts. 2011. Available from https://www.phe.gov/Preparedness/planning/abc/Documents/2011-children-disasters.pdf
Federal Emergency Management Agency. Incident management handbook. 2017a. Available from https://www.fema.gov/media-library-data/1511798700826-e38977943819bb12064e3144c-ca7c576/FnlRvwIMH20171026v1945(508).pdf
Federal Emergency Management Agency. Care of children in disasters. 2017b. Available from https://www.fema.gov/children-and-disasters

Federal Emergency Management Agency. News release home page. 2018a. Available from https://www.ready.gov/kids.

Federal Emergency Management Agency, American Red Cross. Shelter field guide FEMA P-785. 2015. Available from http://www.nationalmasscarestrategy.org/wp-content/uploads/2015/10/Shelter-Field-Guide-508_f3.pdf (FEMA 785).

Institute of Medicine. Preparedness, response, and recovery considerations for children and families: workshop summary. Washington, DC: The National Academies Press; 2014. https://doi.org/10.17226/18550.

Kostelny K, Wessells M. Psychosocial aid to children after the Dec 26 tsunami. Lancet. 2005;366:2066–7.

Nowak M, Adams K. Atlantic County Department of Health: mass shelter handbook for disaster nurses (Internal MRC publication). Newfield, NJ: Atlantic County Department of Health; 2014.

Nowak M, Ashton K, Sayers P. Frontline nurses: ethical and legal considerations of disaster preparedness. J Legal Nurse Consult. 2015;26(3):28.

Pandemic and All Hazard Preparedness Reauthorization Act. Home page. 2018. Available from https://www.fda.gov/EmergencyPreparedness/Counterterrorism/MedicalCountermeasures/MCM.

Schonfeld DJ, Demaria T, Disaster Preparedness Advisory Council & Committee on Psychosocial Aspects of Child and Family Health. Providing psychosocial support to children and families in the aftermath of disasters and crisis. Pediatrics. 2015;136(94):e-1120–e1130.

Shelter Ready. Mass care shelters. 2018. Available from https://www.ready.gov/shelter

Sonntag B. Protecting children from sex off enders in child care. Foster care, and schools report no. 1008110. 2012. Available from https://www.sao.wa.gov/state/Documents/PA_Protect_Children_from_Sex_Offenders_ar1008110.pdf

Soulliere J. Save the children prioritizes recovery of child care centers, schools in Texas in wake of hurricane Harvey. Save the Children Federation. 2017. Available from http://www.savethechildren.org/site/apps/nlnet/content2.aspx?c=8rKLIXGIpI4E&b=9506653&ct=15004131

United States Department of Education. Family Educational Rights and Privacy Act (FERPA) and the disclosure of student information related to emergencies and disasters. Washington, DC: Department of Education. 2010. Available from http://www2.ed.gov/policy/gen/guid/fpco/pdf/ferpa-disaster-guidance.pdf

United States Department of Health and Human Service. Public health emergency: at risk individuals. 2018. Available from https://www.phe.gov/Preparedness/planning/abc/Pages/at-risk.aspx

US Legal. Home page. Good Samaritan rules and legal definitions. 2014. Available from http://definitions.uslegal.com/g/good-samaritan-rule/

Family Reunification

11

Kathleen Stevenson

11.1 Considerations and Planning

Each weekday over 67 million children are in locations away from their primary caregivers either attending school or in child care (Blake and Stevenson 2009). In urban areas, the time or distance that children are separated from primary caregivers continues to grow and can compound the issue. Young children, unable to identify themselves, present unique challenges if they are removed from adults who can identify them or if the adults with them are injured and cannot identify them. Methods used by adults, including social media, telephone calls, and so on, do not translate to children lacking access, and children will rely on the adults and caregivers they are with to assist in reunification with their caregivers.

Large natural disasters as well as smaller events such as bus or train accidents can cause separation of children from their caregivers. During Hurricanes Katrina and Rita in 2005, more than 5000 children were separated from their families, including some who were evacuated to different states. All children were eventually reunited with their families, but this effort took as long as 6 months in some cases (Broughton et al. 2006). Many organizations have worked over the years to review and develop suggested best practices to assist in keeping children with their caregivers if possible or to provide for rapid reunification of families. The complexity of these disasters poses problems with even the most sophisticated plan given the unknowns of what may occur during the event. Potential austere conditions may exist after a disaster and may present a problem for even the best plans. During large-scale events, every effort should be made to try to keep families together in the first place. Unfortunately, during events that occur when children are away from their caregivers, this poses a near-impossible feat. During catastrophic events, the often urgent nature of evacuations may compound the issue resulting in separation of child and caregiver.

K. Stevenson (✉)
Yellowbrick Consulting, Inc., Glendora, CA, USA

© Springer Nature Switzerland AG 2020
C. J. Goodhue, N. Blake (eds.), *Nursing Management of Pediatric Disaster*,
https://doi.org/10.1007/978-3-030-43428-1_11

Best Practices to Limit Child/Caregiver Separation in a Disaster:

- Keep children and parent/legal guardian together and separate as a last resort.
- Evacuations should be to a location as close as possible to the child's original location.
- During evacuations, children should be provided with a method to rapidly identify who the parent or legal guardian is. Consider matching armbands or other means of identification.
- Educate children to be able to provide information about self and family name, age, address, parent name, and so on.
- Communicate plans for tracking children and means for families to access the information.
- When separation is necessary, immediate registration and tracking should occur.
- All agencies tracing children should use the same tracking system.

Local jurisdictions must work in conjunction with regional, state, tribal, and federal partners to ensure this vulnerable population is well planned for and taken care of. It is assumed that the first agencies to deal with the issue are the local agencies and organizations, and they must be ready to make appropriate decisions to ensure the actions they take do not compound the issues of the separation of families. The cooperative effort of these agencies will be key to a successful outcome for reunification.

Key components of this plan should include:

- Identification of lead agency for coordination of the reunification process;
- Identification of location for pediatric safe care centers for children awaiting reunification;
- Reunification procedures and processes for children who become separated from their parents or legal guardians due to the disaster;
- Plans for collection of standard information that can be readily shared among multiple agencies working to reunite families;
- Media plan for communication of information to families as to the resources available and process to locate family members;
- Coordination with law enforcement;
- Coordination with agencies that can provide supplies and equipment for children;
- Implementation of a state mass evacuation and tracking plan that includes a form of tracking;
- Promotion of family reunification planning as part of individual and family preparedness;
- Coordination with schools and child care agencies to include reunification and sheltering with particular attention to children with special health care needs;
- Coordination with hospitals and local public health departments for the care of injured children;
- Plan for testing of current capabilities using drills; and
- Scalability to function at the local level as well as fold into the state and federal response, if applicable.

Evacuation centers must take into account the needs of children both with their families as well as those who have been displaced and are unaccompanied. Often, evacuation centers are not appropriately prepared or have limited resources to care for children. If the location is not prepared for children, there may be a need to separate children from their families that would compound the issue. Staffing considerations should be included in planning for centers to assist with information gathering required to assist in reunification and to provide a safe environment for children. These centers may be staffed by local agencies or NGOs; these staff members should be trained in dealing with children and be prepared to supervise children. Increased focus on preparedness for children has improved the situation; however, ongoing evaluation of plans and increasing training and preparedness should continue at the local, regional, state, and federal level.

Registration or intake information gathering about evacuees should begin as soon in the evacuation continuum as possible. As children present to reunification centers, the registration and intake process should be established to gather as much information as possible to assist in the identification of the child. Minimum data would include pickup location (i.e., cross street, latitude and longitude, facility/school), gender, and name (Children's Hospital Los Angeles 2019). Additional information should include: child's name, parent name, age, description, clothing, location the child came from, any belongings they may have with them, and any information they can provide. Photographs should be taken as quickly as possible, particularly if the child is injured and before bruising or discoloration occurs. Information gathered should be promptly entered into a searchable database such as the Unaccompanied Minors Registry (UMC); the UMC is administered by the National Center for Missing and Exploited Children (NCMEC) and supported by FEMA. Access should be available to all stakeholders to expedite identification and should be as close to real-time information as possible.

Evacuation or holding centers will need to provide strict security access restrictions to ensure the safety of children. Predetermined release policies must be defined and should be carefully followed to ensure children are released to the appropriate caregiver. Release policies should include who can be released and how to assure proper identification for the safety of children, especially for infants and toddlers unable to speak for themselves. Legal considerations should be included in the planning of release policies. Children who can identify both themselves and verbally identify a caregiver can be released to the caregiver; however, if this is not possible, use of other data or technologies may need to be employed. DNA sampling may be a method that can be used definitively but may not be available in austere or remote locations. Question/answer matching with independent questioning may be used or the reunification may need to be turned over to child protective services for ultimate resolution. Once reunification has occurred, a method to allow for easy identification of the child/caregiver pair is suggested. Matching ID bands, photos, name tags, and so on can be of use in centers that have families needing to remain at the location for extended periods of time.

Table 11.1 Suggested Supplies for Pediatric Safe Areas (American Academy of Pediatrics 2019)

Age-appropriate activities	Board games, cards, books, movies, video games, art supplies
Diapers	Available in multiple sizes
Formula	Various brands, including instructions for use and supplies to provide to the infant such as bottles
Age-appropriate food	Baby food, utensils for feeding, and consider allergies
Hand sanitizer	
Clothing	In multiple sizes

Supplies and space that are pediatric safe areas should be planned for; Table 11.1 lists considerations to provide a smooth functioning area for children and their families. In addition to these supplies, sources for age-appropriate sleeping arrangements are important, including cribs or low mats to prevent falls. The area should prevent children from wandering or leaving the secure area by use of separate room or area gated off from any open areas. See Chap. 10 for more information on disaster shelters.

Psychosocial support is a key consideration during the timeframe that families are separated; children should be attentively attended to and as much as possible remain with the same person the entire time they are separated from their families. Children will need someone assigned to helping them navigate the system and who continues to gather information that may assist in reunification. Including mental health professionals in planning and implementation is key to providing appropriate care during this time. Refer to Chap. 12 for more detailed information on postdisaster effects.

11.2   Additional Elements of the Plan

Disaster planners should assess local areas where large numbers of children congregate regularly to determine the potential for reunification needs in the region. These areas include schools and child care centers, as well as museums, churches, amusement parks, and so on. Planners must assess the level of reunification planning that may already exist.

Leadership and an organizational chart for reporting and responsibilities should be established to ensure all essential roles are covered (see Fig. 11.1). The plan should be scalable and able to quickly be enacted to begin the reunification process rapidly. These plans should include the interactions and responsibilities of the various local, regional, state, and federal agencies. Children may arrive at hospitals with injuries; it should not be assumed that hospitals will be equipped to deal with a large influx of children, nor should they be the point that will reunify children with caregivers. Activation of the plan should be coordinated through the agency responsible for local response and escalated to scale. Additional information can be found in Chap. 4.

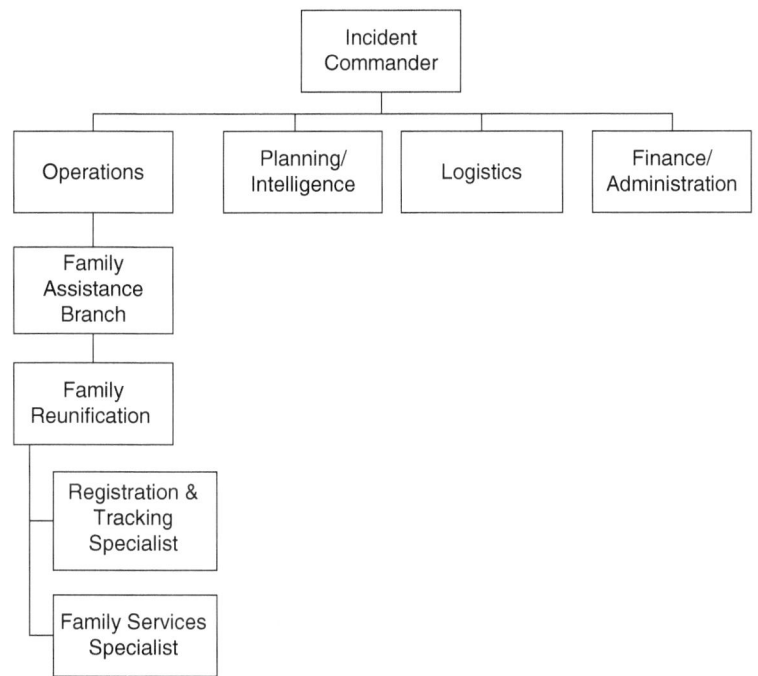

Fig. 11.1 Sample organizational chart

Tracking should continue at every point that the child accesses from pickup at the location of rescue to health care, and if applicable, to a holding location. Unaccompanied children will need to be supervised and cared for until an appropriate caregiver is located, and arrangements made to reunite them. Staff in these areas will need security or prior clearance and appropriate badging, training, and so on. This training should include how to trace children's locations, key information the child or family may provide that can be of assistance in reunification, and a standard method to proceed with the reunification process.

Use of technology will be important in the process of reunification. In many cases, adults are able to track down other members of their families through the use of social media applications with the number and value of these improving continually. With young children, these methods will not be useful due to the lack of information that is available about the child or their ability to provide information about their caregivers. Access to databases and information by all authorities who are working to reunite children is crucial but requires a safe and secure system to prevent the release of information to inappropriate entities (Table 11.2). Automated parental notification systems can assist schools in providing information to families about procedures to pick up children as well as locations that children have been moved to, if needed. The tracking system must have the capacity to be updated by those with authority to do so.

Table 11.2 List of resources in the U.S. that assist with reunification

National Center for Missing and Exploited Children (NCMEC)
Web site: http://www.missingkids.com/home
Phone: 800–843-5678
The Unaccompanied Minors Registry (UMC) is administered by the NCMEC and supported by FEMA
American Red Cross
https://www.redcross.org/get-help/disaster-relief-and-recovery-services/contact-and-locate-loved-ones.html
Restoring Family Links national helpline at 1–844–782-9441
American Red Cross maintains the Safe and Well program to assist in family reunification.
Website: https://www.redcross.org/get-help
Next of Kin Registry
Registry of contact information—registration can be done proactively. Services used to assist during disasters also.
http://nokr.org/
National Emergency Family Registry and Locator System (NEFRLS)
Established in the aftermath of Hurricanes Katrina and Rita, NEFRLS is a nationally accessible, web-based system that facilitates the reunification of families separated or displaced by a disaster.
1–800–588-9822 or at www.disasterassistance.gov.
Lost Person Finder (LPF)
The LPF Project focuses on tools and technologies to enable family, friends, and neighbors to locate missing people during a disaster event. The National Library of Medicine (NLM) initially created this web-based people finder software for finding people who were in hospitals after a disaster. After the Haiti earthquake, it was modified to allow public access for community-wide disasters.
https://lpf.nlm.nih.gov/.
Google Crisis Response
Person Finder and Crisis Map are Google's primary tools that support reunification. Google Person Finder allows individuals to post and search for the status of relatives or friends affected by a disaster.
https://www.google.org/crisisresponse/resources.html.
Facebook Safety Check
Facebook launched its Safety Check feature in 2014 that helps users alert friends and family that they are safe during major disasters.
https://www.facebook.com/about/safetycheck/

A strong media and communication plan is important to aid in reunification. The plan needs to include preparation for large numbers of people looking for loved ones and a method to gather information from them to determine where the person they are looking for is either at the location or which location. Clear and concise messaging to those looking for loved ones will decrease the frustration if reunification is not immediate and can assist those coordinating efforts from having to interact with families multiple times or in the wrong location.

Messaging should include:

- Information about available reunification registries that can be used by survivors and those looking for information about families, friends, and colleagues;
- Reminders to the survivors to contact family and friends via text messaging, telephone, and/or social media sites with status information;
- Appropriate telephone numbers to call, such as a reunification call center number, especially when dispatch centers are overwhelmed with calls from those seeking information about family and friends;
- Locations such as family assistance centers, shelters, and service delivery sites, where reunification services may be provided; and
- Information for institutions and service providers about utilizing common forms of communication and reunification registries to let family members know the status and location of clients/students after a disaster and in cases of evacuation.

11.2.1 Testing of the Plan

Tabletop exercises, once a plan has been established, should be regularly tested with stakeholders to evaluate the plan and adjust as issues are identified. As new technologies or support is available, the plan should be nimble to incorporate the best solutions possible. Once the plans have been vetted, focused or full-scale drills should be incorporated into disaster/emergency preparedness events. Use of actual children to test the intake process, staffing, and accommodation will be useful to identify any additional adjustments or holes in the plan. Los Angeles County current published a pediatric disaster surge plan—https://www.calhospitalprepare.org/sites/main/files/fileattachments/hpp_lac_ems_agency_pediatric_surge_plan_ecopy.pdf.

11.3 Conclusion

Reunification of families following a disaster or major event can be one of the most challenging obstacles for those involved. Ongoing planning and preparation are key to successful reunification of children and their families. Local, regional, state, and federal agencies should be included in planning with local stakeholders and community leaders to build on relationships and strengths already established. Remaining aware of the ongoing efforts to strengthen the ability to reunify families quickly is an important aspect of the plan.

References

American Academy of Pediatrics. Family reunification following disasters: planning tool for health care facilities—American Academy of Pediatrics. 2019. https://www.aap.org/en-us/Documents/AAP-Reunification-Toolkit.pdf. Accessed 30 Mar 2019.

Blake N, Stevenson K. Reunification: keeping families together in crisis. J Trauma. 2009;67(2 Suppl):S147–51.

Broughton DD, Allen EE, Hannemann RD, et al. Reuniting fractured families after a disaster: the role of the national center for missing & exploited children. Pediatrics. 2006;117:S442–5.

Children's Hospital Los Angeles. The issues at hand—Children's Hospital Los Angeles. 2019. https://www.chla.org/sites/default/files/migrated/DisasterReunification.pdf. Accessed 30 Mar 2019.

Supporting Children and Families in the Aftermath of Disasters

12

David J. Schonfeld and Thomas Demaria

12.1 Understanding the Impact of Disaster on Children

Millions of children throughout the world are affected by disasters each year (Penrose and Takaki 2006). Disasters have the potential to cause short- and long-term effects on the psychological functioning, emotional adjustment, health, and developmental trajectory of children (Schonfeld et al. 2015), especially if exposure is prolonged or complicated by other factors (Osofsky et al. 2009). This may have implications for health and psychological functioning in adulthood as well (Institute of Medicine 2003). Children are especially vulnerable to disasters because of their limited coping skills and dependence on social supports that place them at a greater risk for a range of adjustment difficulties, including transitory distress symptoms, bereavement, and symptoms of post-traumatic stress disorder (PTSD) as well of anxiety and depression (Grolnick et al. 2018).

12.1.1 Early Interventions for Adjustment Reactions in Children

Anticipatory guidance and advice can be provided to families by nurses and HCPs in a variety of practice settings on how to identify and address the most common adjustment reactions that can be anticipated among children after a disaster (see Table 12.1). For example, sleep problems are common after a disaster, and

D. J. Schonfeld (✉)
National Center for School Crisis and Bereavement, Children's Hospital Los Angeles,
Los Angeles, CA, USA

Keck School of Medicine of the University of Southern California, Los Angeles, CA, USA
e-mail: schonfel@usc.edu

T. Demaria
National Center for School Crisis and Bereavement, Children's Hospital Los Angeles,
Los Angeles, CA, USA

© Springer Nature Switzerland AG 2020
C. J. Goodhue, N. Blake (eds.), *Nursing Management of Pediatric Disaster*,
https://doi.org/10.1007/978-3-030-43428-1_12

Table 12.1 Common symptoms of adjustment reactions in children after a disaster

- Sleep problems: difficulty falling or staying asleep, interrupted sleep at night or difficulty awakening in the morning, nightmares, or other sleep disruptions.
- Eating problems: loss of appetite or increased eating.
- Sadness or depression: this may result in less participation in previously enjoyed activities or a withdrawal from peers and adults.
- Anxiety, worries, or fears: children may be concerned that the traumatic event may occur again (e.g., children may become afraid during storms after surviving a tornado) or show an increase in unrelated fears (e.g., they become more fearful of the dark even if the disaster occurred during daylight), avoidance, and social withdrawal.
- Difficulties in concentration and attention: this will hamper the child's ability to learn and retain new information or to otherwise progress academically.
- Substance abuse: the new onset or worsening of alcohol, tobacco, or other substance use may be seen in children, adolescents, and adults after a disaster.
- Risk-taking behavior: increased sexual activities or other reactive risk-taking behaviors can occur, especially among older children and adolescents.
- Somatization: children with emotional adjustment difficulties may instead complain of physical symptoms suggesting a physical condition.
- Developmental or social regression: for example, young children may develop secondary enuresis; children may become less patient or tolerant of change, or become irritable and disruptive.
- Post-traumatic reactions and disorders.

Adapted by permission from Springer Nature: Springer-Verlag Textbook of Clinical Pediatrics second ed. by Schonfeld DJ, Gurwitch R.H. Children in disasters. In: Elzouki AY, Stapleton FB, Whitley RJ, Oh W, Harfi HA, Nazer H, eds.; 2012

children who have difficulty sleeping may develop problems with concentration, attention, learning, and academic functioning. Promoting sleep hygiene (e.g., providing a consistent, quiet, and comfortable location and time for sleep that is free of noise or other distractions, preceded by a calming and consistent bedtime ritual) may be challenging in the immediate aftermath of a disaster, especially when families are living in shelters or other temporary sites, but is nonetheless important.

12.1.2 Post-traumatic Stress, Acute Stress Disorder (ASD), and Post-traumatic Stress Disorder (PTSD)

Post-traumatic stress reactions are frequently observed immediately after a disaster and can be best explained to children as the way their body automatically responds after an event frightens them. Most children who are exposed to a traumatic event will experience transitory Post-traumatic Stress (PTS) or an Acute Stress Disorder (ASD). The development of delayed PTSD symptoms after the traumatic event occurred is less common, especially among children.

The diagnostic criteria for PTSD (American Psychiatric Association 2013) specify that a child must be exposed to actual or threatened death, serious injury, or sexual violence, (or learn it occurred to a close family member or friend), and show evidence of persistent reactions for a least 1 month, in all of the following four areas, including:

- intrusive and unwanted memories, dreams, feelings, and detached (dissociative) play activity associated with the traumatic event often activated when the child is reminded of the event;
- avoidance of memories, thoughts, feelings, and external reminders (people, places, conversations, activities, situations) associated with the traumatic event;
- negative thoughts and feelings after the traumatic event, including loss of interest in pleasurable solitary or social activities and blaming of self and/or others;
- change in arousal and reactivity associated with the traumatic event resulting in sleep difficulties, irritability, concentration problems, and hypervigilance.

In the immediate aftermath of a disaster, nurses and HCPs will be involved in the assessment of both the physical and mental health of children. The immediate focus is often medical stabilization and evaluation, but a secondary mental health triage should follow shortly thereafter. Table 12.2 outlines the factors to be assessed during this mental health triage to identify children most in need of mental health services or other immediate attention to their mental health needs.

The following factors, in particular, suggest the need for immediate mental health services:

Table 12.2 Factors associated with an increased risk of adjustment problems after a disaster

1. Preexisting factors
• Previous mental illness and/or substance abuse, significant losses, attachment disturbances, limited coping skills, or exposure to other traumatic events
• Socioeconomic differences that result in lower levels of postdisaster resources and support
2. Nature of disaster experience
• Injury of the child or death or injury of those close to the child
• Nature and extent of actual traumatic exposure, including a greater number of deaths, closer physical proximity to the disaster, and a greater extent of personal loss. Human-made disasters, especially acts of violence that have a high degree of planning and intentionality, generally create reactions that are more prevalent and long lasting.
• Exposure to horrific scenes (including indirect viewing through social media or television)
• Child's perception (at the time of the event) that his or her life was in jeopardy
3. Subsequent factors
• Personal identification in some way with the disaster or victims
• Separation of children from parents or other important caregivers as a result of the event
• Loss of property or belongings; need to relocate or other disruption in daily routine or living environment
• Parental difficulty in coping or impairment because of substance abuse and/or mental illness
• Lack of supportive family communication and support
• Lack of community resources and support.

Adapted by permission from Springer Nature: Springer-Verlag Textbook of Clinical Pediatrics second ed. by Schonfeld DJ, Gurwitch R.H. Children in disasters. In: Elzouki AY, Stapleton FB, Whitley RJ, Oh W, Harfi HA, Nazer H, eds.; 2012

- *dissociative symptoms*, such as detachment, derealization, or depersonalization, which may present in children as appearing confused, daydreaming, or distant; dissociation at the time of exposure has been found to be the most significant predictor of later PTSD,
- *extreme confusion* or inability to concentrate or make even simple decisions,
- evidence of extreme *cognitive impairment* or intrusive thoughts,
- *intense fear, anxiety, panic, helplessness, or horror*,
- *depression* at the time of the event (Lai et al. 2013),
- uncontrollable and *intense grief*,
- *suicidal ideation or intent*,
- *marked physical complaints* resulting from somatization (Schonfeld 2008).

12.1.3 Importance of Social Support

Social support is the main protective factor for children (Lai et al. 2017). When children's caregivers are struggling themselves to cope with the event, helping the caregivers access services for themselves and/or providing a referral to a mental health provider to assist them with children's coping also may be indicated. Parents who are having difficulty coping themselves or who lack the skills to facilitate communication or to provide support to their children are more likely to have children who would benefit from additional mental health or supportive services in the aftermath of disaster or crisis.

12.2 Providing Medical Services to Children Following a Disaster

12.2.1 Creating a Safe Environment With the Medical Home

Sites that provide medical care to children in the aftermath of a disaster should aim to minimize the likelihood of contributing additional stress to children. While this clearly applies to health care sites directly associated with immediate treatment and sheltering of those who are most directly impacted (see Chap. 10 for information on setting up disaster shelters), this also applies to any site that may deliver medical care both in the immediate aftermath of the disaster and during the recovery period. Attempts should be made to minimize the use of invasive or painful procedures or treatments and to provide appropriate sedation or analgesia whenever required. Parents and family members should remain with children to the extent possible throughout the evaluation and treatment process, provided that they are able to cope with their own discomfort or distress. Parents can be guided to support their children, such as advising them to use coping strategies they have found effective in the past (e.g., distraction or attention-refocusing techniques, like a calming touch or use of gentle humor). Parents should be allowed to leave the examination room temporarily if they are feeling overwhelmed, but should notify children before leaving that they will be in an adjacent area and that the nurse or HCP will remain with them for a few minutes until they return.

Practical steps can be taken to minimize children's exposure to frightening images and sounds that may compound their distress or serve as triggers or reminders of a disaster. For example, doors/curtains in the health care setting can be closed to reduce exposure to others who are injured or in pain. Televisions in waiting, examination, and inpatient rooms can be turned off if they are broadcasting coverage of the crisis event. In addition, staff members should be reminded that children can often overhear and understand their conversations.

Nurses and HCPs can provide explanations about medical treatments and care in positive terms that emphasize how these interventions are intended to keep children safe and/or help them feel better. Potential risks may be presented in supportive ways, for example, "We are going to ask you to swallow this medicine that will help you stay healthy" rather than "You need to take this medicine because you were exposed to toxins that may harm you." This advice is relevant even outside the context of a disaster.

Psychological distress may present as signs and symptoms that mimic serious physical conditions—tachypnea, tachycardia, disorientation, confusion, complaints of pain, etc. may emanate from psychological factors rather than physical etiologies. Even if physical etiologies are the primary cause of symptoms, an overlay of psychological distress may worsen symptoms and complicate medical management. Physical and psychosocial factors frequently co-occur and contribute directly to the elaboration, persistence, and/or nature of symptoms.

Individuals who are distressed have difficulty providing accurate and timely historical information, thereby impeding the evaluation and treatment process. Patients who are agitated are less likely to cooperate with necessary treatments and may undermine the provision of emergent care (e.g., an agitated child may refuse to keep an oxygen mask in place or resist having to lay down when their blood pressure is taken).

Time spent on understanding the patient's psychological distress and implementing effective brief interventions may actually shorten the overall time for the encounter and expedite the delivery of appropriate emergency medical care. Better engagement with the patient and family, more efficient acquisition of accurate historical information and description of symptoms, time avoided on unnecessary and ineffective treatments resulting from misattribution of the cause of symptoms, and increased active participation of the patient and family in the treatment process all contribute to the ultimate time savings as well as an improvement in outcome.

12.2.2 Psychological Support in the Aftermath of a Disaster

Evidence for the efficacy of early interventions such as Psychological First Aid (PFA), which involves offering psychoeducation and supportive services to foster effective and normative coping strategies and adjustment and to accelerate the natural healing process, is promising but PFA has not been proven to contribute more to adjustment than the passage of time and natural recovery. There is, however, a strong evidence base for some interventions, particularly those including cognitive–behavioral techniques aimed at ameliorating post-traumatic symptoms and disorders. Far less research has explored the broader range of important adjustment difficulties such as bereavement and loss that are often experienced by children after a disaster (Grolnick et al. 2018).

Nurses and HCPs can play an important role by validating children's (and other family members') feelings and reactions and by encouraging them to express their concerns and seek and accept assistance and support. There is a great deal of stigma associated with mental illness, and it does not go away in the aftermath of a major disaster or crisis, even when many, if not most, individuals are having adjustment difficulties.

12.2.3 Practical Advice for Nurses and Health Care Providers

The following are some practical suggestions on how to communicate and support children after a major disaster (Schonfeld 2008):

- Establish open and honest communication with children and their families. Ask children directly what they know about the disaster and explain to them in simple and direct terms the basic information about the event, without providing unnecessary elaboration or graphic detail. Then ask children what further information they would like and encourage them to share their concerns and questions as they arise. Remember, children may have very different concerns than adults about the crisis event, their health, or the health care interventions. Many of these concerns will be based on misinformation or misunderstandings. Provide clarification and reassurance as appropriate, without providing inaccurate information or false reassurance.
- Ask children and families about how they are coping as well as their personal experiences. Some children will withdraw and many will feel uncomfortable talking directly about what has happened or their personal reactions – do not force the conversations. Validate children's reports of feelings and expressions of concern.
- Allow children to show their distress; do not try to cheer them up or encourage them to hide their distress. Nurses and HCPs should feel free to demonstrate empathy, but should avoid indicating they know exactly what victims are going through (only the victims themselves can know) or telling them how they ought to feel ("Many children that I take care of in emergencies are scared and upset – how are you doing?" is preferable to "You must be scared.").
- Help children to understand the information being provided about the evaluation and treatment process. Use simple and direct explanations, avoid jargon and unnecessary details, and invite and answer questions. Do the same for their par-

ents/caregivers and other family members, since under stress even well-educated adults will have difficulty processing information presented to them.

- Meet children's basic needs for safety, food and drink, and reunification with loved ones as important first steps in meeting their mental health (and by extension their physical health) needs. Let them know that they are safe and what is being done to keep them safe. State actions in positive terms, for example, "I am going to put this belt around your waist so you remain secure and safe in the bed as we move it into the ambulance and drive to the hospital" rather than "I am going to put this belt around your waist, so if we get in a car accident you don't go flying out the window and get even more injured."

- Allow parents and other important caregivers and family members to remain with children to the extent possible as separation can heighten children's distress. Nurses and HCPs can guide adults in how they can be helpful to their children and the health care team. Providing an active and appropriate role for parents in the evaluation and treatment process minimizes the likelihood that their presence will be disruptive. Parents and other caregivers may refuse to be separated from their children in the aftermath of a disaster, even if they themselves are in need of emergency medical care. As a result, HCPs should be prepared to treat families as intact units in the aftermath of a disaster.

- To the extent possible, locate or move children in order to shield them from unnecessary additional exposure to traumatic aspects of the event; be conscious that even young children can and will overhear conversations among members of the health care team, whether related to their own medical care or the disaster. Check to see if televisions or radios may be overheard.

- Help children identify supports and coping techniques that have been effective in the past for other stressors and suggest they try them now. For example, if distraction has worked in the past, consider allowing children to listen to music on their cell phone if that will not interfere with the evaluation or treatment. Nurses and HCPs can also suggest other coping techniques, such as talking with trusted adults, engaging in play activities like drawing, or practicing simple relaxation techniques.

- Consider offering transitional objectives, such as something familiar and comforting from their parents/caregivers or home (e.g., their bedroom pillow or pillow case that has a familiar scent, a picture of a parent who cannot be with the child, one of the child's favorite toys, etc.), being careful not to risk losing something of significant value (monetary or personal) that would be difficult to replace.

- Psychotropic medication is rarely indicated in the immediate aftermath of a crisis and should be prescribed in consultation with a child psychiatrist or other pediatric HCP familiar with the assessment and management of traumatized children. Attempts to use psychotropic medications immediately after an event in order to blunt children's awareness of what is occurring or to reduce typical emotional reactions (e.g., crying) should be discouraged. The opportunity for children to acknowledge their distress and express their feelings is often a helpful first step in their recovery.

12.3   Resiliency and Post-traumatic Growth

Resilience is defined in terms of the positive coping ability demonstrated following serious threats to adaptation and development using "ordinary magic," which is made up of ordinary rather than extraordinary processes (Masten 2001). Resiliency, however, is different from recovery, which may require an extended amount of time. Resilience reflects the ability to maintain stability during the recovery process (Bonanno 2004) that may give caregivers the impression that survivors are no longer suffering. Unfortunately, children demonstrating some resiliency skills who are not able to communicate fully their needs may lead adults to believe that their recovery process and distress has ended. For example, a child may maintain academic performance but have difficulty sleeping at night. An adolescent may maintain peer relationships but begin experimenting with substance use because of intrusive thoughts.

Resilience can be understood as the interplay among personal characteristics, protective contextual factors, and the severity of the stressors faced by the child. Personal characteristics include intellectual ability as well as preexisting mental health, and trauma and loss history. Personal resiliency capacity has been found to include beliefs about personal mastery, a sense of being connected to others, and the capacity for emotional regulation (Cambell-Sills and Stein 2007; Prince-Embury 2011). Contextual or environmental factors include parent and social support networks and secondary stressors that follow an event. Finally, exposure to certain traumatic events (Furr et al. 2010), such as sexual assault or the violent death of a family member, can render most children vulnerable.

The most prevalent post-traumatic stress symptom trajectory among children after exposure to a disaster is characterized by resilience, suggesting that most children do recover following exposure to a traumatic event. It should be noted that even though most children may not necessarily suffer long-term impairment, up to 30% may experience chronic difficulties, especially if social support is not sufficient (Bonanno et al. 2010).

If children receive sufficient and sustained support and have the internal resources to adjust to the event, they may emerge with new skills that they can use to cope with future adversity; shift their life goals to align more with public service; place a higher priority on family, friends, spirituality, and helping others; or become more empathic. In this way, disasters may result in post-traumatic growth among both children and adults. Such post-traumatic growth is more likely to occur when children are provided support of sufficient intensity and duration (Schonfeld et al. 2015).

12.4   Impact of Bereavement and Loss on Recovery

Children, like adults, will struggle with understanding and accepting the death of someone close and the impact it has on them and their family. Parents, teachers, and other caring adults are often reluctant to talk with children who are grieving out of a fear of upsetting children by raising the topic or causing further distress by saying the "wrong thing" (Schonfeld et al. 2016). Avoiding discussion is rarely helpful and often isolates children at a time when they are most in need of support and assistance. Children may also misinterpret silence by adults about a death as an indication that adults are unaware, unconcerned, or unwilling to be of assistance. Children may then conclude that the expression of their intense and complicated feelings is inappropriate, that adults do not feel that the person who died is worthy of being mourned, or that the relationship the children have with the deceased is not considered to be of sufficient value. The common reactions of shame or guilt experienced by grieving children can be intensified by this silence. Children may also demonstrate avoidant behavior by not sharing their feelings for fear of upsetting their caregivers (Schonfeld and Demaria 2018).

Nurses and HCPs can take the following steps to initiate the conversation with grieving children (Schonfeld and Quackenbush 2010):

- Express concern. It is okay to be tearful or simply to let them know you feel sorry someone they care about has died.
- Be genuine; children can tell when adults are authentic and truthful. Do not tell a child you will miss her grandfather if you have never met him; instead, let the child know that you appreciate that he was important to her and you feel sorry she had to experience such a loss.
- Listen and observe; talk less. Simply being present while the child is expressing grief and tolerating the unpleasant affect can be very helpful.
- Invite discussion using open-ended questions such as "How are you doing since your mother died?" or "How is your family coping?"
- Limit the sharing of personal experiences. Keep the focus on the child's loss and feelings.
- Offer practical advice, such as suggestions about how to answer questions that might be asked by peers or how to talk with teachers about learning challenges.
- Offer appropriate reassurance. Do not minimize children's concerns but let them know that over time you do expect that they will become better able to cope with their distress.
- Communicate your availability to provide support over time. Do not require children or families to reach out to you for such support, but rather, make an effort to schedule follow-up appointments and reach out by phone or e-mail periodically.

Adults are often worried that they will say the wrong thing and make matters worse. In the context of talking with a patient who has recently experienced a death, nurses and HCPs may wish to consider the following suggestions (Schonfeld and Quackenbush 2010):

- Although well intentioned, attempts to "cheer up" individuals who are grieving are usually neither effective nor appreciated. Anything that begins with "at least" should be reconsidered (e.g., "at least he isn't in pain anymore," "at least you have another brother"). Such comments may minimize a health care provider's discomfort in being with children who are grieving by encouraging grieving children to reduce their outward distress, but do not help children express and cope with their feelings.

- Do not instruct children to hide their emotions (e.g., "You need to be strong; you are the man of the house now that your father has died.").
- Avoid communicating that you know how they feel (e.g., "I know exactly what you are going through."). Instead, ask them to share their feelings.
- Do not tell them how they ought to feel (e.g., "You must feel angry.").
- Avoid comparisons with personal experiences. When adults share their own experiences in the context of recent loss, it shifts the focus away from the child. If the loss is perceived by the child as less important, the comparison can be insulting (e.g., "I know what you are going through after the death of your father. My cat died this week."). If the experience appears worse (e.g., "I understand your grandfather died. When I was your age, both my mother and father died in a car accident."), the child may feel compelled to provide comfort and be reluctant to ask for help.
- The use of expressive techniques, such as picture drawing or engaging children in an activity while talking with them, may be helpful in some situations in which children appear reluctant to address the topic in direct conversation.

12.4.1 Secondary Losses

Although children generally show a remarkable resiliency and ability to adjust to the death of someone close to them, they do not "get over" a death in 6 months or a year. Rather, they spend the rest of their life accommodating the absence and often maintain their continuing bonds with the deceased. In fact, many find the second year after a death to be more difficult than the first. Unfortunately, by this point in time, the special support they may have received from extended family, teachers, coaches, and others at school and in the community has probably already ended. However, the sense of loss is persistent, and without proper support, it may be perceived as overwhelming.

Maintaining support for children and families is important well beyond the initial period of grief. When children experience a death of someone close to them, they lose not only the person who died (i.e., the primary loss) but also everything that person had contributed or would have contributed to their life (i.e., the secondary losses). Common secondary losses include the following (Schonfeld et al. 2016):

- Change in lifestyle (e.g., altered financial status of the family after the death of a parent).
- Relocation resulting in a change in school and peer group.
- Less interaction with friends or relatives of the person who died (e.g., friends of a child's sister no longer visit after the sister dies).
- Loss of shared memories.

- Decreased special attention (e.g., a child may no longer value participating in sports activities without his parent there to cheer for him).
- Decreased availability of the surviving parent (who may need to work more hours or who becomes less available emotionally because of depression).
- A decreased sense of safety and trust in the world.

12.5 Personal Impact of Disasters on Nurses and Health Care Providers

The disaster and its aftermath impact all members of the affected community, including members of the health care team. Nurses and HCPs should be aware of how their own personal reactions may affect the children they treat. Children and family members are very responsive to the affective tone of the nurse or HCP. HCPs should therefore attempt to convey a sense of control of the situation and respond in a gentle, compassionate, and supportive manner. Panic or anxiety conveyed by a member of the health care team will generally exacerbate the stress reactions of children and their families.

Nurses and HCPs often enter the profession because of a desire to help children grow, develop, and be healthy and happy. Nurses and HCPs who witness children's distress as they grieve the death of someone about whom they care deeply, or who relate a traumatic memory, may experience personal emotional reactions and feelings that may ultimately contribute to the development of compassion fatigue.

The importance of routinely maintaining self-care strategies for health care providers becomes even more critical following a disaster because of the increased emotional and social burdens nurses and HCPs may experience in this context. Developing a comprehensive plan for self-care should include allocating sufficient time to the development of a professional support system, expanding relevant professional knowledge, balancing personal and professional needs, increasing personal awareness and including activities that provide rejuvenation and revitalization on a daily basis (Dorociak et al. 2017).

12.6 Conclusion

Nurses and HCPs should recognize the critical role that they can play to support children and families in the immediate aftermath of a disaster and throughout the long-term recovery process. The strategies and approaches outlined in this chapter are relevant not only in the context of natural and man-made disasters, but also when assisting with a personal or family crisis unrelated to a disaster. Given that significant medical illness and its treatment are often stressful to many children and families and personal and family stressors and adversity are ubiquitous, nurses and HCPs will see great benefit in proactively learning these skills and applying them routinely within their practice settings.

References

Penrose A, Takaki M. Children's rights in emergencies and disasters. Lancet. 2006;367:698–9.

Schonfeld D, Demaria T, Disaster Preparedness Advisory Council, Committee on Psychosocial Aspects of Child and Family Health. Providing psychosocial support to children and families in the aftermath of disaster and crisis: a guide for pediatricians. Pediatrics. 2015;136(4):e1120–30.

Osofsky HJ, Osofsky JD, Kronenberg M, Brennan A, Hansel TC. Posttraumatic stress symptoms in children after Hurricane Katrina: predicting the need for mental health services. Am J Orthopsychiatry. 2009;79(2):212–20.

Institute of Medicine. Preparing for the psychological consequences of terrorism: a public health strategy. Washington, DC: National Academics Press; 2003.

Grolnick WS, Schonfeld DJ, Schreiber M, Cohen J, Cole V, Jaycox L, Zatzick D. Improving adjustment and resilience in children following a disaster: addressing research challenges. Am Psychol. 2018;73(3):215–29.

Schonfeld DJ, Gurwitch RH. Children in disasters. In: Elzouki AY, Stapleton FB, Whitley RJ, Oh W, Harfi HA, Nazer H, editors. Textbook of clinical pediatrics. 2nd ed. New York, NY: Springer-Verlag; 2012. p. 687–98.

American Psychiatric Association. Diagnostic and statistical manual of mental disorders. 5th ed. (DSM-5). Washington, DC: American Psychiatric Association; 2013.

Lai BS, La Greca AM, Auslander BA, Short MB. Children's symptoms of posttraumatic stress and depression after a natural disaster: comorbidity and risk factors. J Affect Disorder. 2013;146(1):71–8.

Schonfeld D. Providing psychological first aid and identifying mental health needs in the aftermath of a disaster or community crisis. In: Foltin G, Tunik M, Treiber M, Cooper A, editors. Pediatric disaster preparedness: a resource for planning, management, and provision of out-of-hospital emergency care. New York, NY: Center Pediatr Emerg Med; 2008.

Lai BS, Lewis R, Livings MS, La Greca AM, Esnard A. Posttraumatic stress symptom trajectories among children after disaster exposure: a review. J Trauma Stress. 2017;30(6):571–82.

Masten AS. Ordinary magic. Resilience processes in development. Am Psychol. 2001;56(3):227–38.

Bonanno GA. Loss, trauma and human resilience: have we underestimated the human capacity to thrive after extremely aversive events? Am Psychol. 2004;59(1):20–8.

Campbell-Sills L, Stein MB. Psychometric analysis and refinement of the Connor-Davidson Resilience Scale (CD-RISC): validation of a 10-item measure of resilience. J Trauma Stress. 2007;20(6):1019–28.

Prince-Embury S. Assessing personal resiliency in the context of school settings: using the resiliency scales for children and adolescents. Psychol Sch. 2011;48(7):672–85.

Furr JM, Comer JS, Edmunds JM, Kendall PC. Disasters and youth: a meta-analytic examination of posttraumatic stress. J Consult Clin Psychol. 2010;78:765–80.

Bonanno GA, Brewin CR, Kaniasty K, La Greca AM. Weighing the costs of disaster: consequences, risks, and resilience in individuals, families, and communities. Psychol Sci Public Interest. 2010;11(1):1–49.

Schonfeld DJ, Demaria T, Committee on Psychosocial Aspects of Child and Family Health, Disaster Preparedness Advisory Council. Supporting the grieving child and family. Pediatrics. 2016;138(3):e2016–147.

Schonfeld DJ, Demaria T. Supporting grieving students in the aftermath of a school crisis. In: Bui E, editor. Clinical handbook of bereavement and grief reactions. Cham: Springer; 2018. p. 217–40.

Schonfeld D, Quackenbush M. The grieving student: a teacher's guide. Baltimore, MD: Brookes Publishing; 2010.

Dorociak K, Rupert P, Bryant F, Zahniser E. Development of a self-care assessment for psychologists. J Couns Psychol. 2017;64(3):325–34.

Hospital Preparedness

Melinda Hirshouer, James Cole Edmonson,
and Kimberly K. Hatchel

13.1 Introduction

This chapter focuses on hospital emergency management with special consider-ations for the pediatric population. While some areas of emergency management have pediatric considerations, like triage and decontamination, there are other areas of emergency management that apply to all populations such as employee safety and memorandums of understanding. This chapter serves as an introduction with an intent to expose and inform the reader of the summary of the main points for hospi-tal emergency preparedness. Appropriate planning and rehearsals will provide opportunities to mitigate risk and eliminate gaps in care before a disaster occurs.

13.1.1 Drills for Pediatrics

Children have distinct and different needs in disaster-related situations and have vulnerabilities that differ from adults. According to the Kaiser Family Foundation in 2017, approximately 24% of the U.S. population was between the ages of 0–18 years (Kaiser Family Foundation 2019). The statistics alone increase the likelihood of pediatric patients being involved in a mass casualty incident (MCI). The types of incidents that have occurred in recent years such as school shootings, hurricanes, infectious disease outbreaks, and mass land fires add an additional layer of concern and complexity. Events involving large numbers of children produce feelings of dread and uneasiness in prehospital and hospital caregivers. Hospital and commu-nity disaster planning drills should focus on communication, coordination, and delivery of pediatric-specific care.

M. Hirshouer (✉) · J. C. Edmonson · K. K. Hatchel
Texas Health Presbyterian Hospital, Dallas, TX, USA
e-mail: MelindaHirshouer@TexasHealth.org; Cole.Edmonson@AMNhealthcare.com;
kimberly.hatchel@hcahealthcare.com

© Springer Nature Switzerland AG 2020   301
C. J. Goodhue, N. Blake (eds.), *Nursing Management of Pediatric Disaster*,
https://doi.org/10.1007/978-3-030-43428-1_13

Collaboration with disaster response coordination (DRC) units increase resources and support during critical times. Preparation, planning, and leadership are integral to building the resiliency to handle high anxiety-provoking infrequent events. The key areas of focus during preparation are:

1. Drills should focus on pediatric-specific treatment scenarios and age-specific developmental reactions to trauma and injuries. Know the pediatric evidence-based guidelines that have been adopted in your region or geography. Drill to them. Children are not little adults.
2. Availability of pediatricians, pediatric advanced practitioners, and pediatric equipment for all phases of care. Consider compacts, agreements, licensure, privileges, and credentialing that expands your coverage availability.
3. Preplan or anticipate surge capacity. Remember a pediatric patient with the family will consume a larger footprint. Furthermore, consider how you will distribute the children in your community to control surge and maximize treatment.
4. Educate the nurses, HCPs, and community on what to anticipate during a disaster including even the littlest community members.
5. Choose your triage tool appropriately and drill on how to use it. Choosing a pediatric tool complimentary to your adult system ensures consistency and reduces error.
6. Consider scenarios that require sheltering large numbers of children in place.
7. Reconnect or reunite children with their families and create situations where a sense of normalcy returns as soon as reasonably possible. See Chap. 11 for more detailed information.
8. Preplan debriefing and counseling resources (Kelly 2010).

Trauma is cumulative and is known to exacerbate preexisting mental health vulnerabilities. Participation in well-planned disaster drills both internally and externally will decrease feelings of apprehension and increase an organization exposure to specialized training, improve response times, efficiency, effectiveness, and resiliency. Ferrer et al. reviewed after-action reports from 34 health care organizations and found that less than one quarter included pediatric victims in their drills and exercises.

13.1.2 Disaster Response Coordination (DRC), Partnerships, and Memorandums of Understanding

MCIs can easily overwhelm any hospital and disaster preparedness plans for health care systems must include planning, mitigation, response, recovery, and collaboration to enhance community resilience. Collaboration has always been part of the nursing process that makes nurses likely participants in the development of coalitions, memorandums of understanding, and in DRC units. Participation in a DRC unit requires a commitment from all parties and can be seen at a local, state, regional, or national level. This is a formal agreement with clearly defined responsibilities for each partner. This agreement is usually executed in a memorandum of understanding (MOU). An example of a DRC unit includes the Chemical Stockpile Emergency Preparedness Program (CSEPP). In this arrangement, the CSEPP provides the medical countermeasures as well as providing the funding for decontamination and personal protective equipment (PPE) supplies while the hospital commits to treating patients exposed to a chemical agent and providing the appropriate training and preparation through drill exercises. Both the participating hospital and the CSEPP are evaluated frequently using predetermined exercise outcomes (Kim 2016).

Coalitions are another form of collaboration and are seen at local or regional levels. Membership is defined by the location that the coalition covers (city, state, region). Coalitions function within an organizational framework and have a defined leader with a specific set of goals and responsibilities. Member organizations also have specific roles and responsibilities that are once again defined through an executed MOU. Coalitions may include additional partnerships outside of the hospital with post-acute, long-term care, and community and public health providers. This type of partnership allows for shared training and educational opportunities among its members. Coalitions may also decide to pursue grants or other funding opportunities to purchase supply caches that can be managed by its members (Kim 2016). An example of a coalition would be a public health department, local hospitals, skilled nursing facilities, and long-term acute care hospitals that have an agreement to participate in disaster drills and also agree to assist in accelerating discharge placements should the hospital experience an MCI. There may be other responsibilities, including the provision of child care, so nurses and HCPs can go to work or affected people in the community can work with governmental or local agencies after the disaster. Coalitions have a unique opportunity to compose themselves in such a way that they can assist their community in recovery or resilience after a large disaster (Kim 2016).

Regardless of the type of collaboration, each member of the team can improve their situational awareness by following the characteristics of highly reliable organizations. Coalitions and DRC units are designed to improve preparedness and response to natural and man-made disasters including acts of terrorism. This means they must be prepared to coordinate critical operations and timely allocate appropriate resources (Autrey and Moss 2006). Communication is crucial, so the DRC unit or coalition will have to fully understand processes while being sensitive to each member's operations to increase the chance of success. They must look for instances where the processes might fail; this aligns with mitigation tasks required in emergency management. Shared disaster exercises provide the opportunity to identify and learn from errors. Finally, subject matter experts from within each member organization should be sought out to provide valuable insight and expertise to make any necessary improvements.

13.1.3 Triage

Children and infants are disproportionately affected by disasters due to their dependency on others to care for them and their anatomical differences from adults. When preparing for disasters, it is advisable that these differences are acknowledged and that the pediatric patient is considered part of a vulnerable population. Physiologic differences, including the rate of respiration and heart rate, increase the susceptibility to both biological and chemical agents (Allen et al. 2007). Size of the child also matters, and not just to determine appropriate medication dosing. Solid organs are proportionately larger and not as well protected due to a smaller percentage of subcutaneous fat (Allen et al. 2007; Gausche-Hill 2009). Vomiting and diarrhea reactions to various chemical agents combined with an overall smaller blood volume increase the likelihood of being seriously affected by volume loss (Gausche-Hill 2009). Head injuries and multisystem injuries from blunt force trauma can be seen as the force applied has a greater impact on smaller body areas (Allen et al. 2007; Gausche-Hill 2009). Immature cognitive abilities, potential lack of coping skills, and possible separation from the child's caregiver may also amplify the effects of trauma (Mace et al. 2012). All of these factors emphasize the need for timely and accurate triage procedures. See Chaps. 5 and 7 for further information on pediatric considerations.

Primary triage may be performed by first responders; however, nurses in hospital settings must also be prepared for patients who self-report and need triaging. Although there is no universal tool for pediatric triage, there is the Model Uniform Core Criteria for Mass Casualty Incident Triage that is agreed upon by many organizations including the National Association of Emergency Medical Services (EMS) Physicians and the American Academy of Pediatrics (AAP) (Federal Interagency Committee on EMS 2014). These criteria focus on using visual markers, like triage tags, simple and quick, easy to apply, and applicable to all age groups. It begins with global sorting into groups of those patients needing lifesaving interventions, those who cannot follow ambulation commands but can follow other simple commands, and those who can ambulate and have no obvious life-threatening injuries (Federal Interagency Committee on EMS 2014). Once patients have been sorted into groups, they must be assessed individually. This is when the visual markers will be applied. There are multiple pediatric triage tools that use the Model Uniform Core Criteria, including JumpSTART, the Pediatric Triage Tape, and Care Flight to assist with this task. These tools take into consideration the physical development stage for ambulation, age-appropriate vital signs, airway positioning/repositioning, and age-appropriate mental status. Pediatric considerations within the Model Uniform Core Criteria can be seen in Table 13.1.

Regardless of the tool, care must be taken to avoid over-prioritization (assessing patients sicker than they are) and under-prioritizing (missing life-threatening injuries in the assessment). Patients must be prioritized into one of five categories and be assigned the corresponding color for that category. These categories can be seen in Table 13.2.

13.1.4 Making Room

Disasters can take on many forms in a health care setting, including surges of patients that can overwhelm the existing resources of hospitals. Resources include space, personnel, equipment, supplies, and pharmaceuticals. The type of disaster or

Table 13.1 Pediatric considerations using the model uniform core criteria (Federal Interagency Committee on EMS 2014)

Model uniform core criteria	Question	Example	Pediatric consideration
Global sorting	Can the victim follow simple commands?	If you can hear me, walk toward the sound of my voice	Has the patient reached physical development for ambulation?
Lifesaving interventions	Are vital signs within normal range?	Is the respiratory rate ≤20 respirations/min	Small children may have normal respiratory rates closer to 30 respirations/min
Lifesaving interventions	Can the intervention be performed quickly	Are multiple attempts needed to open the airway using routine maneuvers?	For children, up to two rescue breaths should be considered in addition to repositioning the airway
Individual assessment	Did the assignment of triage categories use yes or no criteria?	The immediate category includes those that cannot follow simple commands	Is the patient old enough to comprehend simple commands? Purposeful movements may also be used

Table 13.2 Individal Assessment Categories Using model Uniform Core Criteria (Federal Interagency Committee on EMS 2014)

Immediate-First Priority	These patients are unable to follow commands, have respiratory distress, lack of peripheral pulses or a life-threatening hemorrhage.
Delayed	Delayed patients have a pulse and no respiratory distress, but have injuries that are not considered minor.
Minimal	Minimal patients can follow commands and have only minor injuries.
Expectant	Expectant patients have life-threatening injuries that exceed the current available resources. Resuscitation and comfort care should be provided as resources become available.
Expired/Dead-Last Priority	Expired patients should be provided appropriate care to maintain any evidence that may need to be collected at a later point in time.

patients during a surge is somewhat predictive of what area, process, or supply will be in most need. Although facilities are required to have plans in place that generally plan for surge and 96 h of disaster modes, it is a challenge to accomplish this with general community hospitals but especially challenging in tertiary and quaternary pediatric and neonatal services. A robust plan is required to prepare for and maintain a state of readiness. The plan should include a protocol for potentially canceling elective surgeries, prioritization of patients for potential discharge, identified space/equipment/staff for surge patients, and how to create required levels of care for general to critical patients. Plans may include using hallway beds in both inpatient and emergency areas along with consideration of utilizing ambulatory space short-term for lower-risk patients involved in disasters.

Surge situations like disasters can overwhelm the normal processes and routines in hospitals for many reasons. Jen et al. (Jen et al. 2016) found in their planning for relocation of a hospital several learnings that apply to surge situations including:

1. The need to decrease or eliminate elective operative volume through scheduling priorities;
2. Eliminating or reducing nonemergent transfers accepted from outside institutions; and
3. Multidisciplinary discharge planning team including a process and rounds to identify inpatients eligible for expedited discharge and for transfer from high acuity areas to lower acuity.

The authors note clearly "Coordination with ancillary health care services, including nursing homes, rehabilitation centers, and home health services, was intensified during the transition period to overcome various barriers to patient placement and discharge planning encountered at baseline" (Jen et al. 2016).

Testing processes for scalability before surge or disasters is recommended as challenges that have been demonstrated during surge events include registration, identification, staffing capabilities, electronic health record, supply availability/delivery, security, and visitor management. The ability to control access to units during surge events and to locate patients/families can present significant challenges in the pediatric and neonatal critical care settings. Surge can challenge the facility in numerous ways including the number of visitors and extended family members, and in disaster scenarios, entire families who have lost homes or residences may come to the hospital as a safe place. Planning for visitor surge is an important aspect of preparing and creating zones for families and visitors to be accessible for patients and the care teams. Surge can create unforeseen needs for families connected to patients, requiring space for sleeping, eating, bathing, and even storing and identification of breast milk for admitted patients but also their siblings.

13.1.5 Evacuation

The decision to evacuate is a complex one and the abundance of evacuation choices makes it even more complicated. Further complicating the decision is the urgency of the timeline that the evacuation must be completed within. Nursing leadership is responsible for communicating with hospital leadership that care can no longer be provided in a safe environment. Nursing leadership is also responsible for communicating information that has been received from hospital leadership about the current or anticipated status of the facility. The safety of patients, visitors, and staff must be the first priority.

Once it has been determined that care cannot be provided in the current environment and patients, visitors, and staff may be at risk, the next consideration is the time frame in which the evacuation must be completed. Questions to ask include if the evacuation must be immediate as in the case of a fire, whether the evacuation needs to begin within the next few hours as in the case of a utility outage, or if the evacuation can be planned in advance as in the case of a hurricane. Finally, a decision must be made on a location to evacuate to. Is it feasible to stay on the same level if the affected patients are moved past the fire doors or will the patients need to be evacuated to an entirely different floor? If the facility as a whole needs to be evacuated the special needs of the pediatric and neonate populations will drive decisions on transportation needs, travel distance, appropriate placement at a new facility, and reunification measures.

Horizontal or lateral evacuation is the first choice of evacuation options. This can be defined as moving patients from one side of the unit to another, from one unit to another on the same floor, or from one tower to another on the same floor. Vertical evacuation can be defined as moving the patients from the affected floor, up or down, to another floor. Although instinct may be to always descend, all staff should be instructed to follow instructions in their emergency operations plan or from the command center as lower floors may also be affected. Examples of horizontal and vertical evacuations can be seen in Table 13.3. Entire facility evacuations or the evacuation of a special population may necessitate the need for an intrafacility transfer within a large health care system, an interfacility transfer within the local area, an intrastate transfer to a facility that offers similar services, or an interstate transfer to a facility identified from a regional command center that has the capacity to accommodate both volume and acuity of the evacuated patients. Real-life examples of these types of evacuations can be seen in Table 13.4.

Pediatric and neonate populations have special needs that must also be considered when preparing for evacuation. These items include specialty treatment equipment, specialty transportation equipment, developmental age of the patient and communication abilities, the need for specialty transport teams, the distance that must be traveled, and a plan for reunification. Evacuation vests that carry infants may be an acceptable option in the nursery and special care nursery units, while isolettes may be needed in the neonatal intensive care and medical evacuation sleds are needed for older pediatric patients (Espiritu et al. 2014).

Each unit will have its own needs based on the expected patient population and location within the facility. In addition to transporting the patient during the evacuation, special considerations will need to be made for any specialty equipment

Table 13.3 Examples of horizontal and vertical evacuations

	Horizontal	Vertical
One unit to another	3rd floor Tower A West to 3rd floor Tower A East	3rd floor Tower A to 2nd floor Tower A
One side of the unit to the other	3rd floor Tower A West rooms 1–12 to 3rd floor Tower A West rooms 24–36	N/A
One tower to another	3rd floor Tower A to 3rd floor Tower B	3rd floor Tower A to 4th floor Tower B

Table 13.4 Examples of United States Hospital evacuations (Baldwin et al. 2006)

	Sending facility	Receiving facility	Disaster
Intrafacility	Hospitals within the Texas Medical Center	Hospitals within the Texas Medical Center	Tropical Storm Allison
Local-intrastate	New York University Langone Medical Center	New York Presbyterian Hospital Weil Cornell Medical Center Morgan Stanley Children's Hospital at New York Presbyterian Mt. Sinai Hospital St. Luke's Hospital Lenox Hill Hospital Montefiore Medical Center	Hurricane Sandy
Interstate	Children's Hospital of New Orleans	Texas Children's Hospital	Hurricane Katrina

that needs to move with the patients. Items such as ventilators, dialysis equipment, IV pumps, and cardiac equipment will have to be considered for battery versus electrical power, ability to transport with or without use of the elevators, size of the equipment if the patient must be moved by ground or air ambulance, and competence of the staff needed to operate the equipment. If the patient's clinical needs or use of specialty equipment requires the use of specialty staff, as with some neonatal or pediatric intensive care transfers, unit staff should work in collaboration with the incident command team to determine if the facility can spare its own staff to use in transport or if additional accommodations must be made with outside resources (Espiritu et al. 2014).

Tracking of patients and clear communication must occur at each step of evacuation. Being able to locate where each patient is at any moment in time is imperative to provide up to date information on the patient's clinical status, communicate pending test results, and to decrease the anxiety of the parent or guardian who may or may not be able to accompany the patient for an evacuation to another facility (Espiritu et al. 2014). Parental/guardian communication and plans for reunification must be included as part of the disaster plan and rehearsed so that the staff is familiar with the plan and can execute it when the time comes (Espiritu et al. 2014). Tracking tools that provide handoff information and departure checklists can assist departing, transporting, and receiving staff with continuing care while ensuring the patient arrives at the appropriate final destination as well as providing the parents and guardians information necessary for reunification. Tickets to travel, often a form that travels with the patient for tracking and safe handoff purposes, may include sections for departing unit, arriving at ambulance bay, departing ambulance, and arriving at receiving facility and may be combined with tracking data at the incident command center. Additionally, departing checklists that include items such as verifying identification and assigned room, medications packed, diapers changed or restroom needs met, medication list printed, electronic health record printed or transferred, and telemetry monitoring status can be combined with a handoff tool.

Patient Name _____ Age _____

Medical Record Number _____

Parent/Guardian Name #1 _____ Contact Number_____

Parent/Guardian Name #2 _____ Contact Number_____

Sending dept _____ Time departed _____ Signature _____

Time arrived in ambulance bay _____ Signature_____

Handoff to Ambulance Company_____ Time _____ Signature _____

Time arrived at receiving facility _____ Signature_____

Diagnosis _____ History of_____ Attending Physician _____

Allergies/Reaction _____

Procedures (include dates and times)

```
┌──────────────────────────────────────────────────────────────────────────────┐
│                                                                                │
│                                                                                │
│                                                                                │
└──────────────────────────────────────────────────────────────────────────────┘
```

Last set of vital signs HR _____ BP _____ RR _____ SPO2 _____

O2 requirements _____ Mental Status_____

Diet/Formula _____

Last pain medication _____ Date & time _____

Last antibiotic _____ Date & time _____

IV Fluids Currently Infusing _____

Speciality Equipment Needs_____

Fig. 13.1   Evacuation handoff and tracking tool

Ideally, the handoff tool would cover typical shift handoff information such as isolation status, vital signs, pertinent physical assessment findings, oxygen requirements, pain and sedation medication given, and parent/guardian information as well as any last-minute verification of specialty equipment settings (Rozenfeld et al. 2017). An example of a tool that can be used for tracking and handoffs can be seen in Fig. 13.1, a departure checklist can be seen in Fig. 13.2.

13.1.6 Planning

The variation, number, and types of disasters that involve pediatric patients make planning a must-do activity. While there are a few basic national programs like Pediatric Disaster Life Support, none of them deal with the necessary care management specifics (Fox 2008). The treatment nuances that exist with children are more effectively handled when carefully planned out and drilled upon. Planning that begins with the central themes of DRC's, memorandums of understandings, and well thought out inter- and intrafacility partnerships connect hospitals,

Departure Checklist

Patient Name _____ Age _____

Medical Record Number _____

Parent/Guardian Notified _____ Time_____

Personal Belongings Packed   YES   NO

Armband attached   YES   NO

Medication Record Attached   YES   NO

History and Physical Attached   YES   NO

Electronic Health Record Attached   YES   NO

Last Intake _____ Type_____

Last Output _____Type_____

Speciality equipment verified with transport company   YES   NO

Speciality equipment verified at receiving facility   YES   NO

Handoff/Tracking Tool Completed   YES   NO

Fig. 13.2 Evacuation departure checklist

prehospital providers, and community leaders in a pro-active way. These relationships thoughtfully formed will provide the needed foundation for program development. Effective planning should begin with an assessment of city, state, and regional resources. Cities with well-developed hospital districts and children's hospitals may have immediate availability of resources not seen in communities without them.

Planning should begin with what feels like the basics but prove to be crucial: (1) Communication strategies should consider all forms of communication. What types of devices will work even if the cell towers are overwhelmed with traffic in your city? Do your prehospital, hospital, and community leaders agree on what platform will be used if relied upon methods begin to fail? (2) Space consideration must include where your incident command (ICS) will reside, treatment spaces, and housing for those who cannot return home. Reviewing realistic scenarios and predicting pediatric surge should be considered for small- and large-scale events. (3) Pediatric-specific simulation scenarios should be included in all drills. Standard pediatric triage protocols, evidence-based care of the pediatric patient, and pediatric equipment should be as standard as possible across an aligned or prescribed region. Consider partnerships with schools and local physicians' offices and identify areas that can accommodate stockpiling pediatric-specific and disaster-related supplies (Kelly 2010).

13.1.7 Health Care Worker Safety

The safety of health care workers is always paramount; this does not change during disasters. Hospitals are required to follow numerous laws and regulations that are intended to keep the overall safety of the workplace and the individual worker. These include the Occupational Safety and Health Administration (OSHA), The Joint Commission (TJC) accreditation standards, Centers for Disease Control and Prevention, and federal and state regulatory agencies.

TJC requirements (The Joint Commission 2012) for health care worker safety related to disasters are broadly stated that organizations have engaged leadership, safety philosophies, safety policies, training, education, drills, equipment, resources, and measurements. For example, TJC requires specific plans by unit and by the patient population that must be developed, trained on, practiced, monitored, and updated as there are unique differences for certain populations of patients, especially pediatric populations.

Numerous organizations exist to guide the creation of workplace safety including the American Council—Employee Safety (ACES). Eight principles of safety are recommended by ACES (American Council—Employee Safety 2019):

1. Safety is an ethical responsibility.
2. Safety is a culture, not a program.
3. Management is responsible.
4. Employees must be trained to work safely.
5. Safety is a condition of employment.
6. All injuries are preventable.
7. Safety programs must be site specific with recurring audits of the workplace and prompt corrective action.
8. Safety is good business.

Working within a safety framework creates a consistent methodology for achieving workplace and worker safety. In general, plans must be in policy or procedure format, evidence-based, and practiced by affected individuals, departments, and organizations. As ACE notes, it is management's accountability for systems of safety, but individuals are still responsible for their own safety, education, and understanding of how to stay safe in different disaster scenarios.

Physical safety is one aspect of staying safe during disasters; another is emotional and psychological safety. Nurses and HCPs can become victims of disaster themselves and their loved ones as well. The duty to patient and duty to self must be carefully balanced as either can create psychological and emotional distress. Organizations can provide resources for creating safety before, during, and after disaster events through programs like Critical Incident Stress Management, Employee Assistance Programs, etc. Supportive organizations can recognize the daily stress of caregiving and promote resilience by providing self-care programs to nurses and HCPs, as building resilience can help improve well-being and insulate to a degree from the harmful emotional effects of disaster events. In partnership with

Table 13.5 Care for the caregiver websites

Website name	Link
Johnson and Johnson	https://nursing.jnj.com/nursing-news-events/jnj-and-nurses-partnership/innovative-toolkit-empowers-nurses-in-natural-disasters
Texas Organization of Nurse Executives	https://www.texasnurse.org/page/care_for_the_caregiver
Texas Nurses Association	https://www.texasnurses.org/page/c4c

Johnson and Johnson, Texas Organization of Nurse Executives, and Texas Nurses Association created a specific toolkit for nurses who become victims of disasters called "Care for the Caregiver" that can be accessed through all three organizations and the links provided in Table 13.5.

13.1.8 Decontamination

Decontamination is the removal of hazardous substances from the body and other surfaces that may not only harm the affected person but may also be a source of secondary contamination to others that come into contact with the affected person and may be in the forms of solids, liquids, or gasses. The role of the nurse within the hospital is significantly different during the process of decontamination than it is from the first responders on the scene. Cox describes this as the difference between first responders and first receivers (Cox 2016). Contaminated surfaces may remain even after initial decontamination at the scene as often clothing remains and the transportation equipment is also considered contaminated. It is estimated that during a large event involving hazardous material contamination, up to 80% of the victims will self-report to the hospital without primary decontamination at the scene (Cox 2016). For the nurse, this means working with the hospital incident command to safely secure the hospital environment is one of the first priorities to protect existing patients, visitors, and staff. Unauthorized access of contaminated patients can cause extended lockdowns of critical areas and the potential for secondary contamination of key staff members will eliminate them from the available staffing pool. Equally important is early and accurate communication about the known or suspected substance from first responders to the incident command center and from the incident command center to frontline staff to appropriately prepare (Cox 2016).

Appropriate planning and preparation include the purchase and storage of decontamination equipment. Air purified respirators and suits, brushes and soap, must be easily accessible and close to the conveyor belt. Facilities may have a permanent structure for decontamination to protect patients and staff from the elements, but if not, mobile tents will also need to be available. The climate in the storage area must be monitored so that the equipment is not compromised, and there must be enough batteries and they must be charged (Cox 2016).

It is important to note that children may present as unaccompanied minors or with their parents or other caregivers (Freyberg et al. 2008). Although adults and children alike have to undergo the decontamination process, children have additional special needs based on their physical and developmental age that may affect privacy, communication, and airway management. Policies and procedures related to decontamination should include considerations for these needs, in addition to procedures for setting up, performing the decontamination process, and clean up and take down once the MCI has concluded. References to reunification policies to assist with unaccompanied minors, safety and security policies to assist with scene security, and infection control policies to assist with donning and doffing of PPE should also be included. More information on decontamination can be found in Chap. 9 and reunification in Chap. 11.

13.2 Conclusion

Although many disaster preparedness activities apply to all populations, specific considerations for cognitive and physical development, availability of medical, nursing, and other clinical staff with pediatric expertise, and availability of specialized equipment must be taken into account for any hospital that cares for pediatric patients. Hazards and risks should be continuously assessed and emergency drills should incorporate the most likely scenarios the hospital may encounter. Additional considerations should be made for emotional support for employees, patients, and parents during times of trauma, reunification, and overall increased levels of stress.

References

Allen GM, Parrillo SJ, Will J, Mohr JA. Principles of disaster planning for the pediatric population. Prehosp Disaster Med. 2007;22(6):537–40. https://doi.org/10.1017/s1049023x00005392.

American Council—Employee Safety. Eight principles of a safe workplace. 2019. http://www.safetyace.com/eight-principles-of-a-safe-workplace.asp.

Autrey P, Moss J. High-reliability teams and situation awareness. J Nurs Adm. 2006;36(2):67–72. https://doi.org/10.1097/00005110-200602000-00004.

Baldwin S, Robinson A, Barlow P, Fargason CA. Moving hospitalized children all over the southeast: interstate transfer of pediatric patients during Hurricane Katrina. Pediatrics. 2006;117(Suppl 4):S416–20. https://doi.org/10.1542/peds.2006-0099o.

Cox B. Hospital decontamination: what nurses need to know. Nurs Clin North Am. 2016;51(4):663–74. https://doi.org/10.1016/j.cnur.2016.07.010.

Espiritu M, Patil U, Cruz H, Gupta A, Matterson H, Kim Y, et al. Evacuation of a neonatal intensive care unit in a disaster: lessons from Hurricane Sandy. Pediatrics. 2014;134(6):1–8. https://doi.org/10.1542/peds.2014-0936.

Federal Interagency Committee on EMS. National implementation of the model uniform core criteria for mass casualty incident triage (Publication). Federal Interagency Committee on EMS; 2014. p. 1–26. https://www.nhtsa.gov/staticfiles/nti/pdf/811891-Model_UCC_for_Mass_Casualty_Incident_Triage.pdf.

Fox L. Pediatric issues in disaster preparedness: meeting the educational needs of nurses-are we there yet? J Pediatr Nurs. 2008;23(2):145–52.

Freyberg CW, Arquilla B, Fertel BS, Tunik MG, Cooper A, Heon D, et al. Disaster prepared-ness: hospital decontamination and the pediatric patient—guidelines for hospitals and emergency planners. Prehosp Disaster Med. 2008;23(02):166–73. https://doi.org/10.1017/s1049023x0000580x.

Gausche-Hill M. Pediatric disaster preparedness: are we really prepared? J Trauma. 2009;67(2 Suppl):S73–6. https://doi.org/10.1097/ta.0b013e3181af2fff.

Jen H, Shew S, Atkinson J, Rosenthal T, Hiatt J. Creation of inpatient capacity during a major hospital relocation. Accessed JAMA Surg. 2016;151(4):393–4. https://doi.org/10.1001/jamasurg.2015.4417.

Kaiser Family Foundation. 2019. https://www.kff.org/other/state-indicator/distribution-by.age.

Kelly F. Keeping PEDIATRICS in pediatric disaster management: before, during and in the after-math of complex emergencies. Crit Care Nurs Clin North Am. 2010;22(04):465–80.

Kim DH. Emergency preparedness and the development of health care coalitions. Nurs Clin N Am. 2016;51(4):545–54. https://doi.org/10.1016/j.cnur.2016.07.013.

Mace MS, Doyle MC, Fuchs MS, Gausche-Hill MM, Koenig MK, Sorrentino MA, Johnson MR. Pediatric patients in a disaster: part of the all-hazard, comprehensive approach to disaster management. Am J Disaster Med. 2012;7(2):111–25. https://doi.org/10.5055/ajdm.2012.0087.

Rozenfeld R, Reynolds S, Ewing S, Crulcich M, Stephenson M. Development of an evacuation tool to facilitate disaster preparedness: use in a planned evacuation to support a hospital move. Disaster Med Public Health Prep. 2017;11(4):479–86. https://doi.org/10.1017/dmp.2016.154.

The Joint Commission. Improving patient and worker safety: opportunities for synergy, collabora-tion and innovation. Oakbrook Terrace: The Joint Commission; 2012. http://www.jointcom-mission.org/.

Emergency and Disaster Nursing in Schools

14

Robin Adair Shannon

14.1 Introduction

Approximately 56.6 million children attend school in the U.S., spending more waking time during the week at school than at home (National Center for Education Statistics 2018). Parents entrust schools to be safe environments for their children to grow and learn. Yet all schools are at risk for a devastating event. Natural threats include severe events such as tornados, hurricanes, floods, extreme temperatures, wildfires, earthquakes, tsunamis, landslides, and even volcanic eruptions. Potential technical hazards include explosions, accidental release of industrial toxins or hazardous material spills, gas leaks, dam failures, and radiation exposure from a nuclear power station accident. Highly infectious disease outbreaks and pandemics and contaminated food outbreaks represent biological hazards. Human-caused threats can be accidental (e.g., fires) or adversarial such as terrorist attacks, active shooter incidents, gang violence, bomb threats, and other criminal actions (U.S. Department of Education et al. 2013). When an emergency happens or disaster strikes at school, the lives of the students, their families, school staff, and the school community are indelibly altered.

Whether natural or man-made, predicted or unexpected, such crises challenge the school and local emergency medical services (EMS) capacity to respond. Emergency and disaster preparedness minimize injury, destruction, and loss of life. Though emergency and disaster preparedness represent overall readiness principles and strategies, the response to an emergency versus a disaster can differ in scope. In terms of public health, it is generally understood that an *emergency* refers to a dangerous event involving multiple people or casualties that can be handled at the local level. A *disaster* is a dangerous event involving the public that requires a

R. A. Shannon (✉)
Department of Health Systems Science, University of Illinois at Chicago College of Nursing, Chicago, IL, USA
e-mail: rshann2@uic.edu

© Springer Nature Switzerland AG 2020
C. J. Goodhue, N. Blake (eds.), *Nursing Management of Pediatric Disaster*,
https://doi.org/10.1007/978-3-030-43428-1_14

coordinated response by state, and sometimes national governmental agencies. In some instances, emergencies evolve into disasters. For the purposes of this chapter, the terms *critical event* or *incident,* or *crisis*, will be used when referring to any such dangerous event.

The unique needs of children during a crisis are often not prioritized. The Institute of Medicine of the National Academies of Science (Institute of Medicine of the National Academies of Science 2014) advocates for increased coordination between federal, state, regional, and local partner agencies and nurses and health care providers (HCPs) to improve pediatric medical care, care for students with special health care needs (CSHCN), and parent-child reunification during disasters, as well as improve mental health and social services for children and families during recovery. Yet, no coordinated national strategy to achieve these goals is in place, and nearly a third of all states do not meet the minimum standards for emergency planning for child care facilities and schools (Save the Children 2015). Although the majority of schools report that they have emergency policies and plans in place, these plans are insufficient in more than 1 in 4 schools, particularly in smaller and rural districts (Kruger et al. 2018). Schools must do more to protect the health and safety of their students and communities.

Nursing plays a central leadership role in emergency and disaster preparedness in health care and public health systems. School nurses, as public health nurses, are critical to crisis preparedness in the community setting of schools, interfacing with public health, emergency, hospital, and law enforcement agencies. The National Association of School Nurses (NASN) holds the position that "school nurses provide leadership in all phases of emergency preparedness and management and are a vital part of the school team that develops emergency response procedures for the school setting, using an all hazards approach" (National Association of School Nurses 2019) (para 1).

According to the White House, (White House, Office of the Press Secretary 2013) "The term" all-hazards" means a threat or an incident, natural or man-made, that warrants action to protect life, property, the environment, and public health or safety, and to minimize disruptions of government, social, or economic activities." An *all-hazards approach* ensures that schools and communities are ready to mount an effective response in the event of a crisis. This chapter outlines school emergency planning and operations and the role of school nursing in leading schools through all phases of a crisis: prevention/mitigation, preparedness, response, and recovery.

14.2 School Emergency and Disaster Preparedness

School emergency and disaster preparedness should align with *the National Incident Management System*, (U.S. Department of Homeland Security, Federal Emergency Management System 2017) which is a guiding framework for coordinating crisis planning and response across all levels of government through a comprehensive strategy for managing emergencies or disasters. The principles of the National

Incident Management System apply to both public schools as governmental bodies and private/parochial schools as community institutions responsible for the safety of their students and staff. This system lays out the structures of the *Incident Command System* and the roles of the *Incident Management Team* (United States Department of Homeland Security, Federal Emergency Management Agency 2017) in coordinating a unified, rapid, and effective response by partner agencies (e.g., FEMA, public health departments, law enforcement, emergency medical services, HCPs and hospitals, relief agencies, etc.).

14.2.1 The School Emergency Operations Team

The *School Emergency Operations Team* (school EOT) is part of this larger incident command structure. Even when the crisis does not occur on school grounds, schools often play crucial roles as central community institutions, serving as hubs for emergency communications, triage, shelter, food, clothing and resource distribution, immunizations, crisis counseling, and other forms of support.

In a collaborative endeavor, The U.S. Department of Education, Department of Health and Human Services, Department of Homeland Security, Department of Justice, the FBI, and FEMA created A *Guide for Developing High-quality School Emergency Operations Plans* (U.S. Department of Education et al. 2013) to support schools in developing effective preparedness, response, and recovery processes (https://rems.ed.gov/docs/REMS_K-12_Guide_508.pdf). This guide lays out the following principles underlying the development of a comprehensive school Emergency Operations Plan (school EOP).

- Planning must be supported by leadership. At the district and school levels, senior-level officials can help the planning process by demonstrating strong support for the planning team.
- Planning uses assessment to customize plans to the building level. Effective planning is built around a comprehensive, ongoing assessment of the school community. Information gathered through assessment is used to customize plans to the building level, taking into consideration the school's unique circumstances and resources.
- Planning considers all threats and hazards. The planning process takes into account a wide range of possible threats and hazards that may impact the school. Comprehensive school emergency management planning considers all threats and hazards throughout the planning process, addressing safety needs before, during, and after an incident.
- Planning provides for the access and functional needs of the whole school community. The "whole school community" includes children, individuals with disabilities, and others with special health care needs, those from religiously, racially, and ethnically diverse backgrounds, and people with limited English proficiency.

- Planning considers all settings and all times. School EOPs must account for incidents that may occur during and outside the school day as well as on and off campus (e.g., sporting events, field trips).
- Creating and revising a model Emergency Operations Plan is done through a collaborative process. This guide provides a process, plan format, and content guidance that are flexible enough for use by all school Emergency Planning Teams. If a planning team also uses templates, it must first evaluate their usefulness to ensure the tools do not undermine the collaborative initiative and collectively shared plan. There are some jurisdictions that provide templates to schools, and these will reflect state and local mandates, as applicable (U.S. Department of Education et al. 2013).

The composition of the school Emergency Operations Team depends upon the size, unique culture, and potential risks of the school community. School Emergency Operation Team members must be willing to serve and possess area expertise, strong leadership and communication skills, and a steady demeanor in stressful situations. The school nurse assumes a leadership role as the school health expert and serves as a student advocate and liaison between the school, first responders and EMS, HCPs, and public health authorities (National Association of School Nurses 2019). School Emergency Operations Teams also typically include school administrators, administrative assistants, teacher representatives, school psychologists, social workers, counselors, as well as facility, transportation, and food managers. One or more team members should be appointed to represent the school in local/regional interagency emergency operations collaborations.

14.2.2 The School Emergency Operations Plan

The school EOP is based upon an understanding, identification, and likelihood of possible threats and hazards (U.S. Department of Education et al. 2013). Therefore, the school Emergency Operations Team should conduct a thorough risk assessment that carefully examines past critical incidents, current potential threats and hazards, and the probable severity, predictability, and duration of the identified risks. Strengths and weakness should be assessed to address the vulnerabilities of the school grounds, available resources, and functional capacities. Figure 14.1 depicts the steps in developing the school Emergency Operations Plans that are outlined in detail within A *Guide for Developing High-quality School Emergency Operations* (U.S. Department of Education et al. 2013).

The outline for a basic school EOP includes the following sections:

- Introductory Materials: administrative information; approvals, table of contents.
- Purpose and Situation Overview: a statement of the intent of the plan and why it is necessary.
- Concept of Operations: Identifies lines of authority, processes to coordinate with other responding agencies, required resources, and primary actions to be by taken before, during, and after the crisis.

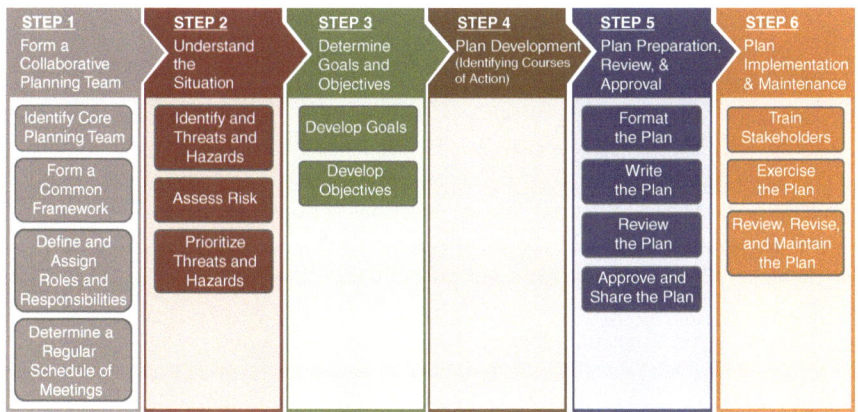

Fig. 14.1   Steps in school Emergency Operations Planning. (*Source:* USDE, USDHHS, USDHS, FBI, FEMA (2013))

- Organization and Assignment of Responsibilities: Outlines the general roles and responsibilities during an emergency of specific school staff (e.g., school district leaders, principals, teachers, nurses, administrative staff, and other student support personnel [counselors, social workers, psychologists, school resource officers, instructional aides, maintenance staff, cafeteria workers, bus drivers]), and school-related community-based organizations or parent-teacher organizations.
- Direction, Control, and Coordination: Describes the school incident command structure; the command and authority structure between the school EOP, the school district, and the emergency management system of the community; and who controls the equipment and supplies.
- Information Collection, Analysis, and Dissemination: Describes how to gather information before, during, and after the crisis that the community needs to know; outlines who will share this information and how.
- Training and Exercises: Outlines the training exercises and drills (e.g., school fire, tornado, shelter-in-place, lockdown, active shooter, wider community disaster with coordinating agencies, etc.) that test the school's EOP and practice readiness; sets the schedule of the frequency of drills and training exercises.
- Plan Development and Maintenance: Details the school EOP-planning process, team roles and responsibilities, and cycle of review and revision.
- Authorities and References: Outlines the school EOP chain of command and next in charge; lists the legal foundations of the EOP (e.g., laws, statutes, rules and regulations, executive orders, and interagency agreements).
- Functional Annexes: Contains documents detailing the emergency operation functions and actions that may be carried out during critical incidents.
  - Evacuation Annex
  - Shelter-in-place Annex
  - Lockdown; Accounting for all Persons Annex
  - Communications and Warning Annex

- Family Reunification Annex (includes family notification of missing, injured, or killed loved one)
- Continuity of School Operations Annex
- Recovery Annex
- Public Health, Medical, and Mental Health Annex
- Security Annex
- Threat and Hazard Specific Annex (describes actions specific to particular critical hazard, e.g., active shooter, bomb threat, explosion, tornado, earthquake, pandemic, etc.) (U.S. Department of Education et al. 2013).

The U.S. Department of Homeland Security and FEMA (n.d.) offers a *Multihazard Emergency Planning for Schools Toolkit* with resources such as training materials, sample forms, checklists, exercises, and drills (https://training.fema.gov/programs/emischool/el361toolkit/start.htm) (United States Department of Homeland Security, Federal Emergency Management Agency n.d.). The National Education Association offers guidance for schools at the local level, *School crisis guide: Help and healing in a time of crisis* (http://www.nea.org/assets/docs/NEA%20School%20Crisis%20Guide%202018.pdf) (National Education Association 2018).

Each school must predetermine a method for clearly and concisely communicating to everyone in the school the nature and location of the threat or hazard and actions that all staff and students should take. Codes and signals that are not universally understood should be avoided (e.g., "Code Gray" for an aggressive person). The announcement should specifically but calmly name the nature and location of the threat (e.g., "Man in a black coat shooting in the library!") (Selekman and Melvin 2017). Schools must collaborate with the agencies in the local incident command system to make sure that shared terminology is adopted. Emergency drills reinforce readiness skills for the students and staff at periodic intervals. The I Love You Guys Foundation (I Love U Guys Foundation 2015) developed uniform school responses to critical incidents for kindergarten through 12th grade schools that represent common crisis procedures commonly used by EMS, police, and schools. This *standard response protocol* stipulates four actions to take immediately:

- LOCKDOWN: Used for a threat inside the school building, such as intruders or active shooters. An announcement is made over the public address system: "Lockdown! Lock doors, Lights off, Out of Sight!".
- LOCKOUT: Used for a threat outside the building such as criminal activity or civil disobedience. The perimeter of the school is secured by the designated school Emergency Operation Team members.
- EVACUATE: Used when school occupants need to move to another location such as in the event of a fire, bomb threat, or internal hazardous material exposure. The secure location to which to evacuate is clearly stated.
- SHELTER: Used in the event of tornados, earthquakes, or external hazardous material exposure. The specific hazard and safety actions are announced. School occupants may need to move to a shelter area in the school, seal the room, seek higher ground, or drop and cover where they are.

14.2.2.1   Active Shooters

Tragically, school shootings have become increasingly and appallingly common in the U.S. As of May 2019, it is calculated that in the 20 years since two students took 19 innocent lives by gunfire at Columbine High School in Colorado in 1999, more than 223,000 children in 234 schools have been exposed to gun violence at school; 144 individuals have died and 302 have been injured (Cox et al. 2019). Sandy Hook Elementary School (26 deaths), Marjory Stoneman Douglas High School (17 lives), and the senseless loss of so many children, teachers, and staff at so many schools have changed the national narrative forever. Since these tragic events, the number of school shootings, casualties, and deaths continues to grow. Now every school community must prepare to avert and respond to the horrific possibility of an active shooter, as well as recover from the subsequent physical and psychological trauma.

For active shooter or dangerous intruder incidents, the U.S. Department of Homeland Security (2017) recommends that schools employ the response protocol: "RUN, HIDE, FIGHT!" More information can be found at www.ready.gov/active-shooter. Some school and law enforcement districts have adopted the response protocol for active shooters, ALICE, (ALICE Training Institute 2019) which stands for "Alert, Lockdown, Inform, Counter, Evacuate." ALICE is a proprietary product that includes fees for blended online and in-person training programs.

The school must be careful that drills adequately prepare the staff and students for the event of an active intruder; however, mock shooter exercises can be upsetting. Drills should not be so realistic as to cause emotional pain. During a mock event, the sight and sounds of guns and gun fire can be traumatic for some individuals, especially for those who have been exposed to gun violence (National Association of School Psychologists and National Association of School Resource Officers 2017). It must be made clear prior to the exercise that it is only a drill. Parents should be notified of the scheduled drill and given an "opt out" choice if they believe it will be too much for their child to handle.

No matter what the critical incident is, it is imperative that schools have a system to account for all students, staff, and visitors during and after the incident. Each teacher should have a roster of the students in their class(es) so that an accurate accounting of who is and is not present with the teacher can be made. Debriefing after drills identifies gaps in preparedness and areas for improvement. Schools must also have a well-thought out means to inform loved ones, school staff, teachers, and the media of the conditions of the ill, injured, or deceased.

14.2.2.2   Pandemics

Pandemics deserve special mention because communicable disease outbreaks can surface rapidly, affect large numbers of people, and can be life-threatening. According to the Centers for Disease Control and Prevention (CDC), (Centers for Disease Control and Prevention 2016) pandemics happen when a novel virus is highly contagious or when a vaccine may not be available or available in large quantities. Populations who have not or choose not to be vaccinated are at risk for serious preventable communicable diseases.

As seen by recent outbreaks in the U.S. of pertussis, measles, varicella, and mumps, unprotected children and the elderly are especially vulnerable to becoming extremely ill or dying. Thousands of people die annually from "the flu." Maria Pappas, a school nurse in New York City, was the first to alert health department officials about large numbers of ill students in her parochial school, which turned out to be the beginning of the H1N1 pandemic in 2009 (Pappas 2011). School communities must be prepared for large numbers of ill students, family members, and school personnel. Normal school operations, as well as the local health care workforce, can quickly become incapacitated.

The CDC's *Pandemic Flu Plan* (Centers for Disease Control and Preventions, U.S. Department of Health and Human Services 2017) informs communities' efforts to prevent and reduce the spread of communicable disease outbreaks. The school nurse takes a lead role as the school health expert and liaison between the school and the public health department in prevention and mitigation efforts (Shannon and Guilday 2019). The school nurse can be charged with collecting disease surveillance data; for example—the number of students presenting or absent with influenza-like illness. During an outbreak, recommendations from the CDC can change rapidly. It is incumbent upon the school nurse to stay updated and present clear and concise information in layman's terms to school administrators, educational staff, families, and students. Pertinent materials and fact sheets can be accessed from the CDC or state health departments.

The school nurse minimizes the risk of outbreaks by instructing students and staff on proper hand hygiene, how to "cover your cough," and when to stay home when ill. When the eruption of a communicable disease is suspected, the school nurse triages and isolates ill individuals and makes referrals for medical evaluation and treatment as indicated. During an outbreak, public health departments may call on schools to be a mass immunization site, in which case the school nurse is integral to organizing this "all hands on deck" approach.

14.3   The Role of the School Nurse in Emergency and Disasters

Nurses will recognize that the steps of the *nursing process* in care planning parallel the steps of Emergency Operations Planning. After the Emergency Operations Team is formed (Step 1), *assessment* guides an understanding (or *diagnosis*) of the situation (Step 2). Goals and objectives *identify the outcomes* of emergency operations (Step 3). *Planning* and preparation (Steps 4 and 5) finalize the plan and get ready to activate the *intervention*. And finally, implementation and maintenance (Step 6) set up a continuous cycle of *evaluation* (Shannon and Guilday 2019). It is the role of school nurses to anticipate and prepare for a worst-case scenario at school. The thought of harm coming to school and injuring innocent children and staff, in what is essentially their second home, is anxiety producing. The nurse has to imagine the unimaginable. The responsibility to be ready before and act quickly during and after a dangerous incident weighs heavily on the minds and hearts of all school nurses. School nurse leadership in emergency and disaster preparedness increases competence and role models' calm and professional conduct. As advocates for student safety, the presence of a school nurse instills in the school community a sense of confidence and trust that they are in capable hands. Unfortunately, one-quarter of schools in the U.S. do not have a school nurse, leaving those school populations even more vulnerable (Willgerodt and Brock 2016).

14.3.1 Preparedness

In addition to being a leading member of the school Emergency Operations Team, the school nurse has many responsibilities to adequately prepare for a critical event. A primary responsibility of the school nurse is to stay up to date with current best practices in prehospital emergency care. Fortunately, there are many relevant resources available. Knowing how to respond to individual emergencies increases readiness to respond to mass casualties. The Illinois Emergency Medical Services for Children's *Guidelines for the nurse in the school setting (3rd ed.)* is an excellent free manual with concise and thorough systematic assessment and triage tools (including mass casualty triage) and school nurse protocols for responding to acute illness and injury at school (Willgerodt and Brock 2016). The school nurse protocols consist of emergency algorithms for *emergent, urgent, and nonurgent* triage categories for a host of emergency conditions (e.g., seizures, respiratory distress, toxic exposure, syncope/unconsciousness, violent behavior) and trauma (e.g., burns, chest, head and spinal cord, hemorrhage, lacerations, musculoskeletal, ear, eye, nose, and throat).

School Emergency Triage Training (SETT) is a live (in-person) or online program offered by the National Association of School Nurses (NASN) (Illinois Emergency Medical Services for Children 2017). "The purpose of SETT is to provide school nurses with the knowledge, skills, and training resources to lead school-based Disaster Response Teams and perform triage in response to mass casualty incident (MCI) events" (National Association of School Nurses 2017a). This continuing education program is designed to give school nurses competency in leading school first aid teams and directing first responders at scenes with multiple victims, and is available at https://www.nasn.org/programs/conferences/sett.

The school nurse should also ensure that a core group of school personnel receive training in first responder skills such as first aid, CPR/AED certification, and stopping severe bleeding. In trauma victims, the leading cause of death is hemorrhagic shock due to uncontrolled bleeding. *Stop the Bleed* is a national campaign to teach as many people as possible "to become trained, equipped, and empowered to help in a bleeding emergency before professional help arrives" (U.S. Department of Homeland Security n.d.). Stop the Bleed actions include: (1) apply pressure with the hands, (2) apply dressing and press, and (3) apply tourniquet(s). Increasingly, schools are making tourniquets part of their rescue equipment, along with automatic external defibrillators.

The school nurse must have the requisite emergency medical triage and treatment supplies at the ready in case of a critical incident. Emergency supplies and equipment must be kept secure but readily accessible in the school health office. On large campuses, extra supplies may need to be appropriated to different parts of the facility. The school nurse maintains a portable *Go Bag* (or rolling *Go Box*) with the essential triage and aid supplies (National Association of School Nurses 2017b) (Box 14.1). Supplies should be checked routinely (at least annually) for integrity and expiration dates. The school EOP should designate a staff member to assist the school nurse if needed supplies cannot be carried alone.

Box 14.1 Recommended Contents for a *School Nurse Emergency Go Bag*

- Ace bandage(s) (various sizes)
- Alcohol wipes
- Band-aids various sizes, latex free
- Biohazard bags
- Blood pressure cuffs (pediatric and adult size)
- Blunt scissors
- Disposable tweezers
- Emesis bags
- Electronic pulse oximetry
- Face masks (N-95 and regular face masks)
- Eye irrigation
- Eye pads
- Eye protection (goggles, face shield)
- First aid tape (various sizes, latex free)
- Gauze (various sizes: 4 × 4, 2 × 2, etc.)
- Glucose monitor with strips
- Hand sanitizer
- Hand soap
- Instant cool/heat packs
- Latex-free gloves
- Normal saline solution
- One-way resuscitation mask
- Pen(s)/Pencil(s)
- Resealable plastic bags
- Source for quick-acting glucose (i.e., glucose tablets, cake-make gel)
- Stethoscope
- Tourniquet(s)
- Triage tags and triage forms for documentation

Source: Adapted from NASN (2017b)

The school nurse should have a portable long-distance radio with a designated frequency to communicate with other school Emergency Operation Team members if land line or cellular telephone communications are disrupted. Schools should have evacuation equipment to safely move injured students or ones with impaired mobility down the stairs or from upper floors if elevators cannot be accessed (National Association of School Nurses 2019). Students who speak English as a second language should be spoken to in their primary language or assigned a trusted adult to assist them. Students should not be assigned the responsibility of other students during a critical event.

14.3.1.1   Students with Special Health Care Needs

All Emergency Operation Plans must be compliant with the Americans with Disabilities Act (1990) (Americans with Disabilities Act of 1990 (P.L. 110-325) n.d.). In case of evacuation or relocation of students, the school nurse maintains a method for retrieving and transporting medications, equipment, and supplies that are prescribed for students with special health care needs. It is essential that a well-thought out plan is in place to ensure students receive necessary medications and treatments, particularly for potentially life-threatening conditions such as diabetes, asthma, anaphylaxis, and seizure disorders. The school nurse maintains an emergency folder with hardcopy lists of students with special health care needs and their medical orders must be kept at the ready. The folder should contain the students' medical orders, individualized health care plans, and emergency action plans, as indicated. Extra copies are advised to share with school administrators and EMS personnel as indicated.

The school nurse should make sure that students always have at least 72 hours of medications and supplies in case of an extended shelter-in-place (National Association of School Nurses 2019). Additionally, the school nurse should collaborate with families to secure HCP orders and medications that are needed around the clock for students with complex medical needs. The function and capacity of oxygen tanks should be regularly checked and maintained. Back-up battery power is required for students who are dependent upon electrical durable medical equipment, such as ventilators, in the event of evacuation or power outage (National Association of School Nurses 2019).

The school nurse is responsible for training the teachers and/or school paraprofessionals or designated school personnel who are designated to care for a student's special health care needs during a crisis (National Association of School Nurses 2019). A student's emergency action plan may stipulate that extra medication, supplies, and special diets or tube feedings be kept by the teacher, carried by the student (if developmentally appropriate), or stored in the school office. Students with significant physical, cognitive, or communication disabilities require individualized evacuation plans. An alarm or communication system should be in place to assist students with visual or auditory impairments (National Association of School Nurses 2019). Special consideration and assistance should be given to students with sensory integration issues, autism, and mental health disorders who are prone to being easily overwhelmed.

14.3.2 Response

The role of the school nurse during a critical event is to triage, treat, and lead the designated school personnel trained to give aid until the scene is controlled by emergency medical services and law enforcement agencies. Once it is safe to do so, the immediate response of the school nurse is to take the *Go Box* to the scene and rapidly triage the ill and injured victims. A quick across-the-scene scan directs the experienced school nurse where to concentrate her/his efforts. The school personnel should be directed to remove the "walking wounded" to a designated safe location. It is prudent for a lead school Emergency Operations Team member to have a bull-horn to help direct the rescue efforts until EMS and the police arrive and have control of the situation (e.g., "REMAIN CALM. STOP THE BLEED").

The school nurse communicates directly with EMS once they are on the scene and communicates the known triage information. As time allows, as much student specific information should be imparted as possible.

The school nurse then begins rapid triage according to the set protocol. In a mass casualty situation, the *START* (Simple Triage and Rapid Treatment) and Jump*START* triage algorithms are effective in the school setting because they are easy to learn, can be performed quickly, and include quick stabilization actions such as opening the airway or stopping hemorrhage (U.S. Department of Health and Human Services 2017a, b). *START* applies to victims who "look like an adult," and Jump*START* is applied to victims who "look like a child." These two different algorithms recognize that in children, respiratory failure typically precedes circulatory failure, whereas respiratory failure usually follows circulatory failure or traumatic brain injury in adults.

Casualties are triaged into one of four categories and assigned a severity level (or color):

- EXPECTANT (BLACK): The victim's injuries are not likely survivable due to severity or level of available treatment (dead or mortally wounded). Provide palliative care and pain relief as possible.
- IMMEDIATE (RED): The victim's injuries (including compromised airway, breathing, and circulation) require immediate intervention and transport (emergent).
- DELAYED (YELLOW): The victim's injuries are serious but not immediately life-threatening or expected to deteriorate. Does not require immediate transport but requires treatment within hours (urgent).
- MINOR (GREEN): The victim's injuries are minor and do not require EMS transport (nonemergent/nonurgent) (U.S. Department of Health and Human Services 2017a, b).

A tagging system can be used to clearly denote each victim's triage category. Triplicate pads can be used to preserve a copy for the school nurses' records, as it may be difficult or impossible to document during a chaotic event. Triage categories can be written in marker on the victim in a place clearly visible to EMS.

At the scene, law enforcement will secure the area. A representative from the school Emergency Operations Team, typically an administrator, interfaces with other agency leaders in the incident command system. School representatives are sent to the hospitals to be with transported victims. The families of the ill or injured are notified as soon as possible. An accounting for all students and staff is priority. Uninjured students or those with minor injuries are reunified with their families. When time allows after the event, the school nurse thoroughly documents the event as accurately as possible to provide continuity of care and facilitate communications. As with any nurse's note in a medical record, the school nurse's documentation is a legal record. Documentation includes an accurate and objective description of the event, the care provided, and follow-up actions.

14.3.3 Recovery

It is essential for the school Emergency Operations Team to debrief as soon as feasible after the crisis to support each other, make an accounting of the event, decide what immediate actions are necessary, and configure next steps toward recovery. Ideally, debriefings are conducted by a school district leader or objective facilitator. Clear messages to the families and school community are crafted. Subsequent debriefings should be held to carefully evaluate the effectiveness of the school EOP and make improvements going forward.

Immediately following the crisis, the school may not be accessible or may be a center for community recovery operations. An alternate physical space for the students to learn may need to be arranged. It is necessary to allow ample time off for students and staff to come together as a community and attend funerals, if necessary. However optimally, the infrastructure and routines of the school should resume to the fullest extent possible, as quickly as possible, to promote a sense of unity and resiliency in students and the school community. Outside crisis and grief counseling should be made immediately available to provide psychological first aid for the students and staff alike. Crisis and grief counseling should be conducted by qualified professionals. It is important to note that neither school nurses nor teachers should not be responsible for immediate post-crisis counseling, nor are they qualified to give therapeutic support to children experiencing severe difficulties with grief, guilt, or other mental health symptoms. Please refer to Chap. 12 for a more detailed discussion on post-disaster effects.

That said, children look to their teachers to give them guidance on how to deal with their stress after the crisis (National Association of School Psychologists 2016). Helping children to recover emotionally should be developmentally appropriate. According to the National Association of School Psychologists, typical reactions experienced by children depend upon the developmental stage:

- Preschool—Regressive behaviors, decreased verbalization, increased anxiety.
- Elementary—Poor attention/concentration, school avoidance, irritability, clinginess, aggression, somatic complaints, nightmares, social withdrawal.
- Middle and High School—Sleeping and eating disturbances, agitation, increase in conflicts, physical complaints, delinquent behavior, and poor concentration (National Association of School Psychologists 2016).

Teachers should be given appropriate shared language to use to help their students cope. School nurses can role model successful strategies to help children heal. Such strategies include: maintain a calm and reassuring demeanor; acknowledge the children's feelings are normal; encourage conversation about the event; teach positive coping skills; and reinforce the student's resiliency. Individuals should make their own needs a priority. Obviously, students and staff should avoid using drugs and alcohol as a coping mechanism (National Association of School Psychologists 2016).

Schools are challenged with the difficult task of acknowledging that things will never quite be the same while working to establish the "new normal." Resources for psychological support for students and staff must be provided indefinitely in recognition that there is no typical timeline for recovery after a traumatic event. The school nurse may anticipate an increased number of health office visits from students with somatic complaints secondary to anxiety, depression, and sleep disturbances in the aftermath of the crisis.

14.4   Conclusion

Students and families expect their schools to be protective and caring, learning environments. But natural or man-made emergencies and disasters can strike any school, potentially endangering lives, causing destruction, disrupting student learning, and changing the lives of everyone touched by the event. Schools must be prepared. A qualified school team is tasked with informed risk assessment and thorough school Emergency Operations Planning as part of the local incident command system. As public nurses and the trusted health professional at school, school nurses play a leadership role in emergency and disaster prevention and mitigation, preparedness, response, and recovery on behalf of the better health and safety of children and school communities.

References

ALICE Training Institute [Internet]. ALICE: alert, lockdown, inform, counter, evacuate. 2019. [Cited 2019 Sept 25]. https://www.alicetraining.com/training-options/organization-certification/.

Americans with Disabilities Act of 1990 (P.L. 110-325) [Internet]. n.d. https://www.gpo.gov/fdsys/pkg/PLAW-110publ325/html/PLAW-110publ325.htm.

Centers for Disease Control and Prevention [Internet]. Pandemic basics. 2016. [Cited 2019 Sept 25]. https://www.cdc.gov/flu/pandemic-resources/basics/index.html.

Centers for Disease Control and Preventions, U.S. Department of Health and Human Services [Internet]. CDC pandemic influenza plan: 2017 update. 2017. [Cited 2019 Sept 25]. https://www.cdc.gov/flu/pandemic-resources/pdf/pan-flu-report-2017v2.pdf.

Cox J, Rich S, Chiu A, Muyskens J, Ulmanu M. [Internet]. More than 228,000 students have experienced gun violence at school since Columbine. The Washington Post. 2019. [Cited 2019 May 8]. https://www.washingtonpost.com/graphics/2018/local/school-shootings-database/?utm_term=.e564d2169cbf.

I Love U Guys Foundation [Internet]. The standard response protocol K12: operational guidance for schools, districts, and agencies. 2015. [Cited 2019 Sept 25]. http://iloveuguys.org/srp/SRP%20K12%20Operation%20Guidelines%202015.pdf.

Illinois Emergency Medical Services for Children [Internet]. Guidelines for the nurse in the school setting. 3rd ed. 2017. https://ssom.luc.edu/media/stritchschoolofmedicine/emergencymedicine/emsforchildren/documents/resources/practiceguidelinestools/Guidelines%20 for%20the%20Nurse%20in%20the%20School%20Setting%203rd%20Edition%20April%20 2017%20Final.pdf.

Institute of Medicine of the National Academies of Science [Internet]. Preparedness, response, and recovery considerations for children and families: workshop summary. 2014. [Cited 2019 Sept 25]. https://www.nap.edu/read/18550/chapter/1.

Kruger J. Brener N, Leeb R, Wolkin A, Avchen RN, Dziuban E. [Internet]. School district crisis preparedness, response, and recovery plans—United States, 2006, 2012, and 2016. Morb Mortal Wkly Rep. 2018;67(30):809–14. [Cited 2019 Sept 25]. https://doi.org/10.15585/mmwr. mm6730a1.

National Association of School Nurses [Internet]. School emergency triage training (SETT). 2017a. [Cited 2019 Sept 25]. https://www.nasn.org/programs/conferences/sett.

National Association of School Nurses. School emergency triage training (SETT): a program for school nurses instructor manual. Silver Springs: Author; 2017b. [Cited 2019 Sept 25].

National Association of School Nurses [Internet]. Position statement: emergency preparedness. 2019. [Cited 2019 Sept 25]. https://www.nasn.org/nasn/advocacy/professional-practice-documents/ position-statements/ps-emergency-preparedness.

National Association of School Psychologists [Internet]. Natural disasters: brief tips and facts. 2016. [Cited 2019 Sept 25]. http://www.nasponline.org/resources-and-publications/resources/ school-safety-and-crisis/natural-disaster/natural-disasters-brief-facts-and-tips.

National Association of School Psychologists and National Association of School Resource Officers [Internet]. Best practice considerations for schools in active shooter and other armed assailant drills. Bethesda: National Association of School Psychologists; 2017. [Cited 2019 Sept 25]. https://www.nasponline.org/resources-and-publications/ resources-and-podcasts/school-climate-safety-and-crisis/systems-level-prevention/ best-practice-considerations-for-schools-in-active-shooter-and-other-armed-assailant-drills.

National Center for Education Statistics [Internet]. Fast facts: back to school statistics. 2018. [Cited 2019 Sept 25]. https://nces.ed.gov/fastfacts/display.asp?id=372.

National Education Association [Internet]. School crisis guide: help and healing in a time of crisis. 2018. [Cited 2019 Sept 25]. http://www.nea.org/assets/docs/NEA%20School%20Crisis%20 Guide%202018.pdf.

Pappas M. From local school nurse to national advocate. NASN Sch Nurse. 2011;26(3):180–2. https://doi.org/10.1177/1942602X11404559.

Save the Children [Internet]. The 2015 National report card on protecting children in disasters. 2015. [Cited Sept 25, 2019]. https://rems.ed.gov/docs/DisasterReport_2015.pdf.

Selekman J, Melvin J. Planning for a violent intruder event. NASN Sch Nurse. 2017;32(3):1–5. https://doi.org/10.1177/1942602X16686140.

Shannon RA, Guilday P. Emergency and disaster preparedness and response for schools. In: Selekman J, Shannon RA, Yonkaitis CF, editors. School nursing: a comprehensive text. 3rd ed. Philadelphia: F.A. Davis Company; 2019. p. 457–77.

U.S Department of Homeland Security [Internet]. Active shooter preparedness. 2017. [Cited 2019 Sept 25]. https://www.dhs.gov/active-shooter-preparedness.

U.S. Department of Education, U.S. Department of Health and Human Services, U.S. Department of Homeland Security, U.S. Department of Justice, Federal Bureau of Investigation, Federal Emergency Management Agency [Internet]. Guide for developing high-quality school emergency operations plans. 2013. [Cited 2019 Sept 25]. http://rems.ed.gov/docs/ REMS_K-12_Guide_508.pdf.

U.S. Department of Health and Human Services [Internet]. START adult triage algorithm. 2017a. [Cited 2019 Sept 25]. https://chemm.nlm.nih.gov/startadult.htm.

U.S. Department of Health and Human Services [Internet]. Chemical hazards emergency medical management, JumpSTART Pediatric Triage Algorithm. 2017b. [Cited 2019 Sept 25]. https:// chemm.nlm.nih.gov/startpediatric.htm#more.

U.S. Department of Homeland Security [Internet]. Stop the Bleed. n.d. [Cited 2019 Sept 25]. https://www.dhs.gov/stopthebleed.

U.S. Department of Homeland Security, Federal Emergency Management System [Internet]. National incident management system. 2017. [Cited 2019 Sept 25]. https://www.fema. gov/media-library-data/1508151197225-ced8c60378c3936adb92c1a3ee6f6564/FINAL_ NIMS_2017.pdf.

U.S. Department of Homeland Security, Federal Emergency Management Agency [Internet]. Incident management team. 2017. [Cited 2019 Sept 25]. https://emilms.fema.gov/IS700aNEW/ NIMS0105summary.htm.

U.S. Department of Homeland Security, Federal Emergency Management Agency [Internet]. Multihazard emergency planning for schools toolkit. n.d. [Cited 2019 Sept 25]. https://training.fema.gov/programs/emischool/el361toolkit/start.htm.

White House, Office of the Press Secretary [Internet]. Presidential policy directive—critical infrastructure security and resilience. 2013. [Cited 2019 Sept 25]. https://obamawhitehouse.archives. gov/the-press-office/2013/02/12/presidential-policy-directive-critical-infrastructure-security-and-resil.

Willgerodt M, Brock D. [Internet]. NASN school nurse workforce study: school nurses in the U.S. 2016. https://www.nasn.org/research/school-nurse-workforce.

Child Care Preparedness

Child Care Preparedness

Laura Prestidge

15.1   Child Care Preparedness

Many families in the U.S. depend on child care services. Access to child care services is vital, so parents/guardians can work and support their families. Other benefits of child care services include early education programs, providing children with nutritious meals/food, and providing social interactions. A significant number of children that are 6 years of age and younger are in the care of someone other than their parents/guardians during the day throughout the work week. It is estimated that approximately 32 million children (61% of children under the age of 6 years) attend some type of child care program during the week (Child Trends 2016). As seen in Table 15.1, there are three basic types of child care options (U.S. Office of Personnel Management n.d.; U.S. Department of Health and Human Services, Maternal and Child Health Bureau 2019). The decision as to which type to access is typically based on a variety of factors such as availability of services, type of staff and educational training, location, cost, the availability of financial assistance or subsidized funding, and for some, the program's ability to care for children with special health care needs (CSHCN), such as chronic medical conditions.

According to the U.S. Census data in 2011, almost 25% of children under the age of 5 years, who are in some type of child care program, attend a child care center, 7.6% are cared for in a child care home, and just under 4% are cared for by a non-relative in their own home (Laughlin 2013; U.S. Census Bureau 2011; Child Care Aware of America n.d.-a).

L. Prestidge (✉)
Mt Sinai Hospital, Emergency Department, Chicago, IL, USA

Texas A&M TEEX Program, College Station, TX, USA

Illinois EMSC, Consultant, Chicago, IL, USA
e-mail: lprestidge@luc.edu

© Springer Nature Switzerland AG 2020   331
C. J. Goodhue, N. Blake (eds.), *Nursing Management of Pediatric Disaster*,
https://doi.org/10.1007/978-3-030-43428-1_15

Table 15.1 Child care options (U.S. Office of Personnel Management n.d.; U.S. Department of Health and Human Services, Maternal and Child Health Bureau 2019)

Type	Description
Child care centers	A center that provides care for a group of children. Some centers also provide education to the children. The centers are staffed by caregivers who may be trained in early childhood education. These centers are either for profit individually owned or part of a chain of centers, or nonprofit agencies such as those associated with religious organizations, public schools, or governmental agencies. The size of the center and the number of children the center can accommodate vary and can range from just a few children to centers with multiple classrooms that can accommodate over a 100 children
Child care homes	In child care homes, a small group of children is cared for in the child care provider's home. Some child care homes also provide education to the children. These programs vary in size. Small child care homes provide care for 1–6 children, while large child care homes provide care to 7–12 children
Child care in the child's home	This type of child care occurs in the home of the child. The parents/guardians employ a caregiver who has experience with young children to care for their child in their own home. Examples of child care in their own home include babysitters, nannies, au pairs, or other types of caregivers

Throughout the remainder of this chapter, the term "child care center/home" will be used to encompass all types of child care centers and child care homes. In addition, it's important to note that disaster/emergency preparedness planning for child care in the child's own home should be addressed within each individual family's preparedness plan. Chapter 6 has additional information on family preparedness planning. Although some of the concepts within this chapter may apply to a family preparedness plan, there are several additional considerations that need to be addressed by child care centers/homes. Therefore, this chapter will focus on disaster/emergency preparedness specific to child care centers and child care homes rather than the components of a family preparedness plan (which would apply when a child care provider is hired to care for a child in their own home).

There are several laws, regulations, and ordinances at the local, state, and federal levels regarding child care preparedness that child care centers/homes need to be aware of and ensure are being addressed in their preparedness activities. Each state authorizes an agency that is responsible for licensing and overseeing child care services, as well as defining licensing criteria and requirements (Child Care Aware of America n.d.-a). Child care centers are usually required to be licensed in each state. An exception may be those child care centers that are affiliated with a religious organization. Child care homes may or may not require licensure, depending on the state requirements, size of the program, and the number of children they care for within their home. Child care in the child's own home does not require a license. Child care centers that serve children and families who qualify for subsidized federal funding through the Child Care and Development Fund (CCDF) program must meet additional standards outlined by the state and federal requirements (U.S. Department of Health and Human Services (HSS), Office of Child Care: An Office of the Administration for Children, and Families 2017). Requiring child care services to be licensed, regardless of their type and size, helps ensure standards are in place for health, safety, staff/child ratios, background checks on all staff members, sleep practices, food preparation, sanitation, and emergency preparedness plans. In addition, licensing allows the state agency to inspect the child care site to ensure compliance with those regulatory standards. For example, a recent study found that licensed child care centers were more likely to have a written disaster/emergency preparedness plan compared to child care homes (Lesser et al. 2019). Child care centers/homes must also consider other laws, ordinances, and regulations that they are required to comply with, such as local building codes and legal jurisdiction for health codes (U.S. Department of Health and Human Services, Maternal and Child Health Bureau 2019). The Individuals with Disabilities Education Act (IDEA), which was initially passed in 1975, ensures children with disabilities (CSHCN) are provided with free public education that is tailored to their individual needs. The Act, which initially addressed children and young adults aged 5–21 years, was expanded in 1983 to include children aged 3–5 years, and then further modified in 1997 to include birth to age two (U.S. Department of Health and Human Services, Maternal and Child Health Bureau 2019). The goal of expanding this Act to include children of all ages aims to improve the services and education for children with CSHCN and their families in child care settings and includes the child in all activities possible unless medically contraindicated (U.S. Department of Health and Human Services, Maternal and Child Health Bureau 2019). Additional information on CSHCN can be found in Chap. 8.

15.1.1 Why Children Are More Vulnerable

Children who attend child care centers/homes are one of the most vulnerable populations during a disaster/emergency. Because of their age (5 years old and younger) and developmental level, they have anatomical, physiological, developmental, and psychological features that increase their vulnerability before, during, and after a disaster/emergency. Note that many of these characteristics that make younger children more vulnerable are also seen in older children. Chapters 5 and 7 review these different characteristics that increase children's vulnerability in greater detail. Those who care for them, such as child care centers/homes, need to be prepared as best as possible, to protect the children they care for should a disaster/emergency occur.

15.1.2 History of Disaster/Emergency Preparedness for Child Care Centers/Homes

Child care centers/homes are responsible for the youngest and one of the most vulnerable populations and may be responsible for protecting these children should a disaster/emergency occur while children are in the care of the center/home. Similar to schools, access to child care is crucial to a community after a disaster/emergency during the recovery phase. Children returning to child care and/or school after a disaster/emergency provides them with a sense of routine and a safe environment that they need in order to begin coping. The availability of child care provides parents/guardians with an opportunity to return to work and conduct other recovery activities (Save the Children 2007; National Commission of Children and Disasters 2010). This contributes to the resiliency, recovery, and rebuilding of the community. In addition, resuming the normal routine of school and/or child care allows the reestablishment of a child's normal routine, which helps their coping mechanisms and mental healing process. The benefits of reestablishing child care as soon as possible after a disaster/emergency occurs help to affirm that child care services in the community are vital and are an essential service to the well-being and recovery of a community. In order for efficient reestablishment of child care services to be possible, child care center/homes disaster plans need to be in place to assist in not only the response to the actual incident but also to reestablish services after a disaster/emergency through their business continuity and recovery planning components.

With so much at risk and such clear benefits that child care services provide before, during, and after a disaster, it could be assumed that disaster/emergency planning is a priority and all child care centers/homes would ensure that these types of plans were in place. However, this is not always the case. Only recently was a federal standard specific to child care center preparedness adopted by Congress. In 2010, less than half of all states required child care centers to have evacuation, relocation, and/or family reunification plans and less than two-thirds of all states did not require a plan to address children with special needs (Save the Children 2010). The National Commission on Children and Disaster's 2010 Report to the President and Congress recommended that Congress and the U.S. Department of Health and Human Services (HHS) require states to include disaster planning and exercises/training in their child care licensure requirement; Congress provides HHS with the authority to require states to develop statewide child care disaster plans; and Congress and federal agencies should improve capacity to provide child care services after a disaster by changing child care to an essential service (National Commission of Children and Disasters 2010). The Child Care Development Block Grant Reauthorization Act of 2014 was passed by Congress and required that by September 2016, all states have a statewide disaster plan that addresses the needs of child care centers and require all regulated (licensed) child care centers to have disaster/emergency plans that address how to respond to emergency situations or natural disasters. The disaster/emergency plans need to include evacuation, lockdown or sheltering-in-place procedures, notification of parents/guardians during and after the disaster, reunification, and exercises/drills/trainings for staff on disaster/emergency plans (National Center on Early Childhood Quality Assurance 2016). The state plans need to address how the state will ensure the availability of safe child care, provision of emergency and temporary child care services, temporary operating standards for child care centers, and recovery of child care services after a disaster (Administration for Children, and Family, Office of Child Care 2017). In 2014, prior to the enactment of the Child Care Development Block Grant Reauthorization Act of 2014, only 57% of the states required staff in licensed child care centers to undergo training in disaster/emergency preparedness and five states required training on acts of violence (e.g., active shooter) or terrorism (National

Center on Early Childhood Quality Assurance 2016). Although 31 states required licensed child care centers to have a disaster plan for natural disasters, only 3 states required plans for acts of violence (e.g., active shooter) (National Center on Early Childhood Quality Assurance 2016).

Although the Child Care Development Block Grant Reauthorization Act of 2014 is leading to increased child care preparedness, as a whole, gaps still exist. The Child Care Development Block Grant requirements only apply to those child care centers/homes that are federally subsidized. Many state child care regulatory requirements do not apply to all types of child care settings. Some state regulations only apply to licensed child care centers and not to child care homes. Due to the number of child care centers/homes that exist in each state, it can be a challenge for state regulatory agencies to verify that all child care centers/homes are compliant with the requirements, the extent that these requirements are met, and that staff at each child care center/home are adequately trained on all of the requirements. In addition, there is no regulatory statute that requires families to have a preparedness plan when their children are cared for within their own home by a nonrelative provider. This leaves many children at risk during and after a disaster.

15.1.3 Emergency Management Process and Child Care Centers/Homes

All child care centers/homes need to be aware of key components that should be incorporated into their disaster plans. These components will be reviewed in this next section. It is important to stress that having a disaster and recovery plan in place is only one small part of the entire emergency management process. It is vital that child care agencies/settings participate in the entire process, not just writing a plan to meet state and federal requirements.

The emergency management process is a cyclical, continuous process that incorporates four components or phases: prevention/mitigation, preparation, response, and recovery. From the child care center/home perspective, the emergency management cycle and everything that is involved in it can be very daunting, intimidating, and difficult to incorporate into the hectic day-to-day responsibilities of owning and operating a child care service agency. Although there are many resources available to assist child care centers/homes with the process, it can still be difficult and challenging since child care providers typically lack any disaster/emergency planning experience. This lack of familiarity along with the complacency of "it won't happen to us, or in our community" are just two of the many contributing factors to the delay or absence of adopting the emergency management process.

15.1.3.1 Prevention/Mitigation
The prevention/mitigation phase includes those steps that the child care center/home should take to reduce their risk and effects of a disaster should one occur in their community or directly within the child care center/home location. Child care centers/homes should perform a hazard assessment to identify what types of

disasters/emergencies the child care center/home is most at risk for experiencing. There are many tools such as a Hazard Vulnerability Analysis (HVA) or a Threat and Hazard Identification and Risk Assessment (THIRA) that can help with the hazard assessment, especially those that are specifically designed and tailored to the uniqueness of the child care setting. Hazards can exist in or immediately surrounding the child care center/home, and/or in the neighborhood, community, and state where the child care center/home is located. It is important to consider all these areas when conducting the hazard assessment because the types of incidents that are most likely to occur will guide the emergency preparedness activities for the individual child care center/home (Administration for Children, and Family, Office of Child Care 2015; National Resource Center for Health and Safety in Child Care and Early Education n.d.-a; Illinois Emergency Medical Services for Children (EMSC) 2016). It is important to consider internal and external threats, natural disasters (e.g., flooding, hurricanes, tornadoes, and winter storms), and unintentional and intentional human-caused disasters (e.g., structure fires, gas leaks, violent intruders, active shooters, and terrorist incidents). This hazard assessment should also include the capabilities that the child care center/home has in place that would lessen or mitigate the effects of a disaster such as safety systems that are in place (e.g., sprinkler system, locked facility), a stockpile of extra supplies, or a van to transport the children.

Other examples of prevention/mitigation tasks for a child care center/home include:

- Review any existing disaster/emergency plans that are in place for the child care center/home to identify any changes that are needed.
- Identify and implement preventative/mitigation strategies for the hazards identified during the hazard assessment.
- Utilize the survey that was conducted during the hazard assessment for the child care center/home to identify any potentially dangerous items such as furniture, blinds, fixtures, outlets, windows, or any unsecure areas. Implement strategies to fix or adapt the environment to make the situation safer. For example, moving cribs, chairs, or other items that children can climb on away from window blinds so that children cannot access the cords within the blinds. Another example of a mitigation activity within the child care center/home is to mount furniture, televisions, book cases, bulletin boards, and other loose and heavy items to the wall to prevent injury.
- Identify resources that would be needed to implement actions within the disaster/ emergency plans and establish relationships within the community that can assist with providing resources during an incident. For example, a nearby child care center/home could contact the local school to determine if the school could serve as its primary or secondary evacuation point. Establishing a memorandum of understanding (MOU) or agreement with a local school bus company to provide transportation during an evacuation is another example of a prevention/mitigation activity for child care centers/homes. Figure 15.1 is an example of an MOU template that child care centers/homes could use.

Appendix 2: MOU Template for Child Care Centers/Child Care Homes

Introduction:

- This agreement will define the relationship, responsibilities, and obligations between the *Click here to enter child care center/ child care home name* and the *Click here to enter company/ agency/facility name that agreement is being made with.*
- The purpose of this MOU is to ensure that, in the event of a natural or human-generated disaster that calls for evacuation, the staff and children in the care of the *Click here to enter child care center/child care home name* may be efficiently evacuated from the *Click here to enter child care center/child care home name* site and tranported to saftey.

Authorities:

- The *Click here to enter child care center/child care home name* (hereinafter referred to as *"Click here to enter abbreviated child care center/child care home name, if applicable"* serves the child care needs of *Click here to enter age range/demographic information for attendees.*
- The *Click here to enter company/agency/facility name that agreement is being made with* (hereinafter referred to as *"click here to enter abbreviated company/agency/facility name that agreement is being made with, if applicable"* works to plan, develop, bulid, and operate *Click here to enter type of service this company provides* system in the *Click here to enter city/town name* area

Areas of Cooperation under the Terms of the Agreement:

- *Click here to enter company/agency/facility name that agreement is being made with* agrees to provide *Click here to enter type of service* for *Click here to enter abbreviated child care center/child care home name, if applicable* staff and children in the event of an evacuation. The management further agrees to provide *Click here to enter additional services.*
- *Click here to enter abbreviated child care center/child care home name, if applicable)* agrees to maintain responsibility for the presence and well-being of *clicks here to enter abbreviated child care center/child care home name, if applicable* staff and children. *Click here to enter abbreviated child care center/child care home name, if applicable* will maintain roll sheets and assemble staff and children for transport. Further, *Click here to enter abbreviated child care center/child care home name, if applicable* agrees to *Click here to enter additional responsibilities.*
- *Click here to enter company/agency/facility name that agreement is being made with* and *click here to enter abbreviated child care center/child care home name, if applicable* agree to mutually determine a list of potential *Click here to enter additional responsibilities and agreements.*

Insurance and Indemnification:

- Each participating organization will maintain independent/individual insurance coverage.
- *Click here to enter company/agency/facility name that agreement is being made with* will insure *Click here to enter coverage and responsibilities.*
- *Click here to enter abbreviated child care center/child care home name. if applicable* will be responsible for *Click here to enter coverage and responsibilities.*

Periodic Review of this Agreement:

- *Click here to enter how the progress of the terms of this MOU will be monitored.*
- *Click here to enter how often the review of this MOU will occur.*

Terms of Enforcement:

- This agreement shall become effective upon the execution by authorized individuals of both organizations. It shall continue with or without subsequent modification until it is terminated.
- Modification shall be by the same means as original execution.

Signature of company/agency/facility that agreement is being made with   Date

---

Signature of director from child care center/child care home   Date

Emergency Preparedness Planning Guide for Child Care Centers & Child Care Homes
2015

Fig. 15.1 MOU template for child care centers/child care homes from the Illinois Emergency Medical Services for Children's *Emergency Preparedness Planning Guide for Child Care Centers/ Child Care Homes* (2016) document

15.1.3.2 Preparedness

The preparedness phase of the emergency management cycle incorporates activities that will assist with responding to disasters/emergencies. It is during the preparedness phase that a disaster/emergency plan would be developed if the child care center/home does not already have such plans in place.

There are several steps that need to occur for a child care center/home to write its disaster/emergency plans.

1. Gather a group who will work on developing the plan. This should include key staff, directors of the child care center/home, nurse consultants (if applicable), and a consultant (if the child care center/home has chosen to hire one) to develop their plans.
2. Perform a hazard assessment to identify what types of disaster the child care center/home is most at risk for experiencing as reviewed in the Prevention/Mitigation section. If the child care center/home does not currently have any disaster/emergency plans in place, the hazard assessment will help prioritize the order in which to start plan development. Those hazards or incidents that the child care center/home are at most risk for experiencing should be the first plans that are developed and gradually expanded to include all hazards, disasters, and emergencies identified in the hazard assessment (National Resource Center for Health and Safety in Child Care and Early Education n.d.-a). See Fig. 15.2 for an example of a hazard assessment for child care centers.
3. Once the determination is made as to which plans need to be developed, the next step is to identify the goals of the response for each incident and build the response steps to meet the goals. The plan would consist of all the steps, procedures, and resources needed to accomplish the goals and objectives for each incident and within each plan. For example, if a child care center/home is developing their plan for an evacuation, the goal would be to evacuate all children and staff safely, obtain important documents to assist with business continuity prior to evacuating, and reunite all children with their parent/guardian. The plan itself would outline all the steps that need to occur in order to accomplish these goals in a safe and efficient manner.
4. After the draft plan is completed, it should be shared with those who will be involved in the response in order to gather feedback on the plan. Examples of who a child care center/home may share the plan with for review include parents/guardians, all child care center personnel/staff, child care referral agencies, regional emergency management agency, the state regulatory agency, and any other group that has identified roles within their plan (e.g., local school district, hospitals, or health care system). Once feedback is obtained, changes would be made to the plan and it can then be finalized. After the plans are developed, they should be reviewed periodically to ensure additional changes are not indicated. Typically, this is on a biannual basis and following any type of incident that led to the activation of any part of the plan (National Resource Center for Health and Safety in Child Care and Early Education n.d.-a). The frequency of this review should be clearly outlined in the plan as well.

Appendix 1: Child Care Center/Child Care Home Hazard Vulnerability Assessment Tool

Overall Assessment Questions:

What types of hazards exists within my building (e.g., heavy furniture that could topple, blocked exits, ordinary glass in windows, etc.) and what could be the consequences?

What types of hazards exist outside my building (e.g., rivers or ponds, open wells, power lines, gas pipelines, dead trees, etc.) and what could be the consequences?

What types of hazards exist in my neighborhood (e.g., rivers and ponds, chemical plants, highways where chemicals are transported, flood plain, power lines, gas pipelines, etc.) and what could be the consequences?

What type of weather extremes may occur in my region (e.g., blizzards, ice storms, high winds, tornadoes, earthquakes, flooding, etc.) and what could be the consequences?

What health issue do my staff/children have (e.g., asthma, diabetes, allergic reactions, limitations in mobility, etc.) and what could be the consequences?

What type of hazards may oocur in child care settings (e.g., missing children, intruders, etc.) and what could be the consequences?

Emergency Preparedness Planning Guide for Child Care Centers & Child Care Homes 2016

Fig. 15.2 Child care center hazard vulnerability assessment from the Illinois Emergency Medical Services for Children's *Emergency Preparedness Planning Guide for Child Care Centers/Child Care Homes* (2016) document

Internal Assessment Checklist

Mitigation Activity	Assessment Date
Are fire extinguishers properly charged, mounted securely, within easy reach?	
Do staff and volunteers know how to use the fire extinguishers properly?	
Are exits clear from obstructions such as locked doors, storage, or possible obstructions such as large nearby objects (i.e. bookcases, filing cabinets) that could fall and block the exit?	
Is a generator needed for back-up power? (A licensed electrician must install a generator)	
Are at least two individuals trained to start and operate the generator?	
Are appliances, cabinets, and shelves attached to the wall with wire or braced by being anchored together?	
Are heavy or sharp items stored on shelves with ledge barriers?	
Are blocks and heavy objects stored on the lowest shelves?	
Are television sets, fish bowls, and similar items restrained so they won't slide?	
Are pictures and other wall hangings attached to the wall with wire and closed screw-eyes?	
Are cribs located away from the tops of stairs and other places where rolling could endanger them or where heavy objects could fall on them?	
Are blackboards and bulletin boards securely mounted to the wall or hung safely from the ceiling?	
Are light weight panels, rather than shelving units or other tall furnishings, used to divide rooms?	
Are large window panes made of shatter resistant glass or covered with safety film?	
Is the street number of the home/building clearly and legibly visible from the roadway?	
In larger centers, is each internal/external door numbered or lettered for indentification?	
Do florescent lights have transparent sleeves to keep broken glass pieces from scattering?	
Are emergency lights in place and are exits clearly marked?	
Are there sign-in and sign-out procedures for everyone entering the building?	
Does the emergency shut off for the water supply and electric service supply have a sign placed next to the control that identifies it as the primary disconnecting/shutoff means?	
Is staff aware of where the emergency shut-offs are, how to operate them, what tools are needed and how to quickly access them?	
Are the building's area(s) of refuge, shelter-in-place locations and evacuation assembly areas marked on your posted floor plan?	
Have savings been set aside in case of a disaster to help financially with re-opening the business?	

Fig. 15.2 (continued)

Once the plans are developed, another key activity or component of the preparedness phase is to test the plans. Staff training on the child care center/home's disaster/emergency plans and procedures should occur through policy review, drills, and exercises. Drills/exercises should be conducted to: test the plans that are in place; identify areas for improvement within the existing plans; address the unique needs of the children at the child care center/home; test communication processes; utilize available supplies and equipment; and engage response partners such as emergency management agencies, fire departments, law enforcement, public health departments, and the state regulatory agency (National Resource Center for Health and Safety in Child Care and Early Education n.d.-a). Each state regulates the type and frequency of drills/exercises that must be conducted by child care centers/homes.

This is the minimum requirement, however, and child care centers/homes should consider conducting more frequent drills/exercises since the more practice that is completed on what to do in a disaster/emergency, the more comfortable and prepared staff will be to respond during a real disaster/emergency. Ideally, drills/exercises should be conducted monthly to ensure staff are familiar with the plans and know how they should respond to various disasters/emergencies (Administration for Children, and Family, Office of Child Care 2015; Illinois Emergency Medical Services for Children (EMSC) 2016). Children who attend the child care center/home and their parents/guardians should be included in the drills/exercises as appropriate. Talking with children in developmentally appropriate language and teaching them how to respond to different types of emergencies can help them respond appropriately during a real incident. Different scenarios should be used each month to ensure staff are prepared to respond to a variety of incidents. Conducting a debriefing session after each exercise can allow those that participated in providing valuable feedback on the plans and procedures that are outlined in the child care centers/homes disaster/emergency plan. Staff who are responsible for updating the plans can take that feedback and integrate changes into the disaster/emergency plans. A log should be maintained by the child care center/home of all the drills/exercises that are conducted, and the lessons learned from each drill (Illinois Emergency Medical Services for Children (EMSC) 2016). This log will help with tracking when and what type of scenarios were used with each drill/exercise in addition to providing documentation for the state regulatory agency that requirements for training are being met.

Child care centers/homes should develop a stockpile of emergency supplies that would be utilized during a disaster to meet the needs and sustain children and staff for an extended period (Illinois Emergency Medical Services for Children (EMSC) 2016; Child Care Aware of America 2018). Supplies should be stored both onsite at the child care center/home as well as at the predetermined relocation/evacuation site (Illinois Emergency Medical Services for Children (EMSC) 2016; Child Care Aware of America 2018; Chang et al. 2018; U.S. Department of Health and Human Services, Office of Administration for Children and Families 2016). For each child and staff member at the child care center/home, there should be at least a 3-day supply of nonperishable age-appropriate food, including formula and one gallon of water per person per day for 3 days (National Resource Center for Health and Safety in Child Care and Early Education n.d.-b). Additional food considerations may be needed for children with chronic medical conditions (CSHCN), those with special dietary requirements, and children with food allergies (National Resource Center for Health and Safety in Child Care and Early Education n.d.-b). In addition to food and water, supplies for sheltering (e.g., blankets), sanitation (e.g., diapers, sanitary wipes, soap), life safety supplies (e.g., flashlights, batteries, tools, duct tape), transportation devices (e.g., car seats), and first aid and medical supplies are examples of other categories of supplies that child care centers/homes should have in their stockpile. Those supplies that will be needed immediately after a disaster should be placed in some type of "go bag" that can easily be taken with staff during incidents such as immediate evacuations. Examples of supplies that may be in the "go bag" include flashlights, child emergency contact information, business continuity documentation, diapers, formula, first aid supplies, and snacks. The remaining items should also be stored in some type of portable container that is accessible by staff. Administrative supplies such as emergency contact information for all children in the child care center/home and important documents for business continuity should also be considered as emergency supplies and need to be able to be accessed quickly during a disaster/emergency. Storage location, transportation of the supplies, and a process to maintain and replenish supplies should all be considered during the development process and incorporated into the disaster/emergency plans.

Other preparedness activities include:

- Develop tools to assist staff with responding to incidents such as response checklists and emergency procedure flip charts.
- Share the basic concepts of the disaster plan with parents/guardians so they know what to expect from the child care center/home during an incident, what the child care center/home expects from the parents/guardians during the incident, and how they will be reunited with their child after an incident.
- Develop and conduct a process to ensure all contact information for parents/guardians is updated on a regular basis to aid in reunification.
- Determine what documents will be needed for reunification and business continuity after a disaster/emergency. Develop a process that makes these documents readily available to take with during an incident, especially during an evacuation.

15.1.3.3 Response

During a real incident, the developed plans are implemented, providing guidance to staff on how to respond. The priority is always to protect children and staff. Staff and children should respond based on the type of incident and the training that they received during drills/exercises. Once the safety and security of the children and staff has been established, key staff and/or administrative staff of the child care center/home should contact the agency overseeing the incident (e.g., incident commander) as well as the agency that provides oversight and regulates child care centers/homes at the state level. Communicating with these different entities allows for situational awareness and status updates on the incident as well as providing an avenue to request additional resources that may be needed to assist the child care center/home with their response.

15.1.3.4 Recovery

The recovery process after a disaster/emergency is dependent on many factors. Recovery and restoration of operations of child care services are directly related to predisaster planning such as mitigation efforts, development of recovery and business continuity plans, and establishment of agreements. Predisaster planning and activities help build the resiliency of a community and its members, including the child care center/home and the children that attend it. Having child care centers/homes in a community return to normal as soon as possible will assist with the overall recovery of a community as well as help children cope with the disaster. Child care services are vital to the economic recovery of a community since, without these services, parents/guardians cannot return to work (Save the Children 2007). Reestablishing child care services and schools early in the disaster provides a safe and stable place for children to attend while their parents/guardians perform recovery actions and/or return to work. These actions help children return to their normal routine and allow them the opportunity to play, both of which help begin their coping process.

Child care centers/homes would implement their business continuity plan that outlines the steps the child care center/home will take to either reestablish services or continue to operate during the disaster and recovery periods. Child care centers/homes need to have a backup copy of all their computer files in order to assist with the reestablishment of services. Ideally, these backup copies are kept off-site, so they cannot be damaged or affected by the incident. Important documents such as insurance papers, staff employment files, and financial records are examples of what should be kept in the backup system/process. Creating backup files that contain the patient/guardian emergency contact information for each child care attendee is crucial to assist with reunification during and after a disaster. These types of documents should be mobile and easy for staff to take during an evacuation (e.g., on a flash drive). This information may also be kept at the off-site location but should be more accessible if reunification occurs before the off-site files can be obtained.

Child care centers/homes need to consider state regulatory requirements and processes for reestablishing services in the existing child care site, operating temporary child care sites, and operating in alternate child care spaces outlined in the recovery plan and through memorandum of understandings (MOUs) or mutual aid agreements. In addition, child care centers/homes may need to consider taking in additional children from families who normally do not attend their child care center/home. Having a plan to temporarily care for additional children can be a tremendous help for families and the community by allowing more members of the community to start their recovery and rebuilding process (U.S. Department of Health and Human Services, Office of Administration for Children and Families 2016).

In order to make the decision on whether to reestablish services in the existing site, depending on the type of incident, a damage assessment of the property needs to be conducted. This assessment should be done as soon as it is safe and secure to do. The purpose of conducting this damage assessment is to (Illinois Emergency Medical Services for Children (EMSC) 2016; U.S. Department of Health and Human Services, Office of Administration for Children and Families 2016; U.S. Department of Health and Human Services (HHS), Office of Administration of Children and Families, Office of Head Start n.d.):

- Assess the extent of the interruptions in child care services;
- Assess the number of staff and children impacted by the incident;

- Determine current operational capacity of the child care community as a whole immediately following the disaster;
- Communicate with community emergency management officials and the state regulatory agency; and
- Record the damage for insurance company claims and disaster financial relief resources.

If a child care center/home is unable to reopen or reestablish services, the center/home should offer to assist parents/guardians in temporary placement of their children in other child care centers/homes until their program can reopen. If an alternative location was determined during the planning phase, it may be as simple as providing families with the alternate center/home's contact information and notifying the alternate center/home about the family's needs. However, this may only be feasible if the child care center/home makes arrangements and establishes agreements or MOUs with other child care centers/homes during the planning phase for this purpose to temporarily care for their children/clients.

To complete the repairs and work needed to open the child care center/home, child care center/home administrators will need to compile damage estimates, prioritize repairs, maintain records of all expenses, notify insurance carriers, and access any disaster resource assistance to assist with the recovery efforts.

The other key component of the recovery phase for child care center/home staff is to assist children with the emotional and mental health effects of the disaster. Children respond differently to the stress of a disaster/emergency as compared to adults. Since they respond based on their age and developmental level, it is important for staff to be aware of normal or common reactions for the different age groups whom they care for, what is considered abnormal or concerning reactions, and how best to help the children cope. Since children spend a significant amount of time each week in the child care center/home, staff can play a significant role in helping these children recover from the disaster.

15.1.4 Common Reactions to Disasters for Children in Child Care Center/Home (Illinois Emergency Medical Services for Children (EMSC) 2018; The National Child Traumatic Stress Network 2012)

Infants and toddlers will not have developed the ability to understand the circumstances of the incident that has occurred, nor can they verbalize their emotions about the incident. Therefore, they express their emotions through their behavior. An infant may have an exaggerated startle response, or a toddler may throw temper tantrums more frequently. Older children who typically attend child care centers/homes (ages 3–6) tend to be magical thinkers. They may not understand everything that has happened and may have false perceptions related to the event. For example, it is common that a child this age may think the event was in some way their fault and that it would not have happened if they had behaved better. A preschool aged child may also not understand that the danger from the incident is over. Overhearing adult conversations or being exposed to the media replaying the incident can add to this confusion. Young children often regress in response to stress, losing developmental abilities that they had previously acquired or skills that they learned. For example, a previously toilet trained child may start having toileting accidents. Toddlers may become aggressive when they are feeling angry or scared. This may be because they are trying to communicate to the adults around them the internal turmoil they are feeling.

Fear of separation is very common in these younger children who completely depend on their parents/guardians to provide for their basic needs and protect them from danger. A toddler may worry excessively that something bad might happen to their parent/guardian. The preschool age child may also have fears of separation and may feel very vulnerable after a disaster. They may cling more to their parents/guardians and child care center/home staff. They may also demonstrate regressive behaviors to elicit nurturance and comforting from adults. Crying and refusing to talk is also common with this age group.

It may be difficult in this younger-aged population to determine when to seek professional assistance for a child who is not coping well after an incident. If a child's reaction appears more severe than other children's reactions or changes in their behaviors are concerning, additional assistance may be necessary. The staff in the child care center/home may recognize these symptoms before the parent/guardian does, and an overwhelmed parent/guardian may require encouragement to seek additional assistance for their child.

There are interventions that child care center/home staff can implement in order to help children cope after a disaster/emergency. Parents/guardians, other caregivers, and trusted adults (i.e., child care center/home staff) need to spend more time with these younger children and provide a lot of physical contact. This can provide the reassurance, a feeling of safety and security, and the comfort that they need. Limiting children's exposure to media and conversations adults are having about the disaster/emergency is also important since young children are not able to understand that the events are not actually recurring when they observe repeat video footage of the incident and hear adults talking about the incident. Reassuring children that they are safe will be very helpful in providing them with a sense of security. Talking to the children in age and developmentally appropriate levels about their feelings and about the events may also help (U.S. Department of Health and Human Services (HHS), Office of Administration of Children and Families, Office of Head Start n.d.; Illinois Emergency Medical Services for Children (EMSC) 2018). It is also important for child care center/home staff to observe a child play and to listen to them to gain a better understanding of what may have occurred to the child during the disaster and their feelings about the incident. Please refer to Chap. 12 for more detailed information on postdisaster effects.

Child care center/home staff should also monitor each other to assess any difficulty coping after a disaster/emergency. Staff should be provided with available resources to assist them with coping after an incident. National resources such as the Substance Abuse and Mental Health Services Administration (SAMHSA) provide immediate, confidential, crisis counseling 24 hours a day through a toll-free, multilingual support line (Substance Abuse and Mental Health Services Administration (SAMHSA) 2019).

One final component in the recovery process for child care centers/homes is to debrief with staff, parents/guardians, and directors about the event. Debriefing provides an opportunity for those involved in the event to share their experiences. This can contribute to their personal recovery. In addition, debriefing provides an avenue to identify lessons learned from the incident, identify what components of the plan worked well and what did not, and develop an action plan to address those components of the plan that need to be changed. This brings the emergency management process full circle for the child care center/home as they begin to implement mitigation strategies to issues that have been identified and make corrections to the plan to reduce the risk and effects of the next disaster/emergency.

15.1.5 Key Components in Child Care Center/Home Disaster/ Emergency Plans (National Center on Early Childhood Quality Assurance 2016; Administration for Children, and Family, Office of Child Care 2015; Illinois Emergency Medical Services for Children (EMSC) 2016; U.S. Department of Health and Human Services (HHS), Office of Administration of Children and Families, Office of Head Start n.d.)

When child care centers/homes are developing their disaster/emergency plans, there are certain components that should be incorporated into the plans. The layout of the plan should follow a simple, clear, and easy-to-understand format with sufficient detail to address what the staff, children, and parents/guardians of the child care center/home will do, when they need to do it, and how it will get accomplished. The plan should include considerations with other key entities and agencies that are directly associated with the child care center/home (e.g., the building the child care center/home is located within if part of a larger building) as well as indirectly associated with (response plans for the community where the child care center/home is located). Ensuring that components within the child care center/home's plans align with other key entities and agencies will contribute to a more unified and coordinated response to a disaster/emergency that impacts the entire community. The timeline/schedule and process for review of the plan and the implementation of revisions of the plan should be included in the plan. The plan and the education provided to the staff on the plans need to stress that employees are expected to remain and provide care to the children within the child care center/home should a disaster/emergency incident occur when they are at work at the child care center/home. It is extremely important that staff be encouraged to develop their own family preparedness plans, so their children and other family members can be cared for if the staff member is unable to leave during the disaster/emergency. Please see Chap. 6 for more information on personal/family disaster planning.

15.1.5.1 Communication Planning

Among the many critical components that should be outlined within the child care center/home disaster/emergency plans, communication procedures are, by far, one of the most important. The communication section of the plan should incorporate how information will be shared internally and externally. Internal communication procedures should outline how information will be shared between staff members, administration, and with the children within the child care center/home. Examples of primary communication methods include automatic notification systems, telephone, email, text messages, and written memos. Alternate communication methods should also be considered in case primary methods are not available. These may include emergency cellular phones or portable two-way radios. It is important that staff receive training on how to use all possible communication methods. Additional internal communication considerations to determine include:

- Process staff will take to notify administration about a disaster/emergency;
- Process to notify staff of a disaster/emergency;
- Process to activate disaster/emergency plans and how the activation of these plans will be shared with staff who are within the child care center/home as well as those who are not present when the plans are activated;
- Location of emergency communication equipment;
- Notification of the "all clear" when the incident has resolved; and
- How, when, and what information should be shared with the children during disasters/emergencies.

External communication procedures outline how information will be shared with parents/guardians, family of staff members, community members (i.e., law enforcement, emergency medical services, emergency management agencies, and public health departments), the state regulatory agency, other agencies in which agreements or MOUs have been made, and the media (National Resource Center for Health and Safety in Child Care and Early Education n.d.-a; Illinois Emergency Medical Services for Children (EMSC) 2016). Examples of external communication methods include phone, text messages, automatic text or email messaging system, automatic phone systems, child care center website and/or social media site, and the local media (e.g., TV and radio stations). A list of emergency phone numbers for community emergency services and other agencies/partners, including the state regulatory agency, should be included in the plan. Although not included directly in the plan, there should be quick access to emergency contact information for the staff's family members. Establishing an out-of-state emergency contact phone number for the child care center/home that parents/guardians can utilize to access information regarding their child (may be used when cellular phones don't operate) can also be helpful. Staff members who will be responsible for external communication should also be outlined in the plan, especially which staff member(s) are designated to speak with the media and what is permitted to be shared on their own social media sites.

Sharing information with parents/guardians will need to occur during and after a disaster/emergency. There are many components to consider for this section of the plan, several of which are listed below (Administration for Children, and Family, Office of Child Care 2015; National Resource Center for Health and Safety in Child Care and Early Education n.d.-a; Illinois Emergency Medical Services for Children (EMSC) 2016):

- Process to obtain parental/guardian contact information and how often this will be updated;
- Process that parents/guardians will be contacted should an illness/injury occur to their child while at the child care center/home. This should include the route that parents will be contacted such as automatic text or email messaging, automatic phone messaging, social media, child care center/home website, and local media;
- Parents/guardians' responsibility to provide and update emergency contact phone numbers as this information changes;
- Identification of alternate preidentified adult(s) who will be designated to pick up the child if the parents/guardians are unavailable;
- Identification of alternate preidentified adult(s) who live in a different town/state/ area and who can be contacted if parents/guardians cannot be reached;
- The process that the child care center/home will take to notify the parents/guardians when a disaster/emergency occurs, including when and how the parents/ guardians should initiate contact so that they do not disrupt or endanger the children or staff during an incident;
- The process that the child care center/home will take regarding the safe release of the children, so the parents/guardians do not endanger themselves or others by attempting to pick up their children before it is safe to do so;
- The process that the child care center/home will take to notify the parents/guardians of where they should pick up their children if an evacuation/relocation occurred as a result of the disaster/emergency;
- The process that parents/guardians should take to notify the child care center/ home staff if they are unable to pick up their children before the close of operations;
- The process that the child care center/home will take to notify the parents/guardians of either limited hours of operation, extended hours of operation, or child care center/home closures due to the disaster/emergencies;
- Process to provide updates after a disaster if the child care center/home is closed due to damage.

15.1.5.2 Reunification Planning

As discussed previously, children of all ages, but especially those less than 5 years of age, are at risk for maltreatment, abduction, and abuse during disasters if they are separated from their parents/guardians during and after a disaster/emergency. Child care centers/homes are responsible for protecting children while they are in their care. They are also responsible for ensuring that each child that is in their care is reunited with their parent/guardian or other adult designated by the parents/guardians. Reunification can be challenging after a disaster/emergency, especially for younger children who are unable to provide any information about themselves or their parents/guardians, and typically do not carry any identification. Depending on the type of incident and extent of the damage to the child care center/home, reunification may be even more difficult if staff are unable to access their emergency contact records from the child care center/home. In addition, if children within the child care center/home sustain injuries as a result of the incident and staff are not available to share information with EMS prior to transportation to a hospital, this further complicates the issue of ensuring the child is reunited with their parent/guardian. Children who are 5 years old and younger may not be able to provide responders with any information regarding who they are or who their parents/guardians are. In addition, information that children this age can provide does not usually help provide insight on possible custodial issues. For example, a 4-year-old child may recognize and be able to tell responders that an adult is their mother or father but more likely will not be able to tell responders that one parent/guardian is not to have contact with them based on court custody rulings. Because reunification is such a high risk and challenging component of disaster response for child care centers/ homes, it is vital that procedures are outlined within the disaster plan for steps staff should take before, during, and after a disaster. Not only does this assist staff with knowing the steps they need to take to ensure the right child is reunited with the right parent/guardian, but it also helps to ensure that all staff are completing the reunification process in a consistent manner.

Before a disaster strikes, many of the components child care centers/homes need to consider for reunification have been outlined in the previous section on communication, including maintaining current contact information for parents/guardians as well as the local and out-of-state alternate preidentified adults. Sharing components of the disaster response plans with the parents/guardians will help them know what to expect and where to go to be reunited with their child after an incident. The child care center/home should have a current digital picture of each child who attends the child care center/home. Taking a picture of the parents/guardians for the center/ home's record may also be beneficial for the reunification process as it assists staff who are not familiar with all the parents/guardians to verify the child is being released to the correct person.

During a disaster, place identification information on the child, especially if an evacuation is anticipated (Illinois Emergency Medical Services for Children (EMSC) 2016). This can be in the form of an identification bracelet or by pinning an information card on the child's back that includes demographic information about the child and their parent/guardian. Having premade information cards for all children who attend the child care center/home will help facilitate this process during a chaotic evacuation incident. Assign staff members to conduct the reunification process and provide those staff members with information about the parents/guardians to assist them in this process. Release children only to those individuals that the parents/guardians have indicated prior to the incident. Staff should require photo identification for all adults that come to pick up a child after a disaster. If the child care center/home has to be evacuated, the location of where children will be reunified with their parents/guardians should only be provided to those listed on the child's emergency contact list. The child care center/home is responsible for caring for that child until they are reunified. If the parent/guardian and other alternate pre-identified adults are unable to be contacted and do not come to the child care center/home to pick up their children, the child care center/home staff will need to contact local law enforcement, local emergency management agency, the state regulatory agency for child care centers/homes, child protection services for the state in which they operate, and the National Emergency Child Locator Center (NECLC) operated by the National Center for Missing & Exploited Children (NCMEC) to file reports and assist with finding placement for the child (Illinois Emergency Medical Services for Children (EMSC) 2016; Federal Emergency Management Agency (FEMA) 2018). If possible, provide the assisting agencies with demographic information on the child and parent/guardian as well as a copy of the photos that are on file for both the child and the parents/guardians. For additional information on reunification, please refer to Chap. 11.

15.1.5.3 Business Continuity Planning

Business continuity planning is a critical component of a child care center/home preparedness. The business continuity components of the plan help protect the child care business. The plan consists of the steps and actions that the child care center/home should take after the immediate threat of the disaster/emergency has passed to address the damage or other threats to the child care center/home being able to continue to operate (Administration for Children, and Family, Office of Child Care 2015; Illinois Emergency Medical Services for Children (EMSC) 2016; U.S. Department of Health and Human Services (HHS), Office of Administration of Children and Families, Office of Head Start n.d.). Insurance policies, disaster relief funds (if available), and a contingency fund (funds set aside by the child care center/home before the disaster that can be utilized after a disaster for repairs, paying staff, or other operating costs) are all possible options that may be available to assist a child care center/home to cover the costs of reestablishing child care services. All documentation that will be needed by a child care center/home to reestablish care services should be kept on site with copies located at an off-site location. Keeping a copy of the business continuity documentations off-site ensures that staff will have access to it, even if the child care center/home sustains significant damage as a result of the incident. Another component that should be included as part of the business continuity plan is the requirements that the state child care regulating agency has for a child care center/home to reopen. If the child care center/home is part of the CCDF program, there may be additional steps that need to be taken and included within the business continuity component of the child care center/home disaster plan (Administration for Children, and Family, Office of Child Care 2015, 2017; U.S. Department of Health and Human Services, Office of Administration for Children and Families 2016).

15.1.5.4 Additional Components of the Disaster/Emergency Plans

The plans need to incorporate the actions that should occur during disaster/emergency incidents that may occur and involve the child care center/home as identified in their hazard assessment. Child care center/homes plans need to address the following types of incidents: illness/injury to a child or staff member, public health emergencies, missing or abducted child, fire, hazardous chemical spill, utility failure, extreme weather, radiological emergencies, violent situations, and terrorism. The specific causes of these incidents would vary for each child care center/home and would be identified during the hazard assessment. Detailed descriptions for evacuation/relocation, shelter-in-place, and lockdown procedures are critical to outline in the plan. These three response procedures would overlap with multiple emergency situations. For example, the shelter-in-place procedure would apply to extreme weather as well as a hazardous chemical leak within the community that the child care center/home is located. Since these procedures are appropriate responses for multiple emergency situations, their general concepts could be included separately instead of repeating the procedures in each applicable emergency situations identified within the plan. These four response procedures as well as the different types of disaster/emergency incidents as they relate to child care centers/homes will be reviewed next. The specific details related to how the child care center/home staff will respond during these procedures and types of situations is the content that should be integrated into the child care center/home's disaster plan.

- **Evacuation/Relocation**

  Evacuation of the child care center/home involves moving all the children and staff out of the area that is either affected or anticipated to be affected by threat and relocating to a safer location. An example when an evacuation would be indicated is if there was a fire inside the child care center/home. The safe area that children and staff relocate/evacuate to can be either on-site (safe staging area on the property of the child care center/home), off-site (designated shelter or other types of areas that are not on the grounds of the child care center/home), or reverse evacuation (movement of children and staff into the child care center/home building from outside). During an evacuation, it is important that attendance is confirmed via roll call before moving the children and again once all staff and children have arrived at the next location. Determining predesignated evacuation routes prior to evacuation may be helpful to staff during an evacuation with the flexibility to alter the route as needed due to impending threats. Identifying a primary and a secondary evacuation site may also be beneficial in case one becomes affected by whatever the disaster threat is. If an off-site evacuation is needed, transportation resources may be needed due to the age of the children in the child care center/home. Where transportation vehicles will be obtained should be outlined in the plan, as well as additional considerations when transporting children such as the need for safety seats in the transportation vehicle(s). Emergency disaster packs may be carried out by staff to include needed supplies for the children, emergency communication devices, and parental/guardian contact information. Other than these emergency supplies, staff should not try to bring their own belongings or the children's belongings during an evacuation. Designated staff members should contact parents/guardian as soon as it is safe to do so and provide them with instructions on being reunited with their children. These instructions would include directing parents/guardians to a reunification point, identifying an alternative time to pick up the child from the child care center/home, or that there are no changes anticipated for the time or location that the parent/guardian normally picks up the child.

- **Shelter-in-place**
  If there is a threat, hazardous condition, or extreme weather occurring outside the child care center/home, sheltering-in-place would be indicated. Children and staff would remain inside the building that would be secured. There are several key differences between shelter-in-place and lockdown. The first is the location of the threat. In a lockdown situation, the threat is typically inside the building where the child center/home is located, while with a shelter-in-place order, the threat is typically outside the child care center/home. In a lockdown, the staff and children typically remain in one area (e.g., a classroom) until there is no longer a threat or the order to immediately evacuate is given. When sheltering-in-place, children and staff may be able to move around inside the building, depending on the cause of the incident. Staff would bring the children into the predesignated areas based on the type of incident. If an interior room with a few or no windows or vents is available, this may be ideal based on the type of incident (e.g., extreme weather or tornado). Sealing the doors, windows, and vents may be indicated if there is a hazardous chemical release outside the center/home. A roll call should be conducted at the start of the shelter-in-place procedures and when all staff and children are in the designated areas. Once the children and staff are safe, staff should notify the parents/guardians and provide them with an update on the situation, instruct them not to come to the child care center/home site due to the identified threat, and inform them that children will not be released until the threat has been cleared. Updates should be provided to the parents/guardians as they become available, including information about where the reunification location will be and when it is anticipated to occur.

- **Lockdown**
  The purpose of a lockdown procedure is to secure the children and staff somewhere inside the child care center/home building to protect against a threat that is typically in the child care center. Violent intruders, active shooters, or hostage incidents are examples of when a lockdown procedure would be indicated. Law enforcement should be notified immediately (when safe to do so). Staff would bring all children into the designated safe areas that are out of view from the presenting threat and remain there until they receive notice that there is no longer a threat. If it is safe to do so, staff should engage the children in activities such as story time during the lockdown to try to keep them calm and quiet. An immediate evacuation may be indicated during a lockdown. Staff may be notified by their

administrator or designee, or law enforcement if there is an opportunity to evacuate the children. While continuing to keep the children calm and quiet, follow the specified route given for the evacuation (which may differ from evacuation routes outlined for other emergencies such as during a fire) and assemble at the designated area outside the building (Child Care Aware of America n.d.-b). All cellular telephones and electronic devices should be placed on silent mode during a lockdown but to aid in communication during and after the incident, staff should try to keep their cellular telephone with them. Once the children and staff are taken to a safe location or there is no longer a threat, staff should notify the parents/guardians and provide them with instructions for how to be reunited with their children.

- **Illness or injury to a child or staff member**
  Staff members who are with the child that is injured or ill would assess the situation, determine what is initially needed, initiate first aid if trained to do so, call for help from other staff members, contact administration, and activate the local emergency medical services (EMS) as indicated. Any available health information for that child should be made available for EMS when they arrive. If the child that is ill or injured is a CSHCN or has other chronic medical conditions, information on their history should be provided to EMS as well. In addition, if the child has an Emergency Information Form (EIF) available, this is crucial to provide to EMS prior to transport to the hospital. The EIF provides a summary of the medical history and needs of children with special health care needs (American College of Emergency Physicians (ACEP), American Academy of Pediatrics (AAP) 2010). After initial first aid and any lifesaving interventions are performed, a staff member should contact the parents/guardians.

- **Public health emergency**
  Child care centers/homes are at risk for infectious disease outbreaks and other public health emergencies such as pandemic influenza. Infants and young children are at an even greater risk for illness during infectious disease outbreaks due to their immature immune systems. Children with chronic medical conditions who are immunocompromised are at a higher risk of infection. Pregnant women are also at higher risk. How a child care center/home will respond to a communitywide public health emergency (e.g., pandemic influenza outbreak) or one directly involving the child care center/home (e.g., rotavirus outbreak that involves numerous child care center/home attendees and/or staff) should be outlined in the child care center/homes' disaster plan. There should be a process on how to contact the local public health department and other reliable sources of information to receive updates on any communitywide outbreaks as well as to report any outbreaks within the child care center/home. The process for communicating with families and staff during outbreaks should be determined. Infection control procedures/measures include: separating ill children if they become ill while at child care; conducting preventative infection control measures to limit the spread of an infection such as frequent hand washing, routine cleaning, sanitizing and disinfecting areas and toys within the child care center/ home; educating and encouraging children on how to follow infectious control

prevention measures in a developmentally appropriate level; ensuring there is availability of supplies to control the spread of infection; educating families and staff about available vaccinations, infection control measures, and about the disease causing an outbreak; using a tracking system to document when children become ill and their symptoms; and maintaining records of children's immunization records (Centers for Disease Control and Prevention (CDC) 2015; Administration of Children and Families 2016). There also needs to be specific criteria regarding when children should be sent home from the child care center/home, when children should not attend child care, and when children can return to the child care center/home after an illness. The criteria for closing the child care center/home along with who makes that decision should also be predetermined in the plans.

- **Missing or abducted child care attendee**
  When a child care attendee is missing, the process may include looking for the child on the premises, checking with other staff for possible known whereabouts, contacting administration, locking down the child care center/home, notifying law enforcement to file a report and activate an Amber Alert, and notifying the parents/guardians. These steps should all be outlined in the plan, along with the specific steps staff would take, which staff would be responsible for contacting outside agencies, and the contact information for those agencies, which should be easily accessible to staff. The child care center/home may develop required documentation for staff to complete about the incident (e.g., incident report form).

- **Fire**
  During a fire within the child care center/home, life safety is the priority. The children should be evacuated prior to any attempts by staff to extinguish the fire or calling the fire department. A roll call of children and staff should be conducted once at a safe location. If there is no threat to children (children are not near where the fire is located), the fire is small, and staff is appropriately trained, a fire extinguisher can be used to attempt to put out the fire. If there is time and it is safe to do so, staff should close the windows and doors in the child care center/home before evacuating to help contain the fire. In addition, if there is time, the designated staff member should grab the emergency backpack with supplies for the children, parental/guardian emergency contact information, emergency communication devices, and business continuity documentation. No staff or children should be allowed to return to the building until cleared to do so by the fire department.

- **Hazardous chemical spill**
  If a hazardous chemical spill occurs inside the child care center/home, the area should be evacuated immediately, preferably uphill and upwind from the location of the spill. Local emergency services should be notified. Electrical switches should be left in their current position, and if it is possible and safe to do so, the ventilation system should be turned off. Anyone (child or staff) with direct contact with the hazardous chemical should wash the area with water immediately. Otherwise, no staff should attempt to contain, identify, or clean up the hazardous materials.

If a hazardous chemical spill occurs outside the child care center/home, a reverse evacuation should occur if children are outside and shelter-in-place procedures should be conducted once all children and staff are inside the center/home. Information should be obtained from local response entities (e.g., fire department, hazmat teams, public health department) on additional procedures that may be needed such as closing off vents and taping doors and windows to create a better seal.

- **Utility emergencies, including gas leaks, electrical power failure, and contaminated water supply**
  When there is a utility failure, the decision has to be made about whether the child care center/home can stay open (if currently open), can delay opening (if closed when a failure occurs), or needs to close or remain closed until the cause of the utility failure can be resolved. If the setting is currently open, staff need to consider the amount of natural light, temperature of the setting, ability to provide water/food/formula, and any risk of health to the children and staff.

  If there is a possible gas leak or if staff in the center smell gas, an immediate evacuation of all children and staff is indicated and once everyone has evacuated to the safer location, notify local emergency services and administration about the issue. No one should reenter the building until cleared by emergency services and the gas company.

  For an electrical power failure, if the child care center/home does not have a backup generator, the decision will need to be made on whether the center/home can stay open.

  If there is a possibility that the water supply is contaminated, discontinue the use of tap water, ice machines, or any other water equipment. A community boil water advisory notice may be issued that indicates the water is safe to drink if it is boiled. If possible, for infants and children with chronic medical conditions (CSHCN), bottled water should be used for feeding and drinking. However, if bottled water is not available, boiled water can be used for infants and children with chronic medical conditions (CSHCN) (Illinois Emergency Medical Services for Children (EMSC) 2016; National Resource Center for Health and Safety in Child Care and Early Education n.d.-b; U.S. Department of Health and Human Services (HHS), Office of Administration of Children and Families, Office of Head Start n.d.; Centers for Disease Control and Prevention (CDC) 2018).

- **Extreme weather**
  The type of extreme weather that child care centers/homes need to plan for will be based on its location and what was identified through the hazard assessment. There are some general concepts that child care centers/homes should consider regardless of the type of extreme weather it may be at risk for. Child care centers/homes should have a weather radio, especially in rural areas where the siren alerts may not be as dependable. Staff members should be assigned to monitor the weather for changes and alerts, indicating a potentially dangerous situation. Flashlights, emergency backpacks, extra batteries, cellular phones, and alternative communication devices should be kept nearby. Determine if closing the child care center/home earlier or staying open later can help ensure the safety

of the children, their parents/guardian, and staff. Staying open later so parents/ guardians can pick up their children safely after a storm has passed can be beneficial for everyone's safety. If the extreme weather emergency causes a need to relocate the children and staff, roll call should be taken before leaving and once everyone arrives in the safer area. A list of vendors to assist with snow/ice removal, debris removal, or repair damages as a result of the storm should be maintained and easily accessible to speed the recovery after an extreme weather incident occurs.

- **Radiological emergencies related to nuclear power plant incidents** (Illinois Emergency Medical Services for Children (EMSC) 2016; U.S. Nuclear Regulatory Commission (U.S. NRC) 2018)

  If a child care center/home is within ten miles of a nuclear power plant, it is important that the child care center/home contacts the local emergency management agency to ensure they are aware of the location of the child care center/ home. By establishing a relationship prior to an incident occurring, the child care center can be informed more quickly of any incidents, including the need to evacuate or shelter-in-place, if indicated.

- **Violent situations, including violent intruder, active shooter, hostage situations, physical and verbal threats, and bomb threats**

  There is a high risk of violent events involving child care centers/homes. Community violence, active shooter, custodial disputes, disgruntled person/staff, or any other type of physical or verbal threats can occur near or in a child care center/home. The assailant may or may not be known to the child care center/ home. Any type of violent situation near or in a child care center/home should prompt the activation of the lockdown procedures and immediate notification of local law enforcement. In certain circumstances such as a bomb threat or if an armed intruder or active shooter is in another part of the building from where the children and staff are, immediate evacuation may be indicated instead of lockdown procedures. Procedures for each type of violent situation should be outlined in the plan. Conduct drills/exercises with a variety of scenarios involving different types of violent situations. Having experience with how to respond to these types of incidents and the ability to remain calm during the incident can help save the lives of children and staff.

- **Terrorism incidents**

  Child care centers/homes need to be just as vigilant as other areas within the community. Report unusual people and/or activities, suspicious items left outside a child care center/home, and anyone who appears to be hanging around without reason. Child care centers/homes should enforce their security measures and restrict visitors. Disaster/emergency response procedures should be shared with only those who need to know them (i.e., staff, emergency medical services, parents/guardians) and not all aspects of the plan need to be shared in their entirety with every person. For example, parents/guardians need to be aware that evacuation areas and secondary locations have been identified should an evacuation be needed. The locations of the primary and secondary evacuation sites do not need to be shared until the incident occurs. If a terrorist incident near the child care center/home involves a weapon of mass destruction, implement the child care center/home's shelter-in-place procedures and follow the instructions provided by local emergency managers.

15.1.6 Conclusion

Child care centers/homes play a vital role in the community on a day-to-day basis as well as during and after a disaster/emergency. Being able to care for and protect the youngest and most vulnerable groups of children requires commitment on behalf of the child care center/home to the entire emergency preparedness process.

References

Administration for Children & Family, Office of Child Care. Resource guide: emergency preparedness and response resources for child care programs. 2015. https://www.acf.hhs.gov/sites/default/files/occ/1306_epr_provider_resource_guide.pdf. Accessed 01 Apr 2019.

Administration for Children & Family, Office of Child Care. What data are needed to support planning, response, and recovery? 2017. https://childcareta.acf.hhs.gov/resource/what-data-are-needed-support-planning-response-and-recovery. Accessed 18 Apr 2019.

Administration of Children & Families. CCDF Health and Safety Requirements Brief #1: prevention and control of infectious diseases. July 2016. https://childcareta.acf.hhs.gov/sites/default/files/public/brief_1_infectious_disease_final.pdf. Accessed 15 Apr 2019.

American College of Emergency Physicians (ACEP), American Academy of Pediatrics (AAP). Emergency information form for children with special health care needs. 2010. https://www.acep.org/by-medical-focus/pediatrics/medical-forms/emergency-information-form-for-children-with-special-health-care-needs/. Accessed 22 May 2019.

Centers for Disease Control and Prevention (CDC). General prevention & control measures: standard cryptosporidiosis (crypto) control measures for the childcare setting. 2015. https://www.cdc.gov/parasites/crypto/childcare/prevent.html. Accessed 18 Apr 2019.

Centers for Disease Control and Prevention (CDC). Disaster planning: infant and child feeding. 2018. https://www.cdc.gov/nccdphp/dnpao/features/disasters-infant-feeding/index.html. Accessed 20 May 2019.

Chang MT, Brandin S, Hashikawa AN. Disaster preparedness among Michigan's licensed child care programs. Pediatr Emerg Care. 2018;34(5):349–56.

Child Care Aware of America. Emergency supply kit. 2018. https://usa.childcareaware.org/wp-content/uploads/2018/06/Emergency-Supply-Kit.pdf. Accessed 05 May 2019.

Child Care Aware of America. Who regulates child care? n.d.-a. https://www.childcareaware.org/who-regulates-child-care/. Accessed 01 Apr 2019.

Child Care Aware of America. Active shooter resources: active shooter response options. n.d.-b. https://usa.childcareaware.org/advocacy-public-policy/crisis-and-disaster-resources/caregiver-and-ccrr-tools-publications-and-resources/active-shooter/. Accessed 25 May 2019.

Child Trends. Child care. 2016. https://www.childtrends.org/?indicators=child-care. Accessed 01 Apr 2019.

Federal Emergency Management Agency (FEMA). National emergency child locator fact sheet. National Center for Missing and Exploited Children. 2018. https://www.fema.gov/media-library/assets/documents/167214. Accessed 25 May 2019.

Illinois Emergency Medical Services for Children (EMSC). Emergency preparedness planning guide for child care centers & child care homes. 2016. https://www.luriechildrens.org/global-assets/documents/emsc/disaster/child-care-centers/emergencepreparednessplanningguidefor-childcarecenters20164.pdf. Accessed 01 Apr 2019.

Illinois Emergency Medical Services for Children (EMSC). Disaster mental health response for children. 3rd ed. 2018. https://www.luriechildrens.org/en/emergency-medical-services-for-children/education/all-healthcare-professionals/disaster-mental-health-response-for-children-2nd-edition/. Accessed 01 May 2019.

Laughlin L. Who's minding the kids? Child care arrangements: Spring 2011. U.S. Census Bureau. 2013. https://www2.census.gov/library/publications/2013/demo/p70-135.pdf. Accessed 01 Apr 2019.

Lesser KA, Coats JL, Roszak AR. Emergency preparedness plans and perceptions among a sample of United States childcare providers (abstract). Disaster Medicine and Public Health Preparedness. 2019. https://www-cambridge-org.archer.luhs.org/core/journals/disaster-medicine-and-public-health-preparedness/article/emergency-preparedness-plans-and-perceptions-among-a-sample-of-united-states-childcare-providers/CE4F0A41728E563EA8E1DDE9BA174788. Accessed 10 Apr 2019.

National Center on Early Childhood Quality Assurance. CCDF health and safety requirements brief #6. July 2016. https://childcareta.acf.hhs.gov/sites/default/files/public/brief_6_emergency-preparedness_final.pdf. Accessed 15 Apr 2019.

National Commission of Children and Disasters. 2010 Report to the President and Congress. 2010. https://archive.ahrq.gov/prep/nccdreport/nccdreport.pdf. Accessed 15 Apr 2019.

National Resource Center for Health and Safety in Child Care and Early Education. Caring for our children (CFOC). Chapter 9: Administration: 9.2.4.3: disaster planning, training, and communication. n.d.-a. https://nrckids.org/CFOC/Database/9.2.4.3. Accessed 05 May 2019.

National Resource Center for Health and Safety in Child Care and Early Education. Caring for our children (CFOC). Chapter 4: Nutrition and food service: 4.9.0.8: supply of food and water for disasters. n.d.-b. https://nrckids.org/CFOC/Database/4.9.0.8. Accessed 15 Apr 2019.

Save the Children. Issue brief: child care: an essential service for disaster recovery. 2007. https://www.savethechildren.org/content/dam/usa/reports/emergency-prep/GRGS-BRIEF-2007.PDF. Accessed 19 May 2019.

Save the Children. The national report card on protecting children during disasters. 2010. https://www.savethechildren.org/content/dam/usa/reports/emergency-prep/disaster-report-2010.pdf. Accessed 15 Apr 2019.

Substance Abuse and Mental Health Services Administration (SAMHSA). Disaster distress hotline. 2019. https://www.samhsa.gov/find-help/disaster-distress-helpline. Accessed 20 May 2019.

The National Child Traumatic Stress Network. PFA: parent tips for helping infants and toddlers after disasters. 2012. https://www.nctsn.org/sites/default/files/resources/pfa_parent_tips_for_helping_infants_and_toddlers_after_disasters.pdf. Accessed 01 May 2019.

U.S. Census Bureau. Who's minding the kids? Child care arrangements, 2011: detailed tables. 2011. https://www.census.gov/data/tables/2008/demo/2011-tables.html. Accessed 01 Apr 2019.

U.S. Department of Health and Human Services (HHS), Office of Administration of Children and Families, Office of Head Start. Emergency preparedness manual for early childhood programs. n.d.. https://eclkc.ohs.acf.hhs.gov/sites/default/files/pdf/emergency-preparedness-manual-early-childhood-programs.pdf. Accessed 01 Apr 2019.

U.S. Department of Health and Human Services (HSS), Office of Child Care: An Office of the Administration for Children & Families. Child care and development fund program plans. 2017. https://www.acf.hhs.gov/occ/plans. Accessed 01 Apr 2019.

U.S. Department of Health and Human Services, Maternal and Child Health Bureau. Caring for our children: National health and safety performance standards guidelines for early care and education programs. 4th ed. A joint collaborative project of the American Academy of Pediatrics, American Public Health Association & National Resource Center for Health and Safety in Child Care and Early Education. 2019. http://nrckids.org/files/CFOC4%20pdf-%20FINAL.pdf. Accessed 01 Apr 2019.

U.S. Department of Health and Human Services, Office of Administration for Children and Families. Post-disaster child care needs and resources. 2016. https://www.acf.hhs.gov/ohsepr/resource/post-disaster-child-care-needs-and-resources. Accessed 05 Apr 2019.

U.S. Nuclear Regulatory Commission (U.S. NRC). Emergency planning zones. 2018. https://www.nrc.gov/about-nrc/emerg-preparedness/about-emerg-preparedness/planning-zones.html. Accessed 20 May 2019.

U.S. Office of Personnel Management. Child care resources handbook. n.d.. https://www.opm.gov/policy-data-oversight/worklife/reference-materials/child-care-resources-handbook/. Accessed 01 Apr 2019.

Office Preparedness

16

Kirsten J. Covec

16.1 Introduction

Infants and children with potentially life-threatening illnesses and injuries are sometimes brought to a primary care office or clinic by caregivers seeking help from health care providers (HCPs) they know and trust. In those cases, the primary care office serves as the entry into the emergency care system, and the office becomes the place for initial evaluation, stabilization, and treatment. Similarly, families view primary HCPs as one of the most trusted sources of information about disasters and may seek care at the primary care office during a disaster, particularly if other emergency care services are unavailable or overwhelmed (AAP Policy Statement 2007; Disaster Preparedness Advisory Council and Committee on Pediatric Emergency Medicine 2015; Jones 2019). Whether for episodic emergencies or full-fledged community disasters, pediatric medical offices that typically emphasize well child care, disease prevention, and continuity services as a child's medical home, may find themselves in an unfamiliar, risky territory when they must stretch beyond their usual scope of practice to care for children when they need it most. Advanced planning can mitigate risk, reduce material and operational losses, improve financial stability, strengthen the medical home, and protect and promote the health of children in the community (AAP Pediatric Preparedness Resource Kit 2013).

Preparing a pediatric primary care office for a disaster requires at least these five components: office self-assessment, effective preparation for more commonplace pediatric emergencies, development of written emergency response and disaster protocols, practice using drills or mock codes, and knowledge and integration of greater local and regional disaster planning and resources (Fuchs 2013; Disaster Preparedness Advisory Council and Committee on Pediatric Emergency Medicine

K. J. Covec (✉)
Santa Rosa Community Health, Santa Rosa, CA, USA

© Springer Nature Switzerland AG 2020
C. J. Goodhue, N. Blake (eds.), *Nursing Management of Pediatric Disaster*,
https://doi.org/10.1007/978-3-030-43428-1_16

2015; Jones 2019). For the purposes of this chapter, an emergency is defined as an episodic event involving one or more children who require equipment and intervention beyond the usual and customary scope of office practice, *in the context of fully functioning office and community resources.* A disaster is defined as similar serious or critical events *in the context of impaired or incapacitated office and community resources.* This chapter will review methods to optimize readiness for episodic pediatric emergencies in the office setting, provide guidance and references for how to adapt and/or develop an emergency response and disaster plan for the office or clinic setting, and considerations for a broader role of the pediatric office in the context of a disaster.

16.2 Pediatric Emergencies in the Office Setting

Pediatric primary HCPs (PPHCPs) regularly assess and manage emergencies in the office setting, including transfer of seriously or critically ill children to emergency departments or for hospital admission (Klig and O'Malley 2007; Heath et al. 2000; AAP Policy Statement, 2007), though reported frequency of these events varies widely. One recent survey of 57 pediatrician respondents in private practice found that 39% reported an average of at least 1 emergency per month; 75% referred a patient to the emergency department or hospital at least monthly (Pendleton and Stevenson 2015). In a much earlier study, 62% of pediatricians and family physicians in an urban setting reported they assessed more than 1 patient per week in their offices who required hospitalization or urgent stabilization (Fuchs et al. 1989).

Despite the frequency of these events, many PPHCPs discount the need for preparation based on the erroneous belief that "emergencies are not very common," because they feel they can rely on a rapid response from emergency medical systems, or because the practice is in close proximity to a hospital. Some office medical administrators or HCPs have interpreted risk management guidelines to mean that simply having emergency equipment and medications on site will increase their liability in emergency situations; however, lack of preparation for emergencies may in fact constitute increased liability (AAP Policy Statement 2007). Whatever the precise reason, most pediatric offices lack adequate systematic preparation (Klig and O'Malley 2007; Kalindi et al. 2018), and the consequences can be serious.

The most common types of pediatric office emergencies are respiratory emergencies, seizures, sepsis or severe infection (primarily in young infants), dehydration, anaphylaxis, choking, head trauma, and cardiac arrest (Fuchs and Weinstock 1996; Pendleton and Stevenson 2015; Mehta and Gupta 2017; Jones 2019). The majority of cardiac arrests in children are secondary to progressive respiratory failure. If respiratory distress is rapidly recognized and prevented from progressing to respiratory failure, a fatal outcome can be prevented. Sepsis, anaphylaxis, and dehydration can all potentially progress to distributive shock. In a child with shock, the compensated state can rapidly progress to decompensated state, requiring equally rapid assessment and intervention.

Preparing PPHCPs and office staff to effectively and efficiently handle these common episodic pediatric emergencies is necessary for effective planning and management of those emergencies in the context of a disaster. Each office will have unique strengths and challenges, so each office needs to do a careful self-assessment.

16.3 Office Self-Assessment

The goal of the office self-assessment is to determine the following (Jones 2019):

- The types of pediatric emergencies most likely to be encountered in the office given the patient population;
- Assessment of office personnel knowledge, skills, and comfort level with pediatric emergencies and resuscitations;
- Office resources available to respond to pediatric emergencies on site;
- Emergency medical services capability (basic life support, advanced life support, or both) and usual response time to the practice;
- The closest facility that can provide a higher level of pediatric resuscitation (e.g., closest general emergency department) along with the best means of communication with that facility and expected transport time;
- The closest facility that can provide definitive pediatric care (e.g., free-standing children's hospital) along with the best means of communication with that facility and expected transport time.

The Massachusetts Emergency Medical Services for Children (EMSC) Task Force (2003) offers an in-depth 27-item questionnaire to help offices better identify areas in which office preparedness for episodic emergencies can be enhanced (Appendix 1).

16.4 Rapid Assessment and Triage

Responding effectively to an emergency can only happen if the emergency is appropriately recognized. It's important to consider: Who has eyes on the waiting room? Are they trained to recognize a child in distress? While patient registration and administrative personnel can be offered periodic training to recognize signs of distress, it is unfair and unrealistic to place that responsibility on busy staff without solid medical training. Periodic surveillance of the waiting room and exam rooms by medical personnel, such as a lead nurse, is advised (AAP Policy Statement 2007; Jones 2019).

16.5   Formal Course-Based Preparation: BLS, PEARS, and PALS

All staff and HCPs at an office are likely required to maintain current Basic Life Support (BLS) certification from the American Heart Association (AHA). HCPs who are first to respond to a child in distress ideally are responsible for activating the appropriate emergency response system, providing basic life support (BLS), and initiating advanced life support (ALS); however, levels of BLS and ALS training among outpatient HCPs are often deficient (Ralston and Zaritsky 2009). Some HCPs in an office may have Pediatric Advanced Life Support (PALS) certification, but it is not common. As any practicing HCP will acknowledge, possessing certification is much different from experience, comfort, or confidence. While PALS is the gold standard for hospital-based care, the level of intervention the course teaches is not realistic for the office setting.

To bridge the gap between BLS and PALS capabilities and interventions, the Pediatric Emergency Assessment, Recognition, and Stabilization Course (PEARS) was cobranded by the AHA and AAP in 2007. This 7-hour course specifically targets outpatient PPHCPs, nurses, dentists, prehospital, and in-hospital personnel who DO NOT practice in pediatric critical care areas; in other words, to those who *may encounter* critically ill or injured children but who do not provide pediatric ALS *in their routine scope* of practice. Core content common to both PEARS and PALS emphasize that rapid, accurate pediatric assessment leads to accurate categorization of illness, and therefore the most appropriate treatments and interventions (Ralston and Zaritsky 2009). The learner taking PEARS will learn: systematic pediatric assessment, recognition, and stabilization of respiratory, shock, and cardiopulmonary arrest emergencies, as well as the resuscitation team concept. The PEARS course is available online via the AHA website in English, Japanese, and Spanish, or via in-person, instructor-led courses available globally (AHA 2019 https://cpr. heart.org/en/courses/pears-course-options). The PEARS course would be an ideal first step in formal training for office HCPs and staff to improve their response processes and capabilities for common pediatric emergencies as well as disaster response.

16.6   Office Resuscitation Equipment and Medications

The AAP Committee on Pediatric Emergency Medicine (AAP Policy Statement 2007) provides lists of recommended equipment and medications for office emergencies. Equipment and supply lists designate items that are considered essential for all offices, and additional supplies that are considered essential if the typical EMS response time to the medical office is greater than 10 min (Table 16.1). Recommended medications for office emergencies are found in Table 16.2.

Utilizing a system that helps clinical staff rapidly determine the appropriate equipment size and emergency medication dosing for children during emergency care is strongly encouraged. The Broselow® Pediatric Emergency Tape and the Broselow™

Table 16.1 Recommended Equipment for Pediatric Office Emergencies

Office Emergency Equipment and Supplies	Priority[a]
Airway management	
Oxygen-delivery system	E
Bag-valve-mask (450 and 1000 mL)	E
Clear oxygen masks, breather and nonrebreather, with reservoirs (infant, child, adult)	E
Suction device, tonsil tip, bulb syringe	E
Nebulizer (or metered-dose inhaler with spacer/mask)	E
Oropharyngeal airways (sizes 00–5)	E
Pulse oximeter	E
Nasopharyngeal airways (sizes 12–30F)	S
Magill forceps (pediatric, adult)	S
Suction catheters (sizes 5–16F) and Yankauer suction tip	S
Nasogastric tubes (sizes 6–14F)	S
Laryngoscope handle (pediatric, adult) with extra batteries, bulbs	S
Laryngoscope blades (0–2 straight and 2–3 curved)	S
Endotracheal tubes (uncuffed 2.5–5.5; cuffed 6.0–8.0)	S
Stylets (pediatric, adult)	S
Esophageal intubation detector or end-tidal carbon dioxide detector	S
Vascular access and fluid management	
Butterfly needles (19–25 gauge)	S
Catheter-over-needle device (14–24 gauge)	S
Arm boards, tape, tourniquet	S
Intraosseous needles (16 and 18 gauge)	S
Intravenous tubing, microdrip	S
Miscellaneous equipment and supplies	
Color-coded tape or preprinted drug doses	E
Cardiac arrest board/backboard	E
Sphygmomanometer (infant, child, adult, thigh cuffs)	E
Splints, sterile dressings	E
Automated external defibrillator with pediatric capabilities	S
Spot glucose test	S
Stiff neck collars (small/large)	S
Heating source (overhead warmer/infrared lamp)	S

- Note that some offices are located at a distance from EMS services. Providers in offices that are located more than 10 min away from the nearest EMS service need equipment that may not be required in the initial minutes of resuscitation but will be required as the resuscitation effort extends past 10 min.
- Adapted from: American Academy of Pediatrics, Committee on Pediatric Emergency Medicine. *Emergency Medical Services for Children: The Role of the Primary Care Provider*. Singer J, Ludwig S, eds. Elk Grove Village, IL: American Academy of Pediatrics; 1992.

Source: AAP Policy Statement: Preparation for emergencies in the offices of pediatricians and pediatric primary care providers. *Pediatrics*. 2007;120(1):200–212. Available at: https://pediatrics.aappublications.org/content/120/1/200. Reaffirmed November 2018
[a]E indicates essential; S, strongly suggested (essential if EMS response time is >10 min)

Table 16.2 Office emergency drugs

	Priority[a]
Drugs	
Oxygen	E
Albuterol for inhalation[b]	E
Epinephrine (1:1000)	E
Activated charcoal	S
Antibiotics	S
Anticonvulsant agents (diazepam, lorazepam)	S
Corticosteroids (parenteral/oral)	S
Dextrose (25%)	S
Diphenhydramine (parenteral, 50 mg/mL)	S
Epinephrine (1:10 000)	S
Atropine sulfate (0.1 mg/mL)	S
Naloxone (0.4 mg/mL)	S
Sodium bicarbonate (4.2%)	S
Fluids	
Normal saline solution or lactated Ringer's solution (500-mL bags)	S
5% Dextrose, 0.45 normal saline (500-mL bags)	S

- Adapted from: American Academy of Pediatrics, Committee on Pediatric Emergency Medicine. *Emergency Medical Services for Children: The Role of the Primary Care Provider.* Singer J, Ludwig S, eds. Elk Grove Village, IL: American Academy of Pediatrics; 1992
[a]E indicates essential; S strongly suggested (essential if EMS response time is more than 10 min)
[b]Metered-dose inhaler with spacer or mask may be substituted

Pediatric Resuscitation System are widely used in the U.S. Correct use of these clinical tools can significantly reduce medication and equipment sizing errors. Charts or manuals with equipment size and medication dosing (including dose in mg/kg, drug formulation, and volume to administer) organized by patient weight are alternative resources that may be useful. Pediatric HCPs may obtain prepackaged emergency kits from commercial medical suppliers (e.g., Armstrong Medical Industries Inc, Banyan International Corporation). An emergency medical services equipment provider or a pediatric hospital may also be able to help with procurement (Jones 2019).

16.7 Response Plan Development

A comprehensive written response plan should be developed for both episodic emergencies and disasters. Emergency response plans should address the following (Jones 2019):

- A system for rapid internal notification
- EMS activation
  - Designated personnel for communication with EMS
  - Scripted instructions to give prompts for clear communication with EMS dispatch

- Office resuscitation procedure
  - Designated exam room or resuscitation area (ideally with enough space for team response, resuscitation kit/equipment, and accessible by EMS stretcher)
  - Predetermined and clearly defined resuscitation roles
- A plan for patient transfer
  - Include a realistic estimate of both BLS- and ALS-capable EMS response time

Once a response plan is developed, all medical personnel who may participate in resuscitation need to be appropriately trained, and assigned responsibilities may not exceed a standard scope of practice. A physician traditionally has the responsibility to lead the resuscitation; however, alternative role assignments should be prepared in the event there is not a physician in the office at all times. Office administration and support staff also need clearly defined roles to interface with Emergency Response services, redirect patient flow, protect patient privacy, and provide proper patient identification and supportive records. Then everyone needs to practice. Together.

16.8 Resuscitation and Response Drills

Compared with well child care and routine sick visits, emergencies and disasters in the outpatient setting are relatively low-frequency, high-risk events. Though it may seem to justify complacency, the fact that outpatient office staff have never performed CPR in the office in the past has *no* bearing on whether or not it could happen in the future. Managing a serious or critical emergency in an office setting is not a matter of "if" but "when," and it can be stressful, frustrating, and frightening without adequate staff, support, tools, and protocols to do so. Any emergency presenting to an office that is not prepared has the potential to go poorly, and the patient and family may suffer as a result (Klig and O'Malley 2007; Jones 2019). Since experience competently managing emergencies is not obtained or integrated through frequent exposure in daily office practice, HCPs and staff need to drill. Despite this logical reasoning, offices, clinics (AAP Policy Statement 2007; Jones 2019), and urgent care centers (Dunnick et al. 2016) rarely drill or practice for these events.

Mock codes and drills have been found to improve skills preparedness as well as staff confidence in responding to emergencies in office practices, and there appears to be little to no difference between high-fidelity (i.e., use of complex electronic simulation equipment meant to mimic real-time patient responses) and low-fidelity (i.e., use of dolls, paper, verbal scenarios) simulation experiences in improving the preparedness and confidence of the office team (Kalindi et al. 2018; Shenoi et al. 2013; Toback et al. 2006). In other words, it's not so much about the complexity of the medical-case scenario simulation, or nailing the rare diagnosis; it's about practicing the team's process.

Carving out time for regular resuscitation drills is no small undertaking for a busy primary care office or clinic. So many other day-to-day things seem to take priority; but both optimizing and expanding everyday office services, and regularly preparing and drilling for episodic emergencies are excellent ways to increase operational resiliency for more severe, large-scale, or surge events (Disaster Preparedness Advisory Council and Committee on Pediatric Emergency Medicine 2015).

16.9   From Emergency Preparedness to Disaster Preparedness

In a large-scale disaster, state and federal relief may take days or weeks to arrive. Supplies to support a minimum of 72 h of self-sufficiency are commonly recommended by leading disaster preparedness organizations, and the office setting is no exception. Look over disaster supply checklists and decide what items to set aside. Keep an inventory list of equipment, consider ways to back up essential files and patient records, and locate and review office insurance policies (AAP Pediatric Preparedness Resource Kit 2013).

Ideally, pediatric offices should be prepared to continue providing services even when normal operations are disrupted. Part of the office disaster response plan should include not only medical service delivery concerns in the immediate response phase but also emergency operations and business continuity plans, such as:

- Is there a telephone or text chain to reach out to clinic staff to check on their safety and well-being, evacuation status, as well as to communicate office status and work plans?
- Is there a backup generator? Do staff members know how to locate and operate emergency shutoff valves for water and gas lines?
- What is the plan for documentation if the server is down and/or electronic medical records (EMRs) are inaccessible?
- Does the practice have financial reserves to make payroll for a week (or more) if the office is closed or damaged, or employees themselves are displaced or otherwise affected by the disaster? Are there ways to support staff who might need help returning to work (i.e., helping organize child care, carpools, or working remotely)?
- If the office site is damaged or threatened and unsafe for operations, can an alternate temporary site be quickly identified and rented? If conditions permit, would a mobile van or tent-style temporary facility be appropriate for short-term operations? If office site damage is more extensive and reconstruction needed, consider lease or purchase of a "Clinic-in-a-Can" http://www.clinicinacan.org/ .

If disaster should strike while the office is open and full of patients, office staff will be well served by their drills and emergency response protocols. In normal circumstances, many offices rely on the quick transfer of patients in fair, serious, or critical condition to a higher level of care, either via EMS services or private/family transport. Since disaster preparedness requires careful planning for impaired or incapacitated office and community resources, consider the following:

- What will be the next steps if a seriously injured or ill child presents to the office, and 911 or other emergency response systems are inoperable or overwhelmed?
- What if the hospitals and response systems are functioning, but the roads are impassable?
- What if the nearest hospitals or referral centers are themselves evacuated, overwhelmed, threatened, or destroyed?

Excellent preparation resources include the AAP Preparedness Checklist for Pediatric Practices available at https://www.aap.org/en-us/advocacy-and-policy/aap-health-initiatives/Children-and-Disasters/Documents/PedPreparednessChecklist1b.pdf, and the Massachusetts Emergency Medical Service for Children (EMSC) Pediatric Disaster Preparedness Toolkit, available at https://emscimprovement.center/education-and-resources/toolkits/pediatric-disaster-preparedness-toolbox/.

A resilient pediatric office adequately prepared to continue delivering services in a disaster becomes a critical community resource. Ideally, this could include expanded pediatric services to share the patient load with local Emergency Department(s) and provide more appropriate child- and family-centered care than are likely to be available from adult-centered or broad community-based service providers. PPHCP expertise managing medically complex children is particularly needed in the disaster context. (Please refer to Chap. 8 for further information on children with special health care needs.) Extensive family communication and case management is involved in caring for medically complex or technology-assisted children in everyday "normal" circumstances; those needs will only intensify in the context of a disaster. With this in mind,

- Is there a roster of high-risk patients for priority outreach?
- How would the clinic staff reach out to families who may be evacuated and depend on multiple medications, or medical technologies requiring electricity?
- Could available office staff/nurses/HCPs organize to do neighborhood or door-to-door outreach for high-risk families?
- If the office or clinic staff is large, could surplus medical staff be deployed to lend help to shelters or overwhelmed emergency response systems? Consider finding a way to pay staff for time spent working remotely doing in-person outreach, working in shelters, telephone follow-up, and/or triage.

16.10 Expanded Role of the Pediatric Office in Family Disaster Preparedness

Encouraging families to prepare for 72-hour self-sufficiency before needing to resupply or seek outside assistance may not only save their lives but will reduce also the impact of minimally or unaffected families on an already-impacted system (AAP Pediatric Preparedness Resource Kit 2013). This should include food, water, clothing, makeshift shelter, and needed personal items. In more rural areas, setting aside food, water, and supplies to shelter in place for 2 weeks may be necessary, as it may take that long for utilities and services to be restored. Many people put off or discount the need for that degree of preparation. For low-resource families, there likely is not enough money leftover in the monthly budget to purchase and set aside extra food, clothing, and prescription medications for an event that may not ever happen. Some ways a pediatric office can help families prepare include:

- Help families build a "Go-Pack," with hard-copy local and regional maps, extra medications, keys, N-95 respirator masks, and other recommended supplies to support 72-hour self-sufficiency. Consider seeking donations or grants to purchase supplies for and assemble basic "shelter-in-place" kits for families who cannot afford to do so.
- Have a "Preparation Party"!
  - Create family identification packets: offer printing and photocopying of electronic or original documents. Take individual color photos of each family member and print a few copies of each to be stored in the family kit. Label with their name, age, and an emergency contact phone number, to be given to reunification service providers if someone is missing. This can be especially crucial for families with preschool children, undocumented immigrant families, and/or non-English-speaking families. Young children may not know their full name, parent's phone number, address; or they may be too frightened or traumatized to accurately identify themselves when pressed.
  - Assemble a small booklet of important names, addresses, and phone numbers of emergency contacts: immediate and extended family, close friends or neighbors, as well as others who might be available to offer transportation, support, or a place to stay, should cellular phones or other electronic address books be destroyed or inaccessible.
  - Assist families with children with complex or special health care needs to complete the Emergency Information Form for Children with Special Health Care Needs (EIF) developed by the American College of Emergency Physicians (ACEP) in conjunction with the American Academy of Pediatrics (AAP). The EIF helps ensure that a child's complicated medical history is concisely summarized and available when it is needed most—when the child presents with an acute health problem at a time when neither parent nor PPHCP is immediately available. Blank as well as a sample prefilled form can be quickly downloaded from https://www.acep.org/by-medical-focus/pediatrics/medical-forms/emergency-information-form-for-children-with-special-health-care-needs/. Along with the EIF, help prepare a kit of duplicate medical equipment, special supplies, prescriptions, and medication lists.
  - Assist with family reunification planning by offering the pediatric primary care office/clinic to serve as a safe predetermined family "meetup" destination. Individuals and families who fear detention, prosecution, or deportation may hesitate to seek help at community shelters or present themselves to law enforcement if they become separated from their families.

Chapter 6 has more detailed information on general disaster preparedness.

Another area where pediatric primary care offices can excel in caring for children in communities impacted by disaster is in child mental health. In everyday life, children are most likely to receive treatment from primary HCPs for symptoms associated with mental disorders, and most psychotropic drug prescriptions for children and adolescents are prescribed by PPHCPs. In a disaster or terrorist event, the need for mental health services will be far greater and the resources even more strained. The AAP Pediatric Disaster Preparedness and Response Topical Collection (2019) is an excellent resource. Chapter 4 highlights the roles of PPHCPs in identifying and addressing the mental health needs of children and families. Available at: https://downloads.aap.org/DOCHW/Topical-Collection-Chapter-4.pdf. Please see Chap. 12 for further information on post-disaster mental health effects.

16.11 Becoming Community Leaders and Advocates

Not all planners or responders in a disaster response system will be appropriately familiar with, or feel capable of, providing for the unique needs of children during a disaster, particularly infants, children separated from their families, and children and youth with special health care needs. PPHCPs can educate emergency and disaster preparedness officials and response teams, and advocate for children to be appropriately served in terms of evacuation and prevention of family separations, sheltering, family reunifications, appropriate feeding/nutrition, mental health, and safety (Disaster Preparedness Advisory Council and Committee on Pediatric Emergency Medicine 2015). Becoming proactively involved with local and regional disaster preparedness groups is an excellent way for a pediatric office to stay abreast of community disaster–planning efforts, as well as to be recognized within a community as a resource for families and children in times of disaster.

A good starting point for PPHCPs interfacing with disaster preparedness officials is the Pediatric and Public Health Preparedness Exercise Resource Kit. This kit provides tools and templates to make it easier for states, communities, hospitals, or health care coalitions to conduct a pediatric tabletop exercise that provides participants with the opportunity to discuss and assess preparedness plans and capabilities for a disaster that affects children.

Available at https://www.aap.org/en-us/Documents/Tabletop_Exercise_Resource_Kit.pdf.

16.12 Recovery and Resilience

Four disaster management cycles are widely recognized throughout the disaster response literature: mitigation through advance planning, preparedness, response, and recovery. Most attention is typically given to the preparedness and response phases. Preparedness includes developing protocols and designating supplies, which usually focus on immediate response activities, and rarely extend to recovery planning. Recovery can be heavily situation dependent, and it isn't possible to create detailed plans to recover from a situation that hasn't happened yet, though geographic and climate patterns and historical natural disasters in a specific area provide good guidance. In most cases, communities that have been struck by a disaster already have strategic plans in place that were created to guide decision-making related to long-term development and investment. Does the office practice or medical services network have a similar strategic plan? Products from previous planning processes—including a shared vision, assessments, and plans—can be optimally leveraged and built upon to guide the recovery-planning process (Institute of Medicine 2015).

Rather like hospital discharge planning, recovery from a specific event should begin as soon as a disaster happens, while the response phase is still in full swing. Unique challenges faced by pediatric practices include preservation of vaccines and readjustment of service types (i.e., reduction of well-child visit scheduling to accommodate more acute visits) (Institute of Medicine 2015). Pediatric offices would be best positioned to support family and community recovery and resiliency by being resilient themselves. Resiliency is all about how quickly and efficiently a practice can respond to adversity and change, and "bounce back" after a disaster. The sooner doors can be reopened for patient visits (even if those doors are makeshift, "canned," or rented from other facilities), lost revenue will be minimized, and patient and staff retention maximized.

After large-scale disasters, many communities look to the Federal Emergency Management Agency (FEMA) as the recovery expert; but really the role of FEMA is to help start the recovery process and provide guidance and resources. One key way FEMA provides assistance is through the National Disaster Recovery Framework, specifically the Community Recovery Management Toolkit. The Community Recovery Management Toolkit (CRMT) is a compilation of guidance, case studies, tools, and training to assist local communities as they are in the midst of managing recovery post-disaster. The CRMT includes a recovery-planning resource guide, a list of disaster recovery–funding resources (by agency), as well as links to a Pre-Disaster Recovery Planning Guide recently published in 2017, available at https://www.fema.gov/community-recovery-management-toolkit.

Loss, grief, and population displacement can create intense pressure from media and community members to "return to normal." But for segments of the affected communities, predisaster conditions were far from optimal. Low-resource populations often suffer from preventable health problems and experience inequitable access to services; a return to "normal" would in fact be shortsighted and inefficient use of recovery resources. We all have basic ideas of how and what could be done better by our office or clinic. We must look with critical eyes at where our faults and shortcomings lie, and develop ideas for how to improve. While unquestionably traumatic and arduous, the disaster recovery process presents unique and valuable opportunities to improve on the status quo. Effective, forward-thinking community and health infrastructure leaders can capitalize on these opportunities to advance the health, resilience, and sustainability of their communities. A visioning process involving key stakeholders in the pediatric practice (including patients and families!) is a vital step (Institute of Medicine 2015).

If a pediatric practice wants to surpass what is currently accepted as "normal," it's helpful to have a "pie in the sky" to aim for. A clean slate can feel intimidating without at least a seed of an idea to get started. Consider the question: "If our pediatric office were destroyed tomorrow, how would we rebuild to be stronger and more resilient?"

- Would you rebuild in the same location, or could there be another that is better suited for patient access or serving marginalized communities? Is there another potential office site you have been eyeballing? Is there a site with less risk of damage from future similar disasters?
- What does your practice do really well right now? Where does it fall short? How would you like to improve?
- What services or programs have you dreamed of offering? What stops you from implementing them now? What changes would open doorways of possibility?
- What would you change about your current office space or layout to improve workflow and efficiency, patient experience, daily staff experience, or simply improve office appearance? Do you need more common space for meetings or patient groups? Consider the more mundane things such as nonclinical office space allocation, supply and equipment storage, patient and staff parking, and heating/ventilation/air conditioning issues; these have a big impact on daily function, accessibility, and comfort, and can greatly affect worker and patient satisfaction.
- You take it from here. What other questions or potential issues arise?

16.13 Conclusion

Considering the time, effort, and resources it would take to adequately prepare a pediatric office for episodic emergencies, planning for disaster response and recovery can seem overwhelming. Feelings of overwhelm can easily lead to paralysis or simple denial. Taken in small decided steps, however, emergency and disaster preparation can build a meaningful investment in prevention and mitigation of serious, long-term negative impacts on patients and families, and support the longevity of a pediatric office in the community. After all, prevention is what is what pediatric primary care practices do best.

Appendix: Office-Based Self-Assessment of Pediatric Emergency Readiness

1. Have you ever experienced emergencies in your office setting? What were they, and how often have they occurred?
2. What is your office setting (free-standing office, clinic-based, health center-based, hospital-based, other)? Are there resources on site but outside of your office that you could call on during an office emergency (security, other medical or dental professionals in the same building, hospital code team)?

3. What are the high and low staffing points during the times when your office is open? Include nights and weekends if applicable.

4. What is the emergency readiness of the staff present during those times? Include any training in:
   (a) First Aid and Cardio-Pulmonary Resuscitation (CPR)
   (b) Basic Life Support (BLS) or Advanced Life Support (ALS)
   (c) Pediatric Advanced Life Support (PALS)
   (d) Advanced Pediatric Life Support (APLS)
   (e) Emergency Nurse Pediatric Course (ENPC)
   (f) Other Continuing Medical Education (CMEs), etc.

5. Have non-clinical staff been trained to recognize a potential or actual emergency?

6. What anticipatory guidance and education do you provide parents regarding injury prevention, first aid and CPR training, recognizing and responding to emergencies, and accessing emergency medical services (EMS)?

7. Is your waiting room under direct observation or screened frequently by a clinical staff member? What child-proofing measures have you implemented?

8. Do all staff know how to access the EMS system? Are staff able to give location of and directions to the office, level of clinical staff present, age and condition of the child (including vital signs if appropriate), desired transport location, and the level of emergency response required (e.g., First Responder [i.e., police or fire department], BLS [basic life support, emergency medical technician] or ALS [advanced life support, paramedic]).

9. Do you have specific telephone triage protocols for non-clinical and clinical staff? Are all staff currently trained in them?

10. How do you ensure getting the closest available ambulance? Is it 911? A private ambulance? How long does it take for EMS to respond to a call from your office?

11. What is the transport time from your office to a site of definitive care, such as the nearest emergency department or the nearest pediatric center?

12. Have your local EMS providers ever been to visit your office for a non-emergency call, or to receive experience in evaluating pediatric patients?

13. What level of provider comes when you call 911? First Responder (i.e., police or fire department), BLS (Basic-Level EMTs), ALS (paramedics)? Does your local EMS have the necessary equipment and expertise to manage children?

14. Do you know the point of entry (hospital of initial destination) for your local 911 response team? (EMS is required by regulation to transport to the closest appropriate hospital, unless they have a state-approved point-of-entry plan to allow a bypass.)

15. If EMS does not go directly to a pediatric center on a 911 call, how do you emergently transport a child to the desired pediatric center when necessary?

16. Does your office use oxygen? If so, how is it supplied? Do all clinical staff know how to operate the oxygen canister? Where is the key kept?

17. What dosage strategy do you use in the office (code card, length-based tape, dosage book, no strategy)?

18. What airway equipment do you stock? Do all clinical staff know how to locate, choose, and use the appropriate size equipment for any given child?

19. What equipment and supplies do you have on site to provide you and your staff with universal precautions?

20. Does your practice care for any children who are technology-dependent or have special health care needs? Do you have need for any additional equipment or expertise, should a technology-dependent child have an emergency in your office?

21. Do you have written office protocols for the common office emergencies, such as respiratory distress, anaphylaxis, sepsis, dehydration, supraventricular tachycardia? Are all clinical staff appropriately and currently trained in them?

22. How do you document events during an office emergency (assigned role, tape recorder, retrospective, other)?

23. How do you and your clinical staff maintain skills and readiness? Examples include attending nursery deliveries, moonlighting in the urgent care or pediatric emergency departments, being a PALS or APLS instructor, holding regular "mock" office codes and scavenger hunts for infrequently used equipment, and providing expert review of pediatric runs for your local EMS.

24. How do you document parent education, staff training, protocols, and stocking for emergencies?

25. What is your risk management company's policy regarding emergency preparedness of your office?

26. Are there other aspects of your office practice that you think could be improved in order to achieve fewer office emergencies and better outcomes?

Reproduced from: Massachusetts EMSC Task Force. Office Preparedness for Pediatric Emergencies, 3rd ed, O'Malley, P (ed), Massachusetts Department of Public Health, Massachusetts 2003

References

American Academy of Pediatrics (AAP) Policy Statement. Preparation for emergencies in the offices of pediatricians and pediatric primary care providers. Pediatrics. 2007;120(1):200–12. Available at: https://pediatrics.aappublications.org/content/120/1/200. Reaffirmed November 2018.

American Academy of Pediatrics, Committee on Pediatric Emergency Medicine. In: Singer J, Ludwig S, editors. Emergency medical services for children: the role of the primary care provider. Elk Grove Village, IL: American Academy of Pediatrics; 1992.

American Heart Association. PEARS (Pediatric Emergency Assessment, Recognition and Stabilization) course. 2019. https://international.heart.org/en/our-courses/pediatric-emergency-assessment-recognition-and-stabilization.

Disaster Preparedness Advisory Council, Committee on Pediatric Emergency Medicine. Ensuring the health of children in disasters. Pediatrics. 2015;136(5):e1407–17. https://doi.org/10.1542/peds.2015-3112.

Dunnick J, Olympia RP, Wilkinson R, Brady J. Low compliance of urgent care centers in the United States with recommendations for office-based disaster preparedness. Pediatr Emerg Care. 2016;32(5):298–302.

Fuchs S. Pediatric office emergencies. Pediatr Clin North Am. 2013;60:1153–61.

Fuchs G, Weinstock DJ. The preparedness of pediatricians for emergencies in the office: what is broken, should we care, and how can we fix it? Arch Pediatr Adolesc Med. 1996;150: 249–56.

Fuchs S, Jaffe DM, Christoffel KK. Pediatric emergencies in office practices: prevalence and office preparedness. Pediatrics. 1989;83(6):931–9.

Heath BW, Coffey JS, Malone P, Courtney J. Pediatric office emergencies and emergency preparedness in a small rural state. Pediatrics. 2000;106(6):1391–6.

Institute of Medicine. Healthy, resilient, and sustainable communities after disasters: strategies, opportunities, and planning for recovery. Washington, DC: The National Academies Press; 2015. https://doi.org/10.17226/18996.

Jones M. Preparing an office practice for pediatric emergencies. 2019. https://www.uptodate.com/contents/preparing-an-office-practice-for-pediatric-emergencies?csi=b38cd7d1-9f98-4b1c-8536-59f8af49960a&source=contentShare.

Kalindi S, Kirk M, Griffith. In-situ simulation enhances emergency preparedness in pediatric care practices. Cureus. 2018;10(10):e3389. https://doi.org/10.7759/cureus.3389.

Klig J, O'Malley P. Pediatric office emergencies. Curr Opin Pediatr. 2007;19:591–6.

Massachusetts Emergency Medical Services for Children (EMSC) Task Force. In: O'Malley P, editor. Office preparedness for pediatric emergencies. 3rd ed. Massachusetts: Massachusetts Department of Public Health; 2003.

Mehta B, Gupta S. Common pediatric medical emergencies in office practice. Indian J Pediatr. 2017;85(1):35–43.

Pediatric Preparedness Resource Kit. Preparedness checklist for pediatric practices. Elk Grove Village, IL: American Academy of Pediatrics (AAP); 2013. Available at: https://www.aap. org/en-us/advocacy-andpolicy/aap-health-initiatives/Children-and-Disasters/Documents/ PedPreparednessKit.pdf.

Pendleton A, Stevenson MD. Outpatient emergency preparedness: a survey of pediatricians. Pediatr Emerg Care. 2015;31(7):493–5.

Ralston M, Zaritsky AL. New opportunity to improve pediatric emergency preparedness: Pediatric Emergency Assessment, Recognition, and Stabilization course. Pediatrics. 2009;123(2):578–80.

Shenoi R, Li J, Jones J, Pereira F. An education program on office medical emergency preparedness for primary care pediatricians. Teaching Learn Med. 2013;25(3):216–24.

Toback S, Fiedor M, Kilpela B, Cohen Reis E. Impact of a primary care office-based mock code program on physician and staff confidence to perform life-saving skills. Pediatr Emerg Care. 2006;22(6):415–21.

Mae de Vera Reyes, Janeen Gaul, and Emily Rodriguez

17.1 Introduction

Due to the unique nutritional, medical, and neurodevelopmental benefits of breast-feeding, the American Academy of Pediatrics (AAP) recommends exclusive breast-feeding for approximately the first 6 months of life and continued breastfeeding for 1 year or longer as other foods are introduced to the infant's diet (American Academy of Pediatrics 2012). Health benefits of breastfeeding include the transfer of antibodies and other immune factors that offer protection for the infant against many diseases and infections (Administration for Children and Families, Office of Human Services Emergency Preparedness & Response 2013; American Academy of Pediatrics 2016). Breastfeeding is a convenient method of infant feeding as extra equipment and preparation are not required, and the milk is provided at a warm temperature. Breastfeeding saves money by eliminating the need to purchase formula, preparation equipment, bottles, and nipples (Administration for Children and Families, Office of Human Services Emergency Preparedness & Response 2013). The AAP has identified increasing the rate of breastfeeding in the U.S. as a key strategy for optimizing infant nutrition in the event of a disaster (American Academy of Pediatrics 2015).

M. de Vera Reyes (✉) · J. Gaul · E. Rodriguez
Neonatal Intensive Care Unit, Mattel Children's Hospital, RR-UCLA Medical Center, Los Angeles, CA, USA

UCLA Health System NICU Emergency Preparedness Committee (EPC), Los Angeles, CA, USA
e-mail: mdvreyes@mednet.ucla.edu; JGaul@mednet.ucla.edu; EHRodriguez@mednet.ucla.edu

17.2   Infant Feeding During Disasters

In the event of an emergency or disaster, breastfeeding is lifesaving. It is the cleanest and safest way to provide infant nutrition (American Academy of Pediatrics 2015). A breastfeeding mother can provide her infant with optimal nutrition during a disaster without the need for additional feeding supplies, refrigeration, or clean water. Additionally, breastfeeding provides milk at a temperature that can help prevent hypothermia. Risks of illness can be higher during a disaster, making the protection from illness that breastfeeding provides even more important (EAPRO, UNICEF 2006). Formula-fed infants are at an increased risk of acquiring a life-threatening infection during a disaster. Formula does not provide the infant with the immune properties that breast milk does, and the risk of contamination of feedings is increased due to a scarcity of resources. Resources required to sustain formula feedings include a source of heat, detergent, boiled water for formula preparation and cleaning of utensils, containers, measuring utensils, bottles, and nipples (Gribble and Berry 2011; IFE Core Group 2017). Refrigeration is required for the safe storage of prepared formula.

It is a false assumption that women under stress cannot breastfeed; in fact, breastfeeding during a disaster can benefit the mother by the release of hormones that help to relieve stress and anxiety (American Academy of Pediatrics 2015; Wellstart International 2005). It is also a myth that a malnourished or hungry woman does not produce enough breast milk to provide adequate nutrition for her infant. Maternal milk comes from the mother's own body stores, so the quantity and quality of maternal milk are not affected in a disaster (Wellstart International 2005; Carothers and Cox 2009). Frequent breastfeedings will help even hungry mothers maintain their milk supply.

If the infant and mother are separated, or if the infant is not able to breastfeed, expressed mother's milk is the next best choice. If a mother has stopped or reduced breastfeeding, it is possible to resume breastfeeding or increase maternal milk supply through a process called relactation. Frequent skin-to-skin contact with the infant suckling can result in a return of maternal milk that will gradually increase. This is usually most successful in younger infants. It can take 2 weeks or more before breast milk is produced with relactation. The infant must be provided supplementation until the mother's milk supply is sufficient (American Academy of Pediatrics 2015; EAPRO, UNICEF 2006; Wellstart International 2005; Gribble 2014; World Health Organization 1998).

When a mother's breast milk is not available, or the supply is insufficient, the next best source for infant nutrition is human donor milk. In the U.S. and Canada, the Human Milk Banking Association of North America (HMBANA) accredits milk banks that follow internationally recognized guidelines for pasteurized donor human milk in consultation with the Centers for Disease Control and Prevention (CDC), U.S. Food and Drug Administration (FDA), and state departments of health. These guidelines ensure that donors are screened appropriately and that the milk is processed properly to provide a safe human milk substitute for mother's milk (Human Milk Banking Association of North America n.d.). The supply of donor milk from milk banks is limited and is therefore provided to infants with a medical need, such as critically ill infants in neonatal intensive care units (NICU) first. A prescription from an HCP may be required for the use of donor human milk from a milk bank in the outpatient setting (Mother's Milk Bank n.d.).

There are disadvantages and risks associated with the provision of formula for infant feeding in a disaster or emergency; therefore, it should be used as a last resort. During a disaster, efforts should be focused on increasing the mother's supply of breast milk. The use of formula may be counterproductive to this effort, and actually decreases the mother's milk supply. The lack of good hygiene, clean water, sterilized equipment and containers, and refrigeration for storage of prepared formula creates risk for contamination and illness, and is therefore dangerous (American Academy of Pediatrics 2015; EAPRO, UNICEF 2006; IFE Core Group 2017). If human milk is not available, ready-to-feed infant formula is preferred to powdered or concentrated liquid formula that would require mixing with water. Premixed and prepackaged ready-to-feed formula can be fed to an infant without the need for any preparation, minimizing the risk of contamination and concentration errors.

If ready-to-feed formula is not available, powdered or concentrated formula should be mixed with bottled or sterile water to prevent any contamination or exposure to harmful bacteria from potentially compromised tap water. The local health department should be contacted to determine the safety of local water (Centers for Disease Control and Prevention 2018a). If tap water is used, it must be boiled and cooled prior to mixing with powdered or concentrated formula to decrease the risk of contamination. Lastly, if neither bottled nor boiled water is available, then treated water can be used.

It is extremely important to follow the directions for preparing powdered or concentrated formula. Adding incorrect amounts of water, making the formula either too concentrated or too dilute, can cause serious harm to an infant. Cleaning and sterilizing the feeding supplies is equally as important as safe formula preparation. Bottle parts and nipples should be thoroughly cleaned with either bottled, boiled, or treated water. Good hand hygiene should be practiced with the handling of all feeding supplies. Hand sanitizer can be used if soap and water are not available (Centers for Disease Control and Prevention 2018b, c). If refrigeration is not available to store prepared formula, only prepare what is needed for immediate use (Centers for Disease Control and Prevention 2018a). Formula must be prepared and stored safely to prevent serious bacterial infections.

The Federal Emergency Management Agency (FEMA) is prepared to deliver either milk-based formula, soy-based formula, or hypoallergenic-hydrolyzed protein ready-to-feed formula during a disaster (United States, Federal Emergency Management Agency 2011). No unsolicited donations of infant formula should be accepted as it is impossible to determine the safety of such products. The use of unsafe products could lead to worse outcomes (IFE Core Group 2017; Gribble 2014). The provision of formula to breastfeeding mothers may result in decreased breastfeeding and increased risks. It is lifesaving to encourage continued and increased breastfeeding rather than the use of formula.

17.3 Supporting Breastfeeding in the Hospital and Community During a Disaster

Due to the lifesaving nature of breastfeeding during disasters, breastfeeding experts should be included as part of health facility and community disaster preparedness plans. Breastfeeding experts should serve on the team to explore ways to incorporate breastfeeding promotion, support, and education into emergency response policies and practice (Carothers & Cox n.d.).

Education in the community can begin during prenatal appointments with nurses and HCPs providing information regarding the benefits of breastfeeding. The best time to learn about the benefits of breastfeeding during a disaster is before it occurs. Education regarding the extensive list of resources required for disaster preparedness for formula-fed infants should be provided to parents before a disaster occurs. This information can be disseminated by obstetricians, nurses, and lactation consultants before and after birth.

At the World Humanitarian Summit in Istanbul in 2016, those involved with funding, planning, and implementing an emergency response were encouraged to prioritize breastfeeding as a key lifesaving intervention during a disaster (Branca and Schultink 2016). The International Lactation Consultant Association (ILCA) provides emergency preparedness checklists for mothers, health care workers, and volunteers that emphasize the lifesaving nature of breastfeeding and strategies for promoting and supporting breastfeeding (Carothers and Cox n.d.).

The lack of privacy, security, comfort, dim lights, and quiet in emergency shelters have been identified as barriers to successful breastfeeding (Administration for Children and Families, Office of Human Services Emergency Preparedness & Response 2013). The AAP urges pediatricians to assist in the support of breastfeeding mothers by using offices, hospitals, and other shelters as secure, safe havens that are conducive to successful breastfeeding (American Academy of Pediatrics 2015). The World Health Organization (WHO) has identified several incidents worldwide in which mother–baby sites were established by the United Nations International Children's Emergency Fund (UNICEF) and its partners to successfully support breastfeeding during disasters. One example was the Save the Children Jordan program in the Syrian refugee camps, in which mother–baby safe havens were provided in the caravans. By providing privacy, support, and daily educational sessions, they helped over 15,000 mothers safely feed their children between December 2012 and May 2014 (Branca and Schultink 2016).

Disaster preparedness plans need to make provisions for keeping families together, providing support for breastfeeding mothers and providing safe, private places for breastfeeding. Strategies to prevent separation of mothers from babies and for family reunification should be incorporated into emergency plans. Prior to a disaster, plans should be in place that include feeding protocols for breastfeeding infants, as well as plans for safe feeding of infant formula as needed. Standards should be in place to ensure that the available formula is safe.

17.4 Support for the Breastfeeding Mother During a Disaster

To encourage, promote, and prioritize breastfeeding, support must be provided for mothers in the form of education, lactation support, counseling, nutrition, and a safe place for mothers to feed their infants. Mothers who have been supplementing breastfeeding with some formula feeding should be encouraged to breastfeed more often to increase the supply of breast milk and reduce the need for formula (Centers for Disease Control and Prevention 2018c). WHO emphasizes the importance of skilled breastfeeding assistance and private places accessible for mothers to feel safe breastfeeding as part of health services (Branca and Schultink 2016).

Lactating mothers have increased nutritional requirements; therefore, special attention should be paid to the nutrition of pregnant and lactating women (Branca and Schultink 2016). Nurses and HCPs should assess the mother's nutritional status and provide food, water, vitamin, and mineral supplements as needed. Hungry or malnourished mothers can produce enough milk to feed their infant. It is better to feed the mother and encourage frequent breastfeeds rather than feeding the infant something other than mother's milk (Wellstart International 2005).

The breastfeeding mother benefits from assistance with positioning, latching, and psychological support (United Nations Children's Fund (UNICEF) and World Health Organization (WHO) 2018). Education on the benefits of breastfeeding and the risks of formula feeding should be provided. Assistance should be provided to help mothers to increase or reestablish their milk supply. With assistance, support, and encouragement, relactation can be achieved (American Academy of Pediatrics 2015). This requires frequent suckling and skin-to-skin contact (Branca and Schultink 2016).

In the NICU setting, infants may not be able to breastfeed. If expressed breast milk is used, mothers may need support with hand expression, particularly if there is no power or clean supplies for electric breast pumps (Centers for Disease Control and Prevention 2018c). Hand hygiene should be done prior to expressing breast milk. A disposable cup or clean jar should be placed underneath the nipple so the milk can be directly collected. If feeding supplies are limited, and an infant can suckle and swallow, then it is possible to provide feedings by the cup. Guidelines from WHO for feeding by cup include holding the infant upright or semi-upright, offering the milk in a small cup and allowing the infant to use the tongue or suck to take the milk from the cup into the mouth (World Health Organization 1998).

17.5 Breast Milk and Formula Storage During Disasters

Safe storage of expressed and donor breast milk is always important but can be challenging during a disaster. Breast milk storage guidelines should be carefully followed as defined by the AAP (DiMaggio 2016). Fresh breast milk can be stored at room temperature up to 77 °F for up to 4 h. Refrigerated breast milk can be kept for up to 4 days at 39 °F or colder. In cases where the breast milk is very cleanly expressed, it may be kept up to 8 days in the refrigerator. Frozen breast milk can be stored in the freezer at zero degrees Fahrenheit or colder for up to 9 months and in a deep freezer at −4 °F for up to 12 months. It is recommended that breast milk be frozen in small batches of 2–4 oz to prevent any waste of milk (DiMaggio 2016). All breast milk must be labeled with the date and time when it was pumped and later defrosted. Particular attention should be paid to the expiration dates noted on bottles of donor milk. Once the donor milk is thawed, note the thaw time and date on the bottle. The thawed donor milk is good for 24 h in the refrigerator at 39 °F or colder (Mother's Milk Bank 2019).

Ready-to-feed infant formula is the safest substitute for human milk. If ready-to-use formula is not available, powdered and liquid concentrate formula should be mixed with bottled or sterile water. Unopened formula must be stored in a cool, dry indoor location. Once opened, formula must be used within 2 h or stored in the refrigerator at 39 °F or less for up to 24 h (Centers for Disease Control and Prevention 2018a).

If a disaster strikes affecting patients in a hospital setting, it is up to the leadership on duty to quickly and effectively assess the situation in order to determine if evacuation is necessary. If possible, establishing an estimate of the duration of the evacuation will help determine how breast milk, donor breast milk, and formula should be stored. If the decision is made to shelter-in-place, it is critical to follow the storage guidelines listed above.

When the mother is present with the baby during an evacuation, the mother and baby should remain together to encourage and support breastfeeding (Centers for Disease Control and Prevention 2018c). If the mother and baby are separated during an evacuation, it is crucial to have access to stored breast milk. If there is safe entry back into the unit that was evacuated, continue to store the breast milk in the evacuated unit and send a runner to obtain the milk when necessary. If the evacuated unit is not safe to return to, necessary steps will need to be taken to keep the milk properly stored for the duration of the evacuation. The location of available freezers and refrigerators should be identified in the emergency evacuation plan. When initially leaving the unit, store breast milk in a plastic bag with ice for transportation to the safe area. Feeding supplies such as bottles and nipples should also be taken to the evacuation area.

If refrigerators and freezers are not available, it is critical to gather ice and place the breast milk in a cooler. Collapsible coolers can be stored with evacuation equipment and supplies for use with ice when refrigeration is unavailable. Ice must be replaced frequently as it melts, to maintain safe temperature for the milk. When ice is not available for the safe storage of breast milk, and the mother is unable to breastfeed, infants will need to be fed formula.

In the event of power outage, generators should be available as a backup power source to maintain refrigeration and freezers. If in flood-prone areas, generators should be safely located high off the ground. Generators need to be well protected in earthquake-prone areas (Barfield et al. 2017). If complete loss of power is anticipated, freeze water in plastic bags or other containers and use them to fill in empty spaces in the freezer. Place breast milk in the middle of the freezer, away from the walls and door opening. Consider using a cooler to store additional breast milk to prevent frequent opening of the freezer. Once power is lost, open the freezer door only when absolutely necessary. The U.S. Department of Agriculture (USDA) states that a full freezer will hold its temperature for approximately 48 h if the door remains closed and 24 h if it is half full. A refrigerator will keep food safely cold for about 4 h if it is not opened. If dry ice is available, 50 lb of dry ice should hold an 18 cubic foot freezer for 2 days (United States Department of Agriculture Food and Safety Inspection Service 2013). Place towels or blankets over the freezer to keep it insulated. If available, snow can be used in coolers or to fill in space inside a freezer. Fill containers with water and leave them outside to freeze for use in the refrigerator, freezer, or coolers (United States Department of Agriculture Food and Safety Inspection Service 2013).

17.6   Case Studies

17.6.1 Tropical Storm Allison, Texas, 2001

Children's Memorial Hermann Hospital, located in the Texas Medical Center in Houston, includes a 118-bed level 4 NICU, with an average daily census of 90–95 patients. In June 2001, southeast Texas was devastated by Tropical Storm Allison. The hospital was shut down for 6–8 weeks due to heavy rains that flooded the basement and generators, causing the entire power grid to go out.

There was total loss of gas, power, and water. Overnight nurses worked with flashlights, able to hand-bag ventilated patients with room air only. Nurses and parents who were present provided kangaroo care to premature infants to keep them warm. Patient evacuations began the following day once a make-shift helicopter landing zone was created. Infants, beginning with the sickest, were evacuated by the Texas National Guard to outside hospitals in San Antonio, Dallas, Austin, and The University of Texas Medical Branch at Galveston, accompanied by staff nurses and respiratory therapists. Patients were transported in the dark, down seven flights of stairs. No NICU patients were lost in the evacuation.

At that time, the unit did not have a formalized plan to refer to and most of the hospital's general evacuation plans were ineffective due to the extreme circumstances. During Allison, only ready-to-feed formula was used. Since then, the hospital has become a Baby Friendly facility and breastfeeding and lactation support has significantly improved. The hospital has since redesigned the facility, with the generators now located on the fourth floor, and the surrounding landscape has been modified to essentially turn the hospital into an island in the event of extreme flooding. The NICU has designated "Storm Teams" with a very effective communication plan in place (Eborde, E., personal communication, May 1, 2019).

17.6.2 Hurricane Sandy, New York, 2012

On October 29, 2012, Hurricane Sandy hit New York City. Electrical power was lost at NYU Langone around 8:00 PM. As a result, all patients had to be evacuated. There were approximately 20 neonates in the NICU. Neonates were triaged for evacuation based upon illness severity and acuity, with the most critical being transported first. Interdisciplinary teams were created to carry each neonate down nine flights of stairs and included a physician, nurse, and respiratory therapist. Intubated neonates were given positive pressure ventilation using an oxygen tank and ambu bag. Patients on noninvasive ventilation were on battery pack units to maintain their current therapy.

Each team with a neonate from the NICU was met by an ambulance at the main entrance. A nurse and a physician accompanied each infant to the receiving hospital. A nurse rode on a stretcher holding a neonate for every transport. Premature infants who were unable to maintain their temperature and required an isolette were provided kangaroo care with a nurse, along with a hat and blanket over both of them to prevent hypothermia. Portable monitors were utilized for transporting the most critical patients. A two registered nurse (RN) handoff was completed at the receiving hospital with an identification band check. Breast milk was brought with the baby when available since the refrigeration stopped working. Breast milk was packed in plastic biohazard bags with a patient label to bring to the receiving hospital. Breast milk was handed off using a two RN check at the receiving hospital.

Babies awaiting transport were given as much routine care as possible using flashlights. Feedings, parenteral nutrition, and medications were prepared, checked, and administered using a two RN check. Vital signs were completed every 15 min to 1 h based upon illness severity. As isolettes cooled, nurses sat close together in circles with their patients holding them chest to chest to perform assessments and maintain body temperature. Parents who were present held their babies. Breast milk remained in refrigerators and freezers, accessing only as needed to maintain cooling. Breast milk remained cold and was able to be warmed by leaving it at room temperature for feeding. Formula was used as needed.

All neonates were safely transported out of the unit throughout the night. Many lessons were learned through the evacuation experience. Emergency supplies on each unit now include additional flashlights, headlamps, and emergency thermal blankets. Clinical teams have regular meetings with the emergency management experts to review evacuation plans, conduct table-top exercises, and revise plans based on testing. Instant ice packs are now stored on the unit, as well as a cooler bag for each patient that parents/caregivers can receive on admission for transporting milk to and from home or another facility. Most importantly, engaging clinical nurses in emergency preparedness activities continues to provide valuable information on improving disaster preparedness (Alessi, S., Condon, M., Gillen, G., Roman, C., personal communication, March 29, 2019).

17.6.3 Camp Fire, Paradise, California, 2018

On November 8, 2018, an emergency was called in Paradise, CA, due to a rapidly approaching wildfire. The Adventist Health Feather River Hospital includes an eight bed Labor and Delivery unit as well as a Level 1 NICU with three to five beds. The morning of the evacuation, all stable mothers and babies were immediately discharged. There was a Cesarean section occurring in the operating room at that time. As soon as the baby was delivered, both the nurse and the father accompanied the neonate to a waiting sheriff's car, and they were safely relocated to another hospital. After her incision was closed, the mother was transported via an ambulance that caught fire on the way. She and the HCPs with her had to shelter-in-place in a cold, smoke-filled garage. Ultimately, the mother and baby were reunited approximately 10 h later. The baby was kept warm and given formula during this time.

There was one patient in the NICU as well, a 35-week premature infant under phototherapy lights and still not able to nipple enough feeds adequately. The parents were present at the bedside and the infant was emergently discharged with them. As mother's breast milk supply was not established, they were provided with formula and feeding supplies and instructed to drive directly to another hospital in nearby Chico, CA, where the baby would be admitted, and mom could continue to work on her supply (Lawton, K. & Rhys, M., personal communication, May 1, 2019).

17.6.4 Lessons Learned

The first priority in any type of disaster is the physical safety of all persons. In all of these scenarios, the emergent threat to life dictated decision-making. Establishing a plan ahead of time, practicing and educating staff regularly, and informing parents and families of the plan is the best way to prepare for a disaster. Keeping families together eases the stress of the situation and also maintains the bond, both physical and emotional, necessary for successful breastfeeding.

All of these hospitals used their experiences to expand and strengthen their evacuation plans at a system level. Using ready-to-feed formula in these situations was the safest option available and proved to be lifesaving. Ultimately, there is only so much one can be prepared for ahead of time and using critical thinking skills in the moment is essential.

17.7 Conclusion

The provision of aid to all infants and young children in an emergency is considerably challenging. For this reason, emergency preparedness is vital to ensure that breastfed and nonbreastfed infants receive adequate and appropriate support necessary for their survival. In an emergency, it is crucial to protect the well-being of breastfed infants and infants who cannot be breastfed. Because of the difficulties of supporting formula-fed infants in emergencies, preparedness plans should stress the importance of protecting, promoting, and supporting breastfeeding prior to as well as during a disaster (Gribble 2014). Community and hospital emergency preparedness plans should include the support of breastfeeding before an emergency should occur as well as an appropriate emergency response. Support of lactating mothers and their nutritional requirements is key in sustaining exclusive and continued breastfeeding in emergent situations. Breastfeeding is the safest, most cost-efficient, and nutritious method of feeding infants and young children both before and during a disaster. Effective guidelines to support and educate mothers on the benefits of breastfeeding/ relactation and preparation for a disaster are of utmost importance. With the expanding interest in nursing management in pediatric disasters, there is an essential necessity for educating nurses, HCPs, the community, and others on skills to support the nutritional needs of infants and young children in a disaster.

Acknowledgements The authors would like to thank UCLA Health-Mattel Children's Hospital NICU Emergency Preparedness Committee (EPC) for their contributions in writing this chapter.
Lindsay Calac, BSN, CCRN.
Renee Cauntay, BSN, CCRN.
Britnie Hanks, BSN, CCRN.
Siyung Kim, ADN, CCRN.
Chandni Patel, BSN, CCRN.
Anahit Sarin-Gulian, MSN, RNC-NIC, NE-BC.
Lauren Muguerza, BSN, CCRN.

References

Administration for Children and Families, Office of Human Services Emergency Preparedness & Response. Infant feeding during disasters [Internet]. 2013. Available from: https://www.acf. hhs.gov/ohsepr/resource/infant-feeding-during-disasters.
American Academy of Pediatrics. Breastfeeding and the use of human milk. Pediatr [Internet]. 2012;129(3):e827–41. Available from: http://pediatrics.aappublications.org/content/129/3/ e827.full.
American Academy of Pediatrics. Infant feeding in disasters and emergencies [Internet]. 2015. Available from: https://www.aap.org/en-us/advocacy-and-policy/aap-health-initiatives/breast-feeding/documents/infantnutritiondisaster.pdf.
American Academy of Pediatrics. Breast feeding benefits your baby's immune system [Internet]. 2016. Available from: https://www.healthychildren.org/English/ages-stages/baby/breastfeed-ing/Pages/Breastfeeding-Benefits-Your-Babys-Immune-System.aspx.
Barfield WD, King SE, COMMITTEE ON FETUS AND NEWBORN, DISASTER PREPAREDNESS ADVISORY COUNCIL. Disaster preparedness in neonatal intensive care units. Pediatr [Internet]. 2017;139(5):e3–e11. Available from: https://pediatrics.aappublica-tions.org/content/139/5/e20170507.
Branca, F, Schultink, W. Breastfeeding in emergencies: a question of survival. 2016. Available from World Health Organization [Internet]: https://www.who.int/mediacentre/commentaries/ breastfeeding-in-emergencies/en/.
Carothers, C, Cox, K. Breastfeeding: a vital emergency response—are you ready? Facts about breastfeeding in an emergency especially for relief workers [Internet]. 2009. Available from

International Lactation Consultant Association: http://portal.ilca.org/files/in_the_news/Emergencies/FACTSforReliefWorkers.pdf.

Carothers, C, Cox, K. Breastfeeding: a vital emergency response—are you ready? Breastfeeding support checklist for relief workers. Breastfed babies are ready for anything! Emergency preparedness checklist for breastfeeding mothers. n.d. Available from International Lactation Consultant Association [Internet]: https://portal.ilca.org/files/in_the_news/Emergencies/Checklists09_PRINT.pdf.

Centers for Disease Control and Prevention. Infant formula preparation and storage [Internet]. 2018a. Available from: https://www.cdc.gov/nutrition/infantandtoddlernutrition/formula-feeding/infant-formula-preparation-and-storage.html.

Centers for Disease Control and Prevention. Food safety for infants after a disaster [Internet]. 2018b. Available from: https://www.cdc.gov/breastfeeding/recommendations/food-safety-for-infants-after-a-disaster.html.

Centers for Disease Control and Prevention. Disaster planning: infant and young child feeding [Internet]. 2018c. Available from: https://www.cdc.gov/features/disasters-infant-feeding/index.html.

DiMaggio, D. Tips for freezing & refrigerating breast milk [Internet]. 2016. Available from: https://www.healthychildren.org/English/ages-stages/baby/breastfeeding/Pages/Storing-and-Preparing-Expressed-Breast-Milk.aspx.

EAPRO, UNICEF. Supporting families to optimally feed infants and young children in emergencies, an important guide for health and relief workers [Internet]. 2006. Available from: https://www.ennonline.net/iycfemergenciesguide.

Gribble K. Formula feeding in emergencies. In: Preedy VW, editor. Handbook of dietary and nutritional aspects of bottle feeding. Wageningen: Wageningen Academic Publishers; 2014. p. 143–61.

Gribble K, Berry NJ. Emergency preparedness for those who care for infants in developed country contexts. Int Breastfeed J. 2011;6(16):1–12.

Human Milk Banking Association of North America. About frequent questions [Internet]. n.d.. Available from: https://www.hmbana.org/about-us/frequent-questions.html.

IFE Core Group. Infant and young child feeding in emergencies operational guidance for emergency staff and programme managers [Internet]. 2017. Available from: https://www.who.int/nutrition/publications/emergencies/operational_guidance/en/.

Mother's Milk Bank. Instructions for the use of processed human milk [Internet]. 2019. Available from: mothersmilk.org.

Mother's Milk Bank. Babies who receive donor milk, when donor milk is prescribed [Internet]. n.d.. Available from: https://www.milkbank.org/milk-banking/babies-who-receive-donor-milk.

United Nations Children's Fund (UNICEF) and World Health Organization (WHO). Advocacy brief: Breastfeeding in emergency situations [Internet]. 2018. Available from: https://www.unicef.org/nutrition/files/8_Advocacy_Brief_on_BF_in_Emergencies.pdf.

United States Department of Agriculture Food and Safety Inspection Service. Keep your food safe during emergencies: Power outages, floods & fires. Retrieved from United States Department of Agriculture Food and Safety Inspection Services [Internet]. 2013. Available from: https://www.fsis.usda.gov/wps/wcm/connect/d3506874-2867-4190-a941-d511d3fcae71/Keep_Your_Food_Safe_During_Emergencies.pdf?MOD=AJPERES.

United States, Federal Emergency Management Agency. Commonly used sheltering items and services listing (CUSI-SL) catalog. 2011. Available from Homeland Security Digital Library [Internet]: https://www.hsdl.org/?view&did=783045.

Wellstart International. Infant and young child feeding in emergency situations [Internet]. 2005. Available from: https://www.wellstart.org/Infant_feeding_emergency.pdf.

World Health Organization. Relactation: Review of experience and recommendations for practice [Internet]. 1998. Available from: https://www.who.int/maternal_child_adolescent/documents/who_chs_cah_98_14/cn/.

Getting Involved: A Practical Approach to Deployment as a Nurse or Health Care Professional Volunteer

18

Sarah Birch and Emily J. Dorosz

18.1 Nurses and Health Care Professionals as Disaster Volunteers

As the majority in the health care workforce, nurses are well positioned to engage in health-related humanitarian service (Dawson et al. 2017). An increase in global education programs also offers nurses a greater understanding of this field and opportunities to serve (Ripp et al. 2012). In order to maximize the impact of their efforts and provide for the safety and well-being of all parties, health-related service opportunities should be thoughtfully planned and evaluated prior to deployment (Ripp et al. 2012).

Volunteering during disasters is an important opportunity for nurses to highlight not only their clinical acumen and organizational skills but also to demonstrate leadership skills, including the organizing of preparedness, response, and recovery efforts (Rudden 2011; Yamashita and Kudo 2014). Their resilience and ability to deal adeptly with an unpredictable work environment prepares them to handle all phases on the disaster continuum (Cooper et al. 2018). There is also an important need for pediatric-trained nurses and health care professionals (HCPs) to be involved in volunteering during disasters. The presence of these individuals allows for the cohorting of pediatric patients and has been shown to improve care for the patients, as well as morale, for the nurses and HCPs (Burnweit and Stylianos 2011).

18.2 Why Nurses and HCPs Want to Volunteer

The decision to volunteer can be a very personal one, and each individual may have a different reason for doing so. Intrinsic motivators could be behind the decision such as beneficence and improving the health and well-being of children in difficult

S. Birch (✉) · E. J. Dorosz
Children's National Hospital, Washington, DC, USA
e-mail: sbirch@childrensnational.org

© Springer Nature Switzerland AG 2020
C. J. Goodhue, N. Blake (eds.), *Nursing Management of Pediatric Disaster*,
https://doi.org/10.1007/978-3-030-43428-1_18

389

circumstances (Dawson et al. 2017; Jachens et al. 2018; Gilbert 2007). Witnessing the hardships of others can offer a different perspective and give nurses a sense of gratitude for the blessings in their own lives (Quevillon et al. 2016). The nursing profession is known for its compassion and care for others. Nurses have knowledge and skills that some feel is an obligation to act or that "doing something is better than doing nothing" (Dawson et al. 2017). The circumstances and geographic location of a disaster could attract those seeking adventure (Dawson et al. 2017). Participating in relief efforts as part of a team can be an opportunity to develop or enhance one's skills such as leadership and organization (Dawson et al. 2017; Rudden 2011). The daily toil of caring for children in a modern health care setting may elicit frustration, burnout, or loss of patient focus (Berger et al. 2015). Several nursing volunteers have reported a reinvigorated passion for the work and love of nursing as a result of their work in disaster settings (Rudden 2011; Gilbert 2007). Extrinsic motivators for nurse volunteers include a desire to improve patient outcomes and quality of life, raise the visibility and value of nursing, and provide an opportunity to advocate for populations who may not be in a position to advocate for themselves (Dawson et al. 2017; Ripp et al. 2012; Rudden 2011).

18.3 Challenges Faced by Nurses and HCP Volunteers

18.3.1 Facing Reality

Nurses and HCPs who wish to volunteer their time and professional skills in a disaster may have to overcome a variety of obstacles along the way. The hypothetical situation a nurse or HCP envisions prior to deployment and the predicted impact of his or her efforts may not line up with the reality of health care in a disaster setting. The rewards and outcomes of the work may not be immediately apparent or may be on a smaller scale than nurse volunteers hope for (Dawson et al. 2017; Quevillon et al. 2016).

18.3.2 Balancing Personal and Professional Responsibilities

Volunteering to aid in a disaster typically requires the nurse or HCP to commit to deploying for a defined period of time. This involves getting approved time off work, finding shift coverage, or asking colleagues to take on additional responsibilities during this absence (Quevillon et al. 2016). Volunteering should not be at the expense of guaranteed continued employment upon return. Friends and family members may also be asked to fill child care, pet care, or other domestic needs while a nurse or HCP is deployed (Quevillon et al. 2016). Employers and families experience an increased burden in the nurse's/HCP's absence that is often difficult to navigate. Humanitarian aid workers have reported difficulty in achieving and maintaining a work–life balance (Jachens et al. 2018). Advanced planning and securing employer support for the program and specific period of deployment are essential for a successful volunteer and reintegration experience.

18.3.3 Culture and Language

Whether the nurse or HCP is working nationally or internationally, there may be local culture or customs of the population that are unfamiliar. A language barrier presents an additional challenge in patient care and navigating the setting in general. Language interpreters who are also familiar with the culture are a priceless resource for nurse or HCP in this situation (Ripp et al. 2012).

18.3.4 Threats to Health and Safety

When volunteering to work as a nurse or HCP in any setting, health and safety is an essential factor that must remain a priority throughout the deployment. The International Federation of Red Cross and Red Crescent Societies published a tool-kit for volunteer safety that includes guidelines for volunteers before, during, and after a disaster as well as a self-assessment to complete prior to field deployment to ensure essential safety and security procedures are in place (International Federation of Red Cross and Red Crescent Societies n.d.).

Conventional infrastructure may be compromised in a disaster so that volunteers may need to plan for alternate means of transportation. Governmental and NGO agencies will remain knowledgeable about the political and social situation of the area to which they are sending volunteers. The presence of civil war, political unrest, rioting, corruption, or ineffectual police forces are challenges that will need to be accounted for in order to guarantee the safety of personnel (Ripp et al. 2012).

There are a number of physical and psychological risks that are encountered by responders from minor ailments to chronic health conditions (Gabern et al. 2016). These vary by the setting and the specific role and functional activities of the volunteer. The volunteer should be aware of any potential environmental hazards that should be planned for such as heat-related injuries, dehydration, environmental exposures, insect bites, trauma, and extreme weather (Ripp et al. 2012; Gabern et al. 2016).

In addition to environmental hazards volunteers may encounter, nurses and HCPs are at high risk of exposure to infectious diseases while caring for patients in resource-limited settings. While this has been reported, proper hand washing and using appropriate personal protective equipment will mitigate these risks (Ripp et al. 2012; Gabern et al. 2016).

The nurse or HCP deploying to aid in a disaster will often experience difficult and taxing working conditions. Working in a humanitarian aid situation has been described as operating in a "constant state of urgency" (Jachens et al. 2018). In an effort to assist the greatest number of people and counteract personnel shortages, work hours are long and performed at a relentless pace, possibly without adequate breaks (Ripp et al. 2012; Burnweit and Stylianos 2011). Volunteer living conditions can be cramped and lacking in the comforts of home, impeding much-needed rest and relaxation. All of these factors compound the inherent stress of the situation that may result in volunteers experiencing exhaustion and burnout (Gabern et al. 2016).

Even to nurses or HCPs with experience working in a disaster setting, each situation is different, presenting a new environment with new challenges (Jachens et al. 2018). The situation could be volatile or unpredictable, resulting in higher or lower patient acuities than predicted or changing the availability of resources (Burnweit and Stylianos 2011). Nurses/HCPs often feel they are working outside their comfort zones, that they are inadequately prepared for these challenges, and/or they experience a general feeling of being stretched (Dawson et al. 2017).

18.3.5 Secondary Trauma

The patients that nurses/HCPs encounter in a disaster setting have experienced life-altering events ranging from the death of loved ones, loss of residence, destruction of community, extreme threat to safety and security, and countless other traumatic experiences. The nurse/HCP caring for these patients at their most vulnerable moment hears their stories and is exposed to their anxiety, emotions, grief, loss, despair, hopelessness, harmful coping mechanisms, or mental health problems in addition to their physical ailments (Dawson et al. 2017; Yamashita and Kudo 2014; Burnweit and Stylianos 2011; Quevillon et al. 2016). Nurses/HCPs may have to witness or participate in rescue efforts that are ultimately unsuccessful (Gabern et al. 2016). Treating these individuals or seeing a large number of affected or deceased people can result in a secondary exposure or vicarious trauma in the volunteers, resulting in adverse psychological effects (Gabern et al. 2016). Disaster volunteers in health care can develop compassion fatigue as well in which they experience such frequent demands on their emotions that it begins to not affect them or they experience numbness related to the suffering of others (Gabern et al. 2016). All pediatric nurses/HCPs are at risk for compassion fatigue due to the potential trauma associated with caring for ill and injured children (Berger et al. 2015). Negative coping mechanisms and emotional responses need to be recognized in the early stages so appropriate intervention can occur. (Table 18.1).

Table 18.1 Examples of negative coping mechanisms and emotional responses (Jachens et al. 2018; Berger et al. 2015; Chan et al. 2017)

- Avoidance, withdrawal
- Psychological distress, anxiety, depression
- Sleeplessness or sleeping all day
- Change in appetite, increase or decrease
- Smoking
- Increased caffeine intake
- Alcohol or other substance abuse, binge drinking
- Sexual misconduct
- Compulsive spending
- Emotional detachment or apathy
- Physical illness

18.3.6 Resource Limitations

A disaster is, by definition, a resource-limited setting. Nurses and HCPs are called upon to be flexible and creative in their utilization of available staff, equipment, medications, and diagnostic testing, resulting in an atypical practice environment for the nurse/HCP (Ripp et al. 2012). When the demand for health care services outweighs the available resources, difficult decisions have to be made about who receives which services and when. The alternate standards of care may be based on the predicted outcome for the patient in the context of the current disaster setting and availability of necessary expertise and treatment to meet the patient's needs (Burnweit and Stylianos 2011). This decision-making process and the execution of the decisions produce an enormous level of stress on the volunteers (Burnweit and Stylianos 2011). In this situation, they may be forced to treat patients under altered standards of care and the outcomes may not always be favorable. Scarce resources (e.g., ventilator) would need to be conserved, reused, and sometimes reallocated to a patient most likely to benefit (Kissoon 2011). Nurses/HCPs may be distressed when patients do not survive, whom they feel may have lived if presenting for care at their home institution or in a nondisaster setting (Ripp et al. 2012). The burden of rationing limited resources may also intensify when treating the pediatric population as allocating versus withholding resources may be the determining factor in the child's fate (Burnweit and Stylianos 2011). Making the transition from fully treating all patients to operating under revised standards of care can cause ethical distress and negative coping mechanisms (Dawson et al. 2017). To take part in this work, volunteers need to recognize the reality of the situation and focus on maximizing the outcomes and survival of the population as a whole, rather than that of each individual (Kissoon 2011).

18.4 Selecting and Applying to an Organization/Group

There are many avenues to volunteerism in disasters, and placements can be short- or long-term. It is best practice to deploy with a reputable disaster group or organization. (Table 18.2) There are many factors to consider when selecting and applying for a volunteer opportunity. (Table 18.3) Spontaneous, unaffiliated, uncoordinated volunteers can compound difficulties experienced at the disaster site, overwhelm a response system, and make things worse instead of better (National Leadership Forum on Disaster Volunteerism n.d.; Merchant et al. 2010).

18.5 Legal Considerations

Scope of Practice describes the "services that a qualified health professional is deemed competent to perform, and permitted to undertake—in keeping with the terms of their professional license" (American Nurses Association n.d.). Registered and Advanced Practice Nurses' Scope of Practice is defined through (1) the state

Table 18.2 Major organizations to consider when volunteering

International Programs
International Red Cross
https://www.icrc.org/en
International Medical Corps
https://internationalmedicalcorps.org/
United Nations
https://www.unv.org
Partners In Health
https://www.pih.org/
Project Hope
https://www.projecthope.org/
Regional, State, and Federal Government-Sponsored Programs
Disaster Medical Assistance Team (DMAT)
https://www.phe.gov/Preparedness/responders/ndms/ndms-teams/Pages/dmat.aspx
Medical Reserve Corps (MRC)
https://www.phe.gov/about/oem/prep/Pages/mrc.aspx
Community Emergency Response Team (CERT)
https://www.ready.gov/community-emergency-response-team
Americorps Disaster Response Team (A-DRT)
https://www.nationalservice.gov/focus-areas/disaster-services/
americorps-disaster-response-teams-drts
Other Nongovernmental (NGOs) Programs
(any agency that is not affiliated with a government):
Employer
Academic
Faith-based
American Red Cross

Table 18.3 Key considerations when evaluating volunteer organizations

1. There should be a clear volunteer position posting available with role expectations and responsibilities, scope of practice, reporting structure, and emergency credentialing process available for review. (Yamashita and Kudo 2014; Burnweit and Stylianos 2011; Fitch 2010)
2. Is there a clear and transparent screening process? (e.g., interviews, background checks, felon and sex offender databases, and criminal background checks). Is there an appeal process if an applicant wants to continue to apply for a postscreening process? (Fitch 2010)
3. Are there appropriate training courses and exercises taught by experts (including the fundamentals of the incident command system)? (Dawson et al. 2017; Rudden 2011)
4. Is personal protective equipment available and is training provided on how to use personal protection (i.e., PPE, safe specimen handling, blood-borne pathogens, and safe patient handling) (Fitch 2010)
5. Is there policy and procedure available if there is an injury while on deployment? Does organization participate in state or another workers' compensation plan and does it cover emotional well-being? (Fitch 2010)
6. Does the organization promote self-care and do they have training in place that includes self-care, measures to maintain safety, methods to assess worker stress, policies on workload and time off, and information on recovery? (Quevillon et al. 2016; Tamburri 2017)
7. How does the organization handle ethical dilemmas in field clinical practice? (Fitch 2010)
8. What methods of communication does the organization use? (Fitch 2010)
9. How long is the duration of assignment? (Fitch 2010)

Nurse Practice Act and (2) the regulatory agency that governs nursing practice in the state (usually the Board of Nursing, but may be jointly governed by the Board of Medicine depending on the state) (American Nurses Association 2019). It is important to consult the licensure requirements for state jurisdiction as there is variability depending on the jurisdiction (American Nurses Association 2019).

Legal protections are provided for nurses and HCPs and institutions that implement crisis standards of care, and nurses/HCPs who follow disaster protocols that have been accepted and vetted in good faith should be protected from civil liability (Kissoon 2011). It is necessary for hospitals to have emergency temporary privileging and credentialing processes in their medical staff bylaws and disaster response plans. The Joint Commission (TJC) requires hospitals to establish procedure for verifying credentials and granting privileges during and after disaster (The Joint Commission 2017a). If a hospital's disaster plan is activated, it may implement a modified process for determining qualifications and competence of volunteers (The Joint Commission 2017b). These are often included in the credentialing and privileging process through the hospital, and the process is delineated in the Medical Staff Bylaws of an organization. Credentialing is the process of obtaining, verifying, and assessing the qualifications of a nurse/HCP to provide care or services in or for a health care organization. Credentials are documented evidence of licensure, education, training, experience, or other qualifications (The Joint Commission 2017c). Privileging is the process whereby a specific scope and content of patient care services (that is clinical privileges) are authorized for a nurse/HCP by a health care organization, based on an evaluation of the individual's credentials and performance (The Joint Commission 2017c). Differences in scopes of practice, standards of care, and regulation have put organizations at risk for negligence as they provide patient care (Rudden 2011).

Nurse and HCP volunteers are often needed during response efforts and are frequently recruited from areas outside the disaster zone including neighboring states and at times from the broader international community. The credentialing and privileging process enables organizations to verify eligibility and provide malpractice insurance and liability coverage (Ripp et al. 2012). It also holds the nurse/HCP to the organizational bylaws and provides the authorization to practice and emergency credentialing. Nurses and HCPs volunteering through agencies that respond outside of the state of residence need to be aware of laws and programs that are set up to benefit them.

18.5.1 Laws

Good Samaritan laws generally provide basic legal protection for those who assist a person who is injured or in danger. All 50 states and the District of Columbia have some type of Good Samaritan law; however, how these laws are implemented varies from state to state (Association of State and Territorial Health Officials (ASTHO) n.d.).

The Volunteer Protection Act 1997 (VPA) applies to medical and nonmedical volunteers (Hershey et al. 2016). The VPA applies to negligence that occurs within the scope of uncompensated volunteer responsibilities. If the volunteer's responsibilities are covered by licensure laws, "the volunteer must be properly licensed, certified, or authorized by the appropriate authorities as required by the law in the state in which the harm occurred" (Association of State and Territorial Health Officials (ASTHO) 2019).

18.5.2 Programs

It is important to be aware of the volunteer organization's credentialing and privileging process. Each organization will vary slightly, but it will guide the volunteer through the process during intake. Volunteering through the Medical Reserve Corps requires preregistration with the Emergency System for Advance Registration of Volunteer Health Professionals (ESAR-VHP). ESAR-VHP is a "federal program created to support states and territories in establishing standardized volunteer registration programs for disasters and public health and medical emergencies. The program, administered on the state level, verifies health professionals' identification and credentials so that they can respond more quickly when disaster strikes. By registering through an ESAR-VHP website, volunteers' identities, licenses, credentials, accreditations, and hospital privileges are all verified in advance, saving valuable time in emergency situations" (Public Health Emergency n.d.). Information collected on the ESAR-VHP site varies from state to state, and some states have an electronic application, some use paper, and others use a combination of both. Specific information related to each state's specific application via the ESAR-VHP registration page can be found at: https://www.phe.gov/esarvhp/Pages/registration.aspx.

The Emergency Management Assistance Compact (EMAC) manages "resources deploy through the state emergency management agencies of their respective states allowing for a coordinated deployment. Deployments are coordinated with the federal response to avoid duplication and overlap" (Emergency Management Assistance Compact n.d.). EMAC provides protections for covered individuals, tort liability protections, workers' compensation, license reciprocity, and reimbursement. Not all nurses and HCPs are covered through EMAC and the provision excludes any "willful misconduct, gross negligence, or recklessness" (Lopez et al. 2013). Worker's compensation and liability protection vary from state to state; it is important to consult the ESAR-VHP state-specific site for guidance related to each specific state.

For the cases in which EMAC does not cover the nurse/HCP providing health or veterinary services, 15 jurisdictions including 13 states and the District of Columbia have approved and recommended that states enact the Uniform Emergency Volunteer Health Practitioner Act (UEVHPA). It allows the nurses/HCPs licensed and in good standing to be recognized in participating states in time of emergency (Lopez et al. 2013).

18.6   Preparing for Deployment

18.6.1 Health Considerations

Prior to deploying to a disaster setting as a nurse/HCP volunteer, there are several elements the nurse/HCP should consider in order to ensure his or her safety and well-being both during and after the experience. First and foremost, maintaining health through recommended vaccinations and other disease prevention methods is of utmost importance for the volunteer. The necessary precautions will vary based on the location of the deployment, length of time, and the nature of the volunteer's role. The Centers for Disease Control and Prevention (CDC) have compiled comprehensive Traveler's Health Guidelines for people traveling to areas outside the United States (Centers for Disease Control n.d.-a).

Health information for international travel is also contained in the CDC Yellow Book, including updated information on infectious disease concerns and recommendations (Centers for Disease Control n.d.-b). An HCP visit should also occur prior to deployment so that any individual health considerations can be discussed in the context of the above recommendations and appropriate prophylaxis medications can be prescribed when appropriate, e.g., antimalarial medication (Ripp et al. 2012; Burnweit and Stylianos 2011). A physical examination and "fitness for duty" determination may also be required prior to volunteering (Centers for Disease Control n.d.-c). As is the case in any health care setting, proper hand washing and sanitation is essential to preventing the spread of disease.

18.6.2 Education and Training

In order to be a safe and effective volunteer in a disaster setting, the nurse/HCP should first ensure baseline knowledge of relevant operations and procedures. Each organization will have a specific predeployment orientation session that covers important preparation and logistics information. The session should include a situation overview, safety and security briefing, health information, relevant cultural information, resource availability, expected care processes, staff competencies, and policies and procedures (Ripp et al. 2012; Quevillon et al. 2016; Kissoon 2011). The nurse/HCP should be informed prior to accepting an assignment, researching the situation, and what the role entails, e.g., practicing in an established hospital as opposed to a temporary field hospital erected for the current crisis (Dawson et al. 2017; Burnweit and Stylianos 2011). If the nurse/HCP is not already practicing concepts of personal, family, and professional preparedness, there are many resources available (Ready.gov Emergency Alerts n.d.).

In addition to attending an orientation session, volunteers should complete online modules or equivalent in-person training, especially if they are new to the field. One of the essential topics to cover is the NIMS Incident Command System (ICS). ICS is a standardized approach to all phases of an incident that is widely

Table 18.4 Disaster applications and alerts

Disaster Information Management Resources Center: Disaster Apps for Your Digital Go Bag
https://disasterinfo.nlm.nih.gov/apps
Ready.gov Emergency Alerts
https://www.ready.gov/alerts
FEMA Emergency Alert System
https://www.fema.gov/emergency-alert-system
FEMA Mobile App
https://www.fema.gov/mobile-app

used to establish common language and processes among responders. It includes important roles, structure, and communication guidelines for Incident Command that are applicable in all-hazards (Federal Emergency Management Agency (FEMA) n.d.). ICS-100 Introduction to the Incident Command System, IS-700 National Incident Management System, An Introduction, and IS-366.A: Planning for the Needs of Children in Disasters are some of the FEMA courses recommended to pediatric disaster volunteers. Understanding the terminology and processes ahead of time will enable the nurse/HCP to speak a common language with other responders and integrate into the system more efficiently. See Chap. 4 for further information.

18.6.3 Alerts and Smart Telephone Applications (Apps)

It is important, especially when traveling abroad, to maintain situational awareness of potential health, weather, security, or political hazards. There are several smart telephone applications and alerts that can be downloaded or registered for ahead of time that provide updates within the United States or in another country (Table 18.4).

18.7   Taking Care of Yourself as a Nurse/HCP Volunteer

Working as a nurse/HCP in a disaster setting and providing for the needs of others leaves the nurse/HCP vulnerable to negative outcomes, as previously discussed. The situation necessitates considering self-care a priority. Taking proper care of one's own needs before, during, and after an assignment in a disaster setting "can reduce negative reactions to stressful emergency work and promote growth, mastery, and self-efficacy after the experience" (Quevillon et al. 2016). This is something that should be understood and promoted by the group membership, leadership, and organization.

> "Indeed, if one consistently does not take care of oneself, then he or she will likely be unable to continue to provide care for others." (Quevillon et al. 2016)

18.7.1 Training

Nurses/HCPs should be aware of the symptoms of burnout and other stress responses so that they are able to recognize them in themselves and others during the deployment. It would also be helpful to complete training in this area prior to the assignment, whether through an organization's orientation program or other means (Burnweit and Stylianos 2011). Nurses/HCPs are vulnerable to the negative effects regardless of experience, but it can be helpful to pair veteran volunteers with those who are less experienced so the veteran can provide mentorship and act as a resource (Burnweit and Stylianos 2011). Nurses/HCPs also have the responsibility to be cognizant of their own baseline stress and triggers to first determine if the timing is right to deploy. Self-awareness of personal limits and boundaries can help guide the establishment of a supportive environment (Quevillon et al. 2016). Self-care is optimized with an individualized approach. Nurses/HCPs should develop their own self-care plans that combine individual efforts with supportive processes from the organization and management (Quevillon et al. 2016; Tamburri 2017).

18.7.2 Physical Health and Well-Being

In their tremendous and often heroic efforts to help others, nurses/HCPs tend to be less concerned with their own welfare. Nurses/HCPs need to be supported and encouraged to look after their own physical health, especially amidst the chaos of a disaster situation (Burnweit and Stylianos 2011). The team should plan time in the schedule for breaks and adequate relief of clinical responsibilities so that nurses/HCPs are actually able to take a real physical and mental break from the toil of disaster relief efforts. Living quarters should be adequate for rest and privacy and made as comfortable as possible given the situation. Workers need to get enough sleep every night so that their bodies have time to recover before the next day's activities. Meditation or relaxation techniques should be utilized. For longer assignments, nurses/HCPs should be allowed to schedule time off or to take an unscheduled day off if it becomes necessary to maintain physical or psychological health. Adequate and consistent nutrition and hydration need to be available to workers so their bodies can maintain high functionality. Above all, nurses/HCPs need to remember their own vulnerability and mortality and provide adequately for their own needs as best they can considering the extreme situation around them (Quevillon et al. 2016).

18.7.3 Communication and Debriefing

Volunteers working within a team have reported that despite difficult living conditions and lack of standard comforts, the group provided a support system for each other (Burnweit and Stylianos 2011). The shared experience of volunteering in a disaster setting can bring individuals together and provide an understanding audience for personal reflection or discussion. Debriefing the experience is a method to share experiences, process activities, and seek a greater understanding (Cooper et al. 2018; Forster and Hafiz 2015). Reflecting and communicating with others can also allow an opportunity for colleagues to intervene if someone is showing signs of distress or fatigue (Burnweit and Stylianos 2011). Exhibiting signs of distress or emotional reactions should not be seen as a sign of weakness, but rather an opportunity to offer support, assist with reflection, and facilitate a time out when necessary (Burnweit and Stylianos 2011; Tamburri 2017). Leadership should plan and support activities that support team building early-on so that this support system can be effective.

18.7.4 Recovery and Reintegration

Regardless of the duration of a disaster assignment, the nurse/HCP may find it difficult to transition back to normal everyday professional and personal life. It is best to allow sufficient time to rest, recover, and reflect upon the life-changing experience (Quevillon et al. 2016). A formal debriefing with the team can be helpful and should occur immediately after the assignment, especially if group members do not routinely work together and will be returning to different locations (Burnweit and Stylianos 2011). Some organizations may offer psychological support or screening on a group or individual basis following a deployment.

It is recommended to engage in pleasurable activities upon returning home such as spending time with family and friends or taking personal time for rest if possible (Quevillon et al. 2016). The absence of the individual has been felt by family and coworkers who have had to take on other responsibilities during the deployment and may have experienced their own stressors as a result. There may be demands placed on the nurse/HCP immediately upon returning from the disaster assignment. Nurses/HCPs may experience fatigue, stress, and a variety of emotions when transitioning back into regular routines. Support from family, friends, and colleagues can be helpful, and nurses/HCPs may also find engaging with a therapist or trained counselor to be an effective method for handling the emotional upheaval (Burnweit and Stylianos 2011; Chan et al. 2017; Forster and Hafiz 2015).

The process of transitioning should not be rushed, and it is important to recognize that the symptoms and emotions of the experience may persist for an extended period of time. One strategy to build psychological resilience is to view events in a more productive and helpful manner by utilizing positive reframing techniques (Quevillon et al. 2016). Not only did the nurse/HCP make a positive impact on individuals through his or her efforts but the nurse/HCP also likely experienced personal growth, professional growth, character building, and strengthened confidence through the experience (Dawson et al. 2017). It is most helpful to focus on all the positive outcomes and emotions associated with the experience and ensure these are the enduring feelings that persist (Table 18.5).

Table 18.5 Examples of self-care practices (Cooper et al. 2018; Burnweit and Stylianos 2011; Quevillon et al. 2016; Chan et al. 2017; Tamburri 2017; Forster and Hafiz 2015)

- Determine if the timing is right to volunteer
- Consider bringing books, games, or exercise equipment
- Set appropriate boundaries
- Take breaks
- Get enough rest
- Utilize meditation and relaxation techniques
- Drink plenty of water
- Do not skip meals; have snacks available
- Recognize and intervene at early signs of stress and burnout
- Speak up if sick or feeling ill
- Engage in religious or spiritual practices as desired
- Talk about the experience
- Attend and actively participate in formal or informal debriefing
- Allow time to reintegrate
- Be patient with yourself; continue self-care practices
- Focus on the positive aspects of the experience

18.8 Conclusion

"Hospitals partnering existing volunteer organizations with functional relief systems already in place is an effective way to make a meaningful contribution in the postdisaster setting" (Ripp et al. 2012). There are "higher risks" associated with working internationally (Dawson et al. 2017). Evaluating risk management strategies available to volunteers is important "to provide a safe, supportive work environment as they serve the program's mission" (Fitch 2010). Volunteers should be aware of risks and make the determination of whether the benefits and potential contributions to the health of the impacted population outweigh the sense of individual risk. Preparation is key for nurse/HCP volunteers. "If one consistently does not take care of oneself, then he or she will likely be unable to continue to provide care for others" (Quevillon et al. 2016). In order to answer the call and meet the demands of their complex and demanding roles, nurse/HCP volunteers need to prioritize their own health and well-being before, during, and after deployments.

References

American Nurses Association. Scope of practice. n.d.. Available at: https://www.nursingworld.org/practice-policy/scope-of-practice/. Accessed 1 May 2019.

Association of State and Territorial Health Officials (ASTHO). ASTHO Legal Preparedness Series Emergency Volunteer Toolkit. n.d.. Available at: http://www.astho.org/Programs/Preparedness/Public-Health-Emergency-Law/Emergency-Volunteer-Toolkit/Volunteer-Protection-Acts-and-Good-Samaritan-Laws-Fact-Sheet/. Accessed 20 Apr 2019.

Berger J, Poliva B, Smoot E, Owens H. Compassion fatigue in pediatric nurses. J Pediatr Nurs. 2015;30(6):e11–7.

Burnweit C, Stylianos S. Disaster response in a pediatric field hospital: lessons learned in Haiti. J Pediatr Surg. 2011;46(6):1131–9.

Centers for Disease Control. Traveler's Health Guidelines. n.d.-a. Available at: https://wwwnc.cdc.gov/travel. Accessed 20 Apr 2019.

Centers for Disease Control. Yellow Book 2018. n.d.-b. Available at: https://wwwnc.cdc.gov/travel/page/yellowbook-home. Accessed 10 May 2019.

Centers for Disease Control. Emergency Responder Health Monitoring and Surveillance. n.d.-c. Available at: https://www.cdc.gov/niosh/erhms/predeploy.html. Accessed 20 Apr 2019.

Chan S, Khong P, Wang W. Psychological responses, coping and supporting needs of healthcare professionals as second victims. Int Nurs Rev. 2017;64(2):242–62.

Cooper L, Briggs L, Bagshaw S. Postdisaster counselling: personal, professional, and ethical issues. Aust Soc Work. 2018;71(4):430–43.

Dawson S, Elliott D, Jackson D. Nurses' contribution to short-term humanitarian care in low- to middle-income countries: an integrative review of the literature. J Clin Nurs. 2017;26(23–24):3950–61.

Emergency Management Assistance Compact. Learn about EMAC. n.d.. Available at: https://www.emacweb.org/index.php/learn-about-emac/what-is-emac. Accessed 20 Apr 2019.

Federal Emergency Management Agency (FEMA). Emergency Alert System. n.d.. Available at: https://www.fema.gov/emergency-alert-system. Accessed 10 May 2019.

Fitch E. Managing the risks of incorporating volunteers into public health emergency response: the other side of the liability issue. Disaster Med Public Health Prep. 2010;4(3):252–4.

Forster E, Hafiz A. Paediatric death and dying: exploring coping strategies of health professionals and perceptions of support provision. Int J Palliat Nurs. 2015;21(6):294–301.

Gabern SC, Ebbeling LG, Bartels SA. A systematic review of health outcomes among disaster and humanitarian responders. Prehosp Disaster Med. 2016;31(6):635–42.

Gilbert L. Where in the world am I? Where should I be? Experiences and exhortation of Itinerant Pediatric Nurse Practitioner. J Pediatr Health Care. 2007;21(6):381–4.

Hershey TB, Van Nostrand E, Sood RK, Potter M. Legal considerations for health care practitioners after superstorm sandy. Disaster Med Public Health Prep. 2016;10(3):518–24.

International Federation of Red Cross and Red Crescent Societies. Volunteers, stay safe! A security guide for volunteers. n.d.. Available at: https://media.ifrc.org/ifrc/wp-content/uploads/sites/5/2018/03/Volunteer-Security-manualENGLISH.pdf. Accessed 10 May 2019.

Jachens L, Houdmont J, Thomas R. Work-related stress in a humanitarian context: a qualitative investigation. Disasters. 2018;42(4):619–34.

Kissoon N. Task force for pediatric emergency mass critical care. Deliberations and recommendations of the Pediatric Emergency Mass Critical Care Task Force: executive summary. Pediatric Crit Care Med. 2011;12(6):S103–8.

Lopez W, Kershner SP, Penn MS. EMAC volunteers: liability and workers' compensation. Biosecur Bioterror. 2013;11(3):217–25.

Merchant R, Leigh J, Lurie N. Health care volunteers and disaster response--first be prepared. N Engl J Med. 2010;362(10):872–3.

National Leadership Forum on Disaster Volunteerism. Preventing a disaster within a disaster: the effective use of management of unaffiliated volunteers. n.d.. Available at: https://www.ncjrs.gov/pdffiles1/Archive/202852NCJRS.pdf. Accessed 20 Apr 2019.

Public Health Emergency. The Emergency System of Advance Registration of Volunteer Health Professionals. n.d.. Available at: https://www.phe.gov/esarvhp/Pages/About.aspx. Accessed 20 Apr 2019.

Quevillon RP, Gray BL, Erickson SE, Gonzalez ED, Jacobs GA. Helping the helpers: assisting staff and volunteer workers before, during, and after disaster relief operations. J Clin Psycol. 2016;72(12):1348–63.

Ready.gov Emergency Alerts. n.d.. Available at: https://www.ready.gov/alerts. Accessed 10 May 2019.

Ripp J, Bork J, Koncicki H, Asgary R. The response of academic medical centers to the 2010 Haiti earthquake: the Mount Sinai School of Medicine experience. Am J Trop Med Hyg. 2012;86(1):32–5.

Rudden P. Volunteering for service: the role of emergency nurses. Emerg Nurse. 2011;19(4):18–9.

Tamburri LM. Creating healthy work environments for second victims of adverse events. AACN Adv Crit Care. 2017;28(4):366–74.

The Joint Commission. Standard EM 02.02.13. Comprehensive Accreditation Manual for Hospitals; 2017a:EM-34.

The Joint Commission. Standard EM 02.02.15. Comprehensive Accreditation Manual for Hospitals; 2017b:EM-34.

The Joint Commission. Standard MS.06.01.05. Comprehensive Accreditation Manual for Hospitals; 2017c:MS-28-MS-36.

Yamashita M, Kudo C. How differently should we prepare for the next disaster? Nurs Health Sci. 2014;16(1):56–9.

Appendix: Resources

Catherine J. Goodhue

Web-based resources, including toolkits, checklists, and newsletters/listserves, continue to expand and evolve over time. Revised documents following major disasters also continue to grow. Unfortunately, many links change rapidly and may not be current at publication. However, this appendix has a wealth of information that the nurse/HCP may find helpful.

Listservs

Name of Network	Website	Contact
National Pediatric Disaster Coalition	www.npdcoalition.org	nationalpedicoalition@gmail.com
National Library of Medicine	https://disasterinfo.nlm.nih.gov/stay-connected	https://public.govdelivery.com/accounts/USNLMDIMRC/subscriber/new

Health Care Organizations with Disaster-Related Websites

Organization	Website
American Academy of Pediatrics	https://www.aap.org/en-us/advocacy-and-policy/aap-health-initiatives/Children-and-Disasters/Pages/default.aspx
National Association of Pediatric Nurse Practitioners—Children in Disasters Special Interest Group	https://www.napnap.org/be-prepared
TRACIE	https://asprtracie.hhs.gov/technical-resources/31/pediatric-children/0
National Mass Violence Victimization Resource Center (NMVVRC)	http://www.nmvvrc.org/

C. J. Goodhue
Division of Pediatric Surgery/Trauma Program, Children's Hospital Los Angeles,
Los Angeles, CA, USA
e-mail: cgoodhue@chla.usc.edu

© Springer Nature Switzerland AG 2020
C. J. Goodhue, N. Blake (eds.), *Nursing Management of Pediatric Disaster*,
https://doi.org/10.1007/978-3-030-43428-1

Organization	Website
EMSC Innovation and Improvement Center	https://emscimprovement.center/
Centers for Disease Control and Prevention	https://emergency.cdc.gov/
Centers for Disease Control and Prevention Center for Preparedness and Response	https://www.cdc.gov/cpr/index.htm
CDC Caring for Children in Disasters	https://www.cdc.gov/childrenindisasters/index.html
National Center for Disaster Preparedness	https://ncdp.columbia.edu/
Save the Children	https://www.savethechildren.org/us/what-we-do/us-programs/disaster-relief-in-america/preparedness
National Child Traumatic Stress Network	https://www.nctsn.org/

Position Statements

Organization	Website
American Academy of Pediatrics	https://pediatrics.aappublications.org/content/pediatrics/early/2015/10/13/peds.2015-3112.full.pdf
National Association of Pediatric Nurse Practitioners	https://www.jpedhc.org/article/S0891-5245(18)30506-6/pdf
Society of Pediatric Nurses	http://www.pedsnurses.org/p/cm/ld/fid=220&tid=28&sid=3311

Policy Statements

Organization	Website
AAP—Understanding Liability Risks and Protections for Pediatric Providers During Disasters	https://pediatrics.aappublications.org/content/143/3/e20183892 https://pediatrics.aappublications.org/content/143/3/e20183893
AAP Emergency Department Preparedness for Pediatrics	https://pediatrics.aappublications.org/content/142/5/e20182459
AAP Children with Special Health Care Needs	https://pediatrics.aappublications.org/content/125/4/829
AAP Pediatric Readiness in Emergency Medical Services Systems	https://pediatrics.aappublications.org/content/pediatrics/early/2019/12/17/peds.2019-3308.full.pdf

Games for Health Care Professionals

Name	Website	Description
Survival Disaster Triage	http://disastertriagegame.org/help.html	Combines START/JUMPSTART
Surge World	http://surgeworld.lachildrenshospital.net/	

Disaster Exercises, Resources, and Training

Organization	Website
State of OHIO Hospital and Health Care System	https://odh.ohio.gov/wps/portal/gov/odh/about-us/offices-bureaus-and-departments/bhp/resources/hospital-preparedness-program
World Health Organization	https://openwho.org/
Minnesota State Burn Surge Plan	http://www.cwchealthcarecoalitions.org/wp-content/uploads/2016/10/BurnSurgePlan_Final_October_2016.pdf
Pediatric Scenarios—Montana	https://onedrive.live.com/?authkey=%21ABFqx6pOVbGfVSY&id=310BEE72CB77CC98%2152739&cid=310BEE72CB77CC98
NACCHO MRC Team MRC Deployment Ready Guide 2019	https://www.naccho.org/uploads/downloadable-resources/MRC-Deployment-Ready-Guide_August-2019_082719.pdf
Hospital Evacuation During Wildfire	https://files.asprtracie.hhs.gov/documents/aspr-tracie-the-last-stand-evacuating-a-hospital-in-the-middle-of-a-wildfire.pdf
Safe Transport of Children	https://nasemso.org/committees/safe-transport-of-children/
Family Information Centers	https://www.calhospitalprepare.org/FIC
Family Reunification Resources	https://asprtracie.s3.amazonaws.com/documents/family-reunification-annotations.pdf
LA County Pediatric Surge Guide	https://www.calhospitalprepare.org/sites/main/files/file-attachments/hpp_lac_ems_agency_pediatric_surge_plan_ecopy.pdf
CDC	https://emergency.cdc.gov/coca/trainingresources.asp
Drug and Lactation Guide	https://www.ncbi.nlm.nih.gov/books/NBK501922/
NICU Evacuation Guide	https://www.calhospitalprepare.org/sites/main/files/file-attachments/nicu_evac_guidelines.pdf
Pediatric Trauma Basics—Training	https://www.openpediatrics.org/assets/video/basics-pediatric-trauma-assessment-and-management
Special Needs Training	https://www.openpediatrics.org/course/virtual-home-visit-child-medical-complexity
Decontamination Resources for Hospitals	https://www.massgeneral.org/assets/MGH/pdf/emergency-medicine/MDPH-Hospital-Based-Decontamination-Resources-June-2014.pdf
CHEMM ASPIRE	https://chemm.nlm.nih.gov/aspire.htm
Helping Others Radiation Exposure Decon	https://www.cdc.gov/nceh/radiation/emergencies/selfdecon_helpothers.htm?CDC_AA_refVal=https%3A%2F%2Femergency.cdc.gov%2Fradiation%2Fselfdecon_helpothers.asp
Radiation Emergency Medical Management	https://www.remm.nlm.gov/radiation_children.htm
Pediatric Disaster Preparedness Guidelines for Hospitals	https://www.luriechildrens.org/globalassets/documents/emsc/resourcesguidelines/guidelines-tool-and-other-resources/practice-guidelinestools/00_peddisasterguide3ed_jan2019final.pdf
First Responder Treatment Protocols	https://www.umchealthsystem.com/docs/default-source/for-ems/umc-ems-lubbock-fd-protocols-17.pdf?sfvrsn=a8c64061_2
Disaster Recovery Tracking Tool	http://www.trackyourrecovery.org/
Minnesota Pediatric Surge video	https://www.health.state.mn.us/communities/ep/surge/pediatric/video.html

Checklists

Organization	Type	Website
AAP	Postdisaster Considerations for Pediatricians in Practice	https://www.aap.org/en-us/Documents/AAP_Disaster_Recovery_Checklist.pdf
State of Illinois	Pediatric Decontamination Checklist	https://www.luriechildrens.org/globalassets/documents/emsc/disaster/other/pediatricdecontaminationchecklistjune2017.pdf

Evaluation Guides

Type	Website
Pediatric Medical Surge Exercise Evaluation Guide	https://urldefense.proofpoint.com/v2/url?u=http-3A__www.cidrap.umn.edu_sites_default_files_public_php_26947_Exercise-2520Evaluation-2520Guide-2520Sample-2520-2D-2520Pediatric-2520Medical-2520Surge.doc&d=DwIFAg&c=RpR9LiQNIoGO8A8CMgA1NQ&r=M4dd6PEEcUJfOmHzoAF68thjTBNvkd_8ER8lcCzEAsQ&m=L2tu0oUoUuz189Nix531aMwqCFXSE1ZPYXrY_FXM6yA&s=fIE3SCrHYTapgqg1cN4lq709m904-8xz3wGlKxL1dQc&e=

Toolkits

Name	Website
Association of State and Territorial Health Officials Tool kit	http://www.astho.org/Programs/Preparedness/Public-Health-Emergency-Law/Emergency-Authority-and-Immunity-Toolkit/Pandemic-and-All-Hazards-Preparedness-Act-Fact-Sheet/
Mass Violence Toolkit	www.ovc.gov/pubs/mvt-toolkit
Vicarious Trauma Toolkit	www.ovc.gov/vtt
Exercise and Evaluation Toolkits for NICU, PICU, and Non-PICU patients	http://www.programinfosite.com/pdc/hospital-toolkit/
MCIs and Toolkit Overview	https://hazards.colorado.edu/resources/suggested-tools
Create a Child-Friendly Space in a Humanitarian Setting	https://resourcecentre.savethechildren.net/library/toolkit-child-friendly-spaces-humanitarian-settings
Greater New York Hospital Association Mass Casualty Incident Toolkit	https://www.gnyha.org/tool/mass-casualty-incident-response-toolkit/
Pediatric Disaster Preparedness Toolkit	https://emscimprovement.center/education-and-resources/toolkits/pediatric-disaster-preparedness-toolbox/
NYC Pandemic Flu Pediatric Toolkit	https://www.omh.ny.gov/omhweb/disaster_resources/pandemic_influenza/hospitals/bhpp_focus_ped_toolkit.html
NICU Disaster Preparedness Toolkit	http://cdphready.org/wp-content/uploads/2015/06/NICU-Disaster-Preparedness-Toolkit.pdf
NICU Evacuation Tabletop Exercise Toolkit	https://www.luriechildrens.org/globalassets/documents/emsc/resourcesguidelines/guidelines-tool-and-other-resources/practice-guidelinestools/nicunurseryevacuationttxtoolkit3.pdf
Toolkit for EMS Providers to Engage Children Affected by Crisis	https://www.colorado.gov/pacific/cdphe/engage-calm-distract

Specific Disaster Types

Name/Type of Disaster	Website
Wildfires	https://www.pehsu.net/_Library/facts/wildfire_acute_2011_health_prof.pdf https://www.aap.org/en-us/advocacy-and-policy/aap-health-initiatives/Children-and-Disasters/Pages/Wildfires.aspx
Blast Injuries	https://www.savethechildren.org.uk/content/dam/gb/reports/pbip_blastinjurymanual_2019.pdf
Radiation	https://www.cdc.gov/childrenindisasters/radiation-emergencies.html https://emergency.cdc.gov/radiation/getinside.asp https://emergency.cdc.gov/radiation/stayinside.asp https://emergency.cdc.gov/radiation/staytuned.asp
Radiation and Pregnancy	https://emergency.cdc.gov/radiation/pdf/infographic_radiation_and_pregnancy.pdf
Radiation and Breastfeeding	https://emergency.cdc.gov/radiation/breastfeeding.asp
Active Shooter	https://www.childhoodpreparedness.org/post/lessons-learned-el-paso-and-dayton-shootings

Resources for Families

Type	Website
Power Outage Preparedness	https://www.ready.gov/power-outages
Preparing the Home	https://www.redcross.org/content/dam/redcross/atg/PDF_s/Preparedness___Disaster_Recovery/General_Preparedness___Recovery/Home/A4497.pdf
Digital Go Bag	https://disasterinfo.nlm.nih.gov/content/files/apps_flyer_2018.pdf
Checklist	https://www.cdc.gov/childrenindisasters/checklists/index.html
Talking to Children about Disaster or Trauma	https://store.samhsa.gov/product/tips-talking-helping-children-youth-cope-after-disaster-or-traumatic-event-guide-parents/sma12-4732
General Disaster Preparedness	https://www.nctsn.org/sites/default/files/resources/tip-sheet/family_preparedness_thinking_ahead.pdf
Wallet Card for Family Contacts	https://www.nctsn.org/sites/default/files/resources/special-resource/family_preparedness_wallet_card.pdf
Pictorial of Family Preparedness	https://www.aap.org/en-us/PublishingImages/disasters_disaster_preparedness_month.png

Resources for Children

Name	Website
STEP and TEEN CERT Programs	https://www.ready.gov/kids/curriculum
FEMA's Youth Preparedness Council	https://www.ready.gov/kids/youth-preparedness-council
FEMA Podcast: Teaching Children What to Do in an Emergency	https://www.fema.gov/podcast
Ready Kids	https://www.ready.gov/kids
Sesame Street	https://www.sesamestreet.org/toolkits/ready
Wrigley Book	https://www.cdc.gov/cpr/readywrigley/books.htm

Child Care Center Preparedness

Name	Website
CDC: Caring for Children in Disaster: Teachers and Childcare	https://www.cdc.gov/childrenindisasters/schools.html
California Child Care Disaster Plan	https://cchp.ucsf.edu/content/disaster-preparedness
FEMA	https://emilms.fema.gov/is36/assets/EAP_Sample.pdf
State of Minnesota	https://mn.gov/dhs/assets/KeepingKidsSafe_tcm1053-317025.pdf
State of Illinois	https://ssom.luc.edu/media/stritchschoolofmedicine/emergencymedicine/emsforchildren/documents/disasterpreparedness/organizationalresources/childcarecenters/Emergence%20Preparedness%20Planning%20Guide%20for%20Child%20Care%20Centers%202016(2).pdf
Child Care Aware	https://usa.childcareaware.org/advocacy-public-policy/crisis-and-disaster-resources/
OHSEPR	https://www.acf.hhs.gov/ohsepr/information-for-providers
AAP Pennsylvania Chapter	http://ecels-healthychildcarepa.org/tools/checklists.html
Managing Infectious Diseases	https://www.aap.org/en-us/advocacy-and-policy/aap-health-initiatives/healthy-child-care/Pages/Curriculum-for-Managing-Infectious-Diseases.aspx
Building Stronger Child Care Plans	https://www.collabforchildren.org/harveyrelief

Children with Special Health Care Needs

Name	Website
Training	https://www.openpediatrics.org/course/virtual-home-visit-child-medical-complexity
Evacuation	https://hazards.colorado.edu/news/research-counts/special-collection/evacuating-under-fire-children-with-special-healthcare-needs-in-disaster
Phoenix Children's Hospital Autism and First Response	https://youtu.be/fkFplizD8No
Autism and First Response Awareness	https://youtu.be/zjRUeAlC8xw
American Academy of Pediatrics	https://www.aap.org/en-us/advocacy-and-policy/aap-health-initiatives/Children-and-Disasters/Pages/CYWSN.aspx
Resources for Hurricane Preparedness	https://www.phe.gov/Preparedness/planning/abc/Pages/kids-spcl-hc-needs-hurcn-resp17.aspx
Preparing for Emergencies for CSHCN—Domestic Preparedness	https://www.domesticpreparedness.com/updates/preparing-children-with-special-healthcare-needs-for-an-emergency/?utm_source=DomesticPreparedness&utm_campaign=b30b67becb-EMAIL_CAMPAIGN_2019_12_11&utm_medium=email&utm_term=0_9a091366ad-b30b67becb-254122053
American Red Cross	https://www.redcross.org/get-help/how-to-prepare-for-emergencies/disaster-safety-for-people-with-disabilities.html
Emergency Information Form	https://www.acep.org/globalassets/uploads/uploaded-files/acep/clinical-and-practice-management/resources/pediatrics/medical-forms/eifspecialneeds.pdf

School Preparedness

Name	Website
SETT	https://www.nasn.org/programs/conferences/sett/sett-live
National Association of School Psychologists—School Violence	https://www.nasponline.org/resources-and-publications/resources-and-podcasts/school-climate-safety-and-crisis/school-violence-resources/recovery-from-large-scale-crises-guidelines-for-crisis-teams-and-administrators
Federal Report on School Safety	https://www.hsdl.org/?abstract&did=819607
AAP Resources for School Preparedness	https://www.aap.org/en-us/advocacy-and-policy/aap-health-initiatives/Children-and-Disasters/Pages/Schools.aspx
Building Resilience in Children	https://hazards.colorado.edu/news/research-counts/special-collection/new-school-a-modern-approach-to-disaster-risk-reduction-and-resilience-education-for-children

Shelters

Name	Website
Breastfeeding in Shelters	https://hazards.colorado.edu/news/research-counts/special-collection/safe-spaces-creating-a-culture-to-support-infant-feeding-in-shelters
Infant Feeding in Shelters	https://www.cdc.gov/features/disasters-infant-feeding/

Foster Family Preparedness

Websites/Resources
https://www.slideshare.net/jpkids/disaster-emergency-plan-template-for-families
https://www.childwelfare.gov/pubPDFs/disasterplanning.pdf
https://rcrctoolbox.org/wp-content/uploads/2018/05/Best-Practices-Checklist-for-Foster-Care.pdf
https://www.childwelfare.gov/topics/management/disaster-preparedness/

Reunification

Organization/Type of Resource	Website
Multiagency Reunification Template	https://www.nationalmasscarestrategy.org/wp-content/uploads/2016/01/Multi-Agency_Reunification_Services_Plan_Template_508_final_v1.pdf

Mental Health

Organization/Type of Resource	Website
PTSD in Children and Teens	https://www.ptsd.va.gov/professional/treat/specific/ptsd_child_teens.asp
Substance Abuse and Mental Health Services Administration (SAMHSA) Disaster Distress Helpline	https://www.samhsa.gov/find-help/disaster-distress-helpline
National Hazards Center	https://hazards.colorado.edu/news/research-counts/special-collection/how-parent-mental-health-can-affect-children-after-disaster